From Ptolemaus to Copernicus: The Evolving System of Gluten-Related Disorder

Special Issue Editors

Carlo Catassi
Alessio Fasano

MDPI • Basel • Beijing • Wuhan • Barcelona • Belgrade

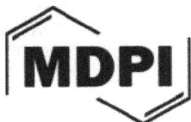

MDPI

Special Issue Editors
Carlo Catassi
Università Politecnica delle Marche
Italy

Alessio Fasano
Massachusetts General Hospital East
USA

Editorial Office
MDPI AG
St. Alban-Anlage 66
Basel, Switzerland

This edition is a reprint of the Special Issue published online in the open access journal *Nutrients* (ISSN 2072-6643) from 2016–2017 (available at: http://www.mdpi.com/journal/nutrients/special_issues/evolving_system_gluten_disorders).

For citation purposes, cite each article independently as indicated on the article page online and as indicated below:

Lastname, F.M.; Lastname, F.M. Article title. *Journal Name*. **Year**. *Article number*, page range.

First Edition 2018

ISBN 978-3-03842-731-5 (Pbk)
ISBN 978-3-03842-732-2 (PDF)

Table of Contents

About the Special Issue Editors

Carlo Catassi is the Head of the Department of Pediatrics and full professor of pediatrics at the Universit Politecnica delle Marche, Ancona, Italy and the President of the Italian Society for Pediatric Gastroenterology, Hepatology and Nutrition during the years 2013–2016. By training he is MD with specialization in Pediatrics (1980), Human Nutrition (1987)and Biostatistics (1997). Since 2001 he joined the Center for Celiac Disease (CFCR) at the University of Maryland School of Medicine, Baltimore (USA), and was appointed as Co-Director of the CFCR in 2003, Adjunct Professor of Pediatrics at the University of Maryland School of Medicine in 2012. Prof. Carlo Catassi has been appointed Visiting Scientist at the Massachusetts General Hospital for Children in 2014. Prof. Catassis research expertise is focused on the world epidemiology, clinical spectrum and primary prevention of celiac disease, gluten sensitivity and other gluten-related disorders. Prof. Catassi is considered one of the world leader experts in the area of gluten-related disorders.

Alessio Fasano is the W. Allan Walker Chair of Pediatric Gastroenterology and Nutrition at Massachusetts General Hospital for Children and Professor of Pediatrics at Harvard Medical School. He is Division Chief of Pediatric Gastroentrology and Nutrition, Director of the Mucosal Immunology and Biology Research Center and Associate Chief for Basic, Clinical and Translational Research for the Department of Pediatrics at at the same Institution. Dr. Fasanos research expertise encompasses both basic science focused on bacterial pathogenesis, gut microbiome, and translational science focused on the role of impaired intestinal barrier function in the pathogenesis of autoimmune and inflammatory diseases, including celiac disease. Dr. Fasano is author of more than 280 peer reviewed manuscripts, he has been funded continuously by the National Institute of Health since 1996, is inventor of more than 160 patents, and has received several awards, including the Shwachman award, the Linus Pauling Award, and the Entrepreneur of the year award and the Researcher of the year award.

Preface to "From Ptolemaus to Copernicus: The Evolving System of Gluten-Related Disorder"

At the time we launched the Nutrients Special Issue "From Ptolemaus to Copernicus: The Evolving System of Gluten-Related Disorders", our call for papers stated that "Gluten is the major protein of wheat and other cereals (rye and barley), which is responsible for triggering celiac disease (CD) in genetically predisposed individuals. Until a few years ago, CD was the major (if not the only) well-known gluten-related disorder. However, in recent years it has become clear that gluten proteins may activate different pathological mechanisms, leading to a wide spectrum of human diseases, including non-celiac gluten sensitivity (NCGS), gluten ataxia, neuro-psychiatric disorders, and may others. Conceptually, we have therefore moved from a Ptolemaic to a Copernican system, i.e., CD is no longer the "center of the universe", but is just one of the possible worlds of gluten intolerance. Many other gluten planets do indeed exist and deserve the attention of researchers and clinicians alike. Although different gluten-related disorders show specific epidemiological, pathophysiological, and clinical aspects, these conditions share a trigger and treatment, the gluten-free diet. For a very long time, awareness of these disorders has been limited and, therefore, the epidemiology of gluten-related disorders is still a "work in progress". Current research strives to clarify the boundaries between these entities, their disease mechanisms, and how a proper diagnosis can be implemented".

This was a broad introduction for a Special Issue that proved to be extremely successful, given that 18 papers were eventually selected for publication. By glancing at the titles of the published articles we can identify some leitmotivs of current research on gluten-related disorders. The epidemiology of gluten-related disorders is still a primary area for research, but nowadays there is a growing interest in evaluating the diffusion of non-celiac gluten/wheat-induced clinical conditions, e.g., the poorly defined situation of self-reported gluten intolerance (two papers here). As for celiac disease, it is obvious that the area of unmet need is shifting from diagnosis and clinical presentation to follow-up of treated patients and adherence to treatment with the gluten-free diet (8 papers). The Copernican system of gluten-related disorders is still under exploration (2 papers), while the issues of dietary trigger/s and role of the intestinal microbiome continue to attract the interest of researchers (4 articles). The review paper authored by Michael Marsh, one of the greatest experts in the history of celiac disease, on the evolving role of the small intestinal biopsy and its interpretation and misinterpretations deserves a special mention.

This book capitalizes on the contribution of opinion leader experts in the multidisciplinary ramifications of gluten-related disorders. We want to take the opportunity to thank all the contributors of this book. This project is the third printed collection of papers on gluten-related disorders that we had the pleasure to edit first as Special Issues of Nutrients and then as books. This enterprise would not have been possible without the enthusiasm, the expertise and the invaluable contribution and technical support of the Nutrients editorial team.

Carlo Catassi, Alessio Fasano
Special Issue Editors

nutrients

MDPI

Article

Supplementation of Reduced Gluten Barley Diet with Oral Prolyl Endopeptidase Effectively Abrogates Enteropathy-Associated Changes in Gluten-Sensitive Macaques

Karol Sestak [1,2,]*, Hazel Thwin [1], Jason Dufour [3], David X. Liu [4], Xavier Alvarez [4], David Laine [5], Adam Clarke [5], Anthony Doyle [5], Pyone P. Aye [3,4], James Blanchard [3] and Charles P. Moehs [6,]*

[1]   Division of Microbiology, Tulane National Primate Research Center, Covington, LA 70433, USA;
      hthwin@tulane.edu
[2]   PreCliniTria, LLC., Mandeville, LA 70471, USA
[3]   Division of Veterinary Medicine, Tulane National Primate Research Center, Covington, LA 70433, USA;
      jdufour@tulane.edu (J.D.); paye@tulane.edu (P.P.A.); jblanch1@tulane.edu (J.B.)
[4]   Division of Comparative Pathology, Tulane National Primate Research Center, Covington, LA 70433, USA;
      dliu1@tulane.edu (D.X.L.); Xavier@tulane.edu (X.A.)
[5]   TEVA Biologics, Discovery & Development, Sydney, Macquarie Park 2113, NSW, Australia;
      David.Laine@tevapharm.com (D.L.); Adam.Clarke@tevapharm.com (A.C.);
      Anthony.Doyle@tevapharm.com (A.D.)
[6]   Arcadia Biosciences Inc., Seattle, WA 98119, USA
*   Correspondence: ksestak@tulane.edu (K.S.); max.moehs@arcadiabio.com (C.P.M.);
      Tel.: +1-985-871-6409 (K.S.); +1-206-903-0262 (C.P.M.)

Received: 17 May 2016; Accepted: 23 June 2016; Published: 28 June 2016

Abstract: Celiac disease (CD) is an autoimmune disorder that affects approximately three million people in the United States. Furthermore, non-celiac gluten sensitivity (NCGS) affects an estimated additional 6% of the population, e.g., 20 million in the U.S. The only effective treatment of CD and NCGS requires complete removal of gluten sources from the diet. While required adherence to a gluten-free diet (GFD) is extremely difficult to accomplish, efforts to develop additional supportive treatments are needed. To facilitate these efforts, we developed a gluten-sensitive (GS) rhesus macaque model to study the effects of novel therapies. Recently reported results from phase one of this project suggest that partial improvement—but not remission—of gluten-induced disease can be accomplished by 100-fold reduction of dietary gluten, i.e., 200 ppm—by replacement of conventional dietary sources of gluten with a mutant, reduced gluten (RG) barley (*lys3a*)-derived source. The main focus of this (phase two) study was to determine if the inflammatory effects of the residual gluten in *lys3a* mutant barley grain could be further reduced by oral supplementation with a prolylendopeptidase (PE). Results reveal that PE supplementation of RG barley diet induces more complete immunological, histopathological and clinical remission than RG barley diet alone. The combined effects of RG barley diet and PE supplementation resulted in a further decrease of inflammatory mediators IFN-γ and TNF secretion by peripheral lymphocytes, as well as decreased plasma anti-gliadin and anti-intestinal tissue transglutaminase (TG2) antibodies, diminished active caspase production in small intestinal mucosa, and eliminated clinical diarrhea—all comparable with a gluten-free diet induced remission. In summary, the beneficial results of a combined RG barley and PE administration in GS macaques may warrant the investigation of similar synergistic approaches.

Keywords: celiac; gluten; protease; IL-15; oral supplement; gluten-free; rhesus macaque; glutenase; gluten-sensitive enteropathy

1. Introduction

Any future alternative to the gluten-free diet (GFD) will need to meet a high threshold of safety and efficacy. There is a number of celiac disease (CD) treatments currently in development, including glutenases, enzymes that degrade gluten [1–3]. Nevertheless, none of the glutenases are intended to allow celiac patients to deviate from GFD. These are only intended to degrade low quantities of inadvertently ingested gluten. Similarly, low gluten versions of cereals such as barley and wheat are being engineered by transgenic or mutagenic means while most retain sufficient gluten levels to make them incompatible with a GFD [4–6]. Several studies have been conducted which focus on the ability of glutenases such as prolylendopeptidase (PE) to help proteolytically degrade those gluten peptides with high content of proline residues that are known to be immunotoxic in celiac and/or gluten-sensitive (GS) patients [1–3].

During phase one of this project, we showed that novel varieties of cereal grains with low gluten content such as reduced gluten (RG) barley can have beneficial health effects in GS macaques [7]. In particular, feeding the RG barley diet led to improvement in the villous architecture of the small intestine as well as reduced inflammatory responses in peripheral blood and intestine. Due to the residual amounts of gluten present in RG barley (~1% of that contained in the parental cultivar), feeding of RG barley-derived chow to GS macaques still triggers intermediate inflammatory responses while no such responses could be found in healthy control macaques or GS macaques fed a GFD [7]. Due to the high sensitivity of GS individuals to even minute quantities of dietary gluten, it is important to formulate effective new strategies. Because of its ability to degrade proline-rich residues in immunotoxic gluten peptides [1–3,8–12], a PE was added to the RG barley diet, in the current study. The main goal was to determine if such supplementation would lead to a more complete disease remission in GS macaques than that induced by the RG barley diet alone.

2. Experimental Section

2.1. Ethics Approval

This study was performed with non-human primates. Ethics approval for veterinary procedures was obtained from the Tulane University Animal Care and Use Committee, Animal Welfare Assurance (Ethic approval code: A-4499-01). All procedures were in accordance with the recommendations of the Guide to the Care and Use of Laboratory Animals (NIH) 78-23.

2.2. Pre-Screening and Selection of GS Macaques

Pre-screening and identification of candidate macaques for this study (phase two) was done consistent with the methodology described for phase one [7]. After pre-screening, six GS juvenile (<3 years-old) rhesus macaques were assigned to the study based on simultaneous presence of anti-gliadin plasma antibodies (AGA) and anti-tissue transglutaminase (TG2) plasma (IgG) antibodies. Since baseline data with three negative control macaques were already generated under phase one, only GS macaques were used in phase two. All six macaques were free of rhesus-specific enteric pathogens [13].

2.3. Diets and Oral Glutenase (PE) Supplement

Three gluten-modified diets were formulated: (1) GFD; (2) conventional (cultivar Bomi) barley diet; and (3) reduced gluten barley (RGB, i.e., Risø 1508 (lys3a) derived from Bomi by mutagenesis) diet, consistent with the phase one experiment [7]. The 160–320 g of chow was consumed daily by juvenile macaques. It was estimated that Bomi chow delivered a dose of 2.5–5 g of gluten/day, while the RGB chows delivered approximately 32–64 mg of gluten/day. In order to accelerate progression of disease relapse, Bomi diet was fed to macaques together with a slice of wheat bread per day for each animal (Bomi + B). Based on past experiments [7], each diet was administered for at least one month to induce disease remission (GFD), relapse (Bomi + B), followed by RGB, and RGB orally supplemented with PE

(RGB + PE) regimens, to evaluate if RGB + PE regimen induces more complete remission than RGB diet alone. GFD started two weeks after the macaques were assigned to the study, i.e., switched from regular, gluten-containing monkey chow (GD) to GFD. A distinct feature of the phase two experiment was that the RG diet was not only used alone, but also in conjunction with PE oral supplementation, i.e., 580,000 Protease Picomol International (PPI) per animal, consistent with manufacturer's recommended dose (Tolerase® G, DSM Nutritional Products, Heerlen, The Netherlands). Individual doses of PE (1 g each per day given with chow) were mixed and dissolved in 50 mL of Gatorade every morning and provided using feeding bottles to each of the six macaques for one month. Evaluating whether inclusion of PE into a RGB diet would further ameliorate symptoms of GS in juvenile macaques was the main purpose of this (phase two) study.

2.4. Samples and Data Collected

All six macaques were evaluated daily for the symptoms of clinical diarrhea and dehydration ranging between 1 (normal, formed stool), 1.5 (pasty), 2.0 (semi-liquid), 2.5 (liquid), and 3 (liquid, dehydrated). Once every two weeks, animals were bled (5 mL EDTA) and rectally swabbed in order to obtain plasma, peripheral blood mononuclear cells (PBMCs), and gut microbiome samples. At four selected time points, small intestinal biopsies were collected to evaluate the impacts of four dietary regimens (GFD, Bomi + B, RGB and RGB + PE) on intestinal tissue architecture, as described [14,15].

2.5. Histopathological Evaluation, AGA, TG2 Antibody Responses and Fluorescent-Activated Cell Sorting (FACS)

Histopathological evaluation of small intestinal biopsies representing each of the four dietary periods (GFD, Bomi + B, RGB and RGB + PE) was done via microscopic evaluation of hematoxylin and eosin (H&E)-stained tissue sections, as described [14]. In addition, AGA and TG2 plasma antibodies were measured every two weeks (July 2015–January 2016). Briefly, pepsin-trypsin digested gliadin was prepared as described [16] and used at a concentration of 20 μg/mL to coat the 96-well plates (Corning, NY, USA). For anti-TG2 test, 10 μg/mL of recombinant human TG2 was used. Antigen-coated plates were washed $3\times$ with $1\times$ PBS, pH 7.4, 0.05% Tween-20 prior to blocking and between all subsequent steps. Plasma samples were diluted 1:1000 in blocking buffer and 100 μL/well was incubated overnight at 4 °C. Secondary, alkaline phosphatase-conjugated antibodies (rabbit anti-monkey IgG, Sigma-Aldrich, St. Louis, MO, USA) were diluted 1:250 in blocking buffer and 100 μL/well was incubated at 3 h at room temperature. Para-Nitrophenylphosphate (pNPP) substrate (Sigma-Aldrich) was used to develop the color reaction in 3 wells, i.e., 3 absorbance values/sample were recorded at 405 nm as described in [16]. The expression of PBMC inflammatory and inhibitory markers—including interferon-gamma (IFN-γ) by CD3+CD8+ T cells, tumor necrosis factor (TNF) by CD20+ B and CD3+CD4+ T cells, and cytotoxic T-lymphocyte-associated protein 4 (CTLA-4 also known as CD152) expression by CD3+CD4+ T cells—was monitored at time points representing the four dietary periods by Fluorescent-Activated Cell Sorting (FACS) [7]. Briefly, PBMCs were stained with a mix of fluorescently-labeled antibodies specific for extracellular antigens first (CD3, CD4, CD8, CD20, and CD152) first, according to the manufacturer's instructions (BD Pharmingen, San Diego, CA, USA). In order to detect intracellular antigens (TNF and IFN-γ), cells were stimulated with 0.1 μM phorbol miristate acetate (PMA) and 0.5 μg/mL ionomycin (Sigma) and processed according to instructions (BD Pharmingen). Samples were resuspended in BD Stabilizing Fixative (BD Biosciences, San Jose, CA, USA) and data were acquired on FACSAria flow cytometer (BD Biosciences). Data were analyzed by Flowjo software (Tree star, Ashland, OR, USA).

2.6. Confocal and Morphometric Evaluation of Small Intestinal Biopsies

Proximal jejunum biopsy tissues collected at time points representing the four dietary periods (GFD, Bomi + B, RGB, and RGB + PE) were used to evaluate gluten-sensitive enteropathy (GSE)-associated changes within the intestinal mucosa. Biopsies were collected and processed as described [14,15]. Briefly, tissues were embedded in paraffin and 7 µm sections were stained first with unconjugated primary antibodies, including: (1) antibodies to tight junction protein Zonula Occludens-1 (ZO-1) as a marker of epithelial integrity; (2) active caspase as a marker of cell apoptosis; and (3) cytokeratin 1 as an epithelial cell marker: (ZO-1, 33-9100, Life Technol. Invitrogen, Waltham, MA, USA; IgA, 617-101-006, Rockland, Inc., Pottstown, PA, USA; Active Caspase, Ab13847, Abcam; Cytokeratin 1, CKLMW 8/18, Biocare Medical; Villin, 2369 S, Cell Signaling Technol. and DAPI nuclear DNA stain, D1306, ThermoFisher Scientific, Waltham, MA, USA). Primary antibodies were followed by appropriate secondary fluorochrome-conjugated antibodies. Confocal microscopy with a Leica TCS SP8 laser scanning confocal microscope system equipped with four lasers, with eight laser lines available, capable of simultaneously collecting information in six channels (five fluorescent and one for differential interference contrast) was used to collect images. Image analysis was performed with Volocity software (version 6.3, PerkinElmer, Waltham, MA, USA) to count the apoptotic cells on a software-generated grid (Supplementary Materials Figure S1). Epithelium and lamina propria from biopsied animals were evaluated for the extent of apoptosis.

2.7. Immunohistochemistry of IL-15 in Rhesus Small Intestine

To develop the immunohistochemistry procedure, antigen-positive and negative control samples were generated. Expi 293F (a derivative of HEK-293) cell lines were transiently transfected with either rhesus IL-15 (GenBank, U19843.1) or mock plasmid according to manufacturer's instructions (Life Technologies, ExpiFectamine™ 293 Transfection Kit A14526, Carlsbad, CA, USA). After 48 hours, cells were harvested and assessed for expression of rhesus IL-15 by flow cytometry on live cells or on 4% paraformaldehyde (PFA)-fixed cells using anti-human IL-15 antibody (R & D Systems, MAB647) and an IgG1k isotype control (Abcam, AB18443) mouse monoclonal antibody. It was established that MAB647 antibody reacts with rhesus IL-15 (Supplementary Materials Figure S2). Transfected PFA-fixed cells were then used to identify optimal conditions for the positive immunohistochemistry tissue staining including antibody concentrations that would result in minimal background.

To perform small intestinal tissue analysis, MAB647 and an IgG1k isotype control antibody were used as the primary antibodies at 20 µg/mL on 4% PFA-fixed small intestine tissue samples from GS and healthy control rhesus monkeys. The detection system consisted of anti-mouse secondary (Vector, BA-2000) and ABC-Peroxidase kit (Vector, PK-4000) with a DAB + chromagen substrate kit (DAKO, K3468), yielding the brown-colored deposit. Slides were imaged with a DVC 1310C digital camera coupled to a Nikon microscope. The entire immunohistochemistry procedure was also performed on an adjacent section of the 4% PFA-fixed control tissue in the absence of primary antibody to serve as a negative control. Brown color intensity was recorded on a 0–4 scale (0 = negative, 1 = blush, 2 = faint, 3 = moderate, 4 = strong).

2.8. Statistical Analysis

Graphical representation and statistical analysis of the cytokine-producing, apoptotic cell, CTLA-4 data and clinical diarrhea scores were performed using the GraphPad Prism 6.0 (GraphPad Software, San Diego, CA, USA). Comparisons between the time-points corresponding to each diet were done for each measurement (plasma AGA and TG2 antibodies, clinical diarrhea scores, and cytokine/apoptotic cells) by Mann-Whitney U-test. Values of $p < 0.05$ were considered statistically significant.

3. Results

3.1. Peripheral AGA and TG2 Antibody Responses

Withdrawal of dietary gluten (GFD) resulted in complete remission of plasma AGA and TG2 antibody levels within one month (Figure 1). Elevated AGA and TG2 antibody responses reflected administration and re-introduction of dietary gluten (GD and Bomi + B diets, respectively) while its removal (GFD) or replacement with RGB diet were followed by lowered levels of both antibodies.

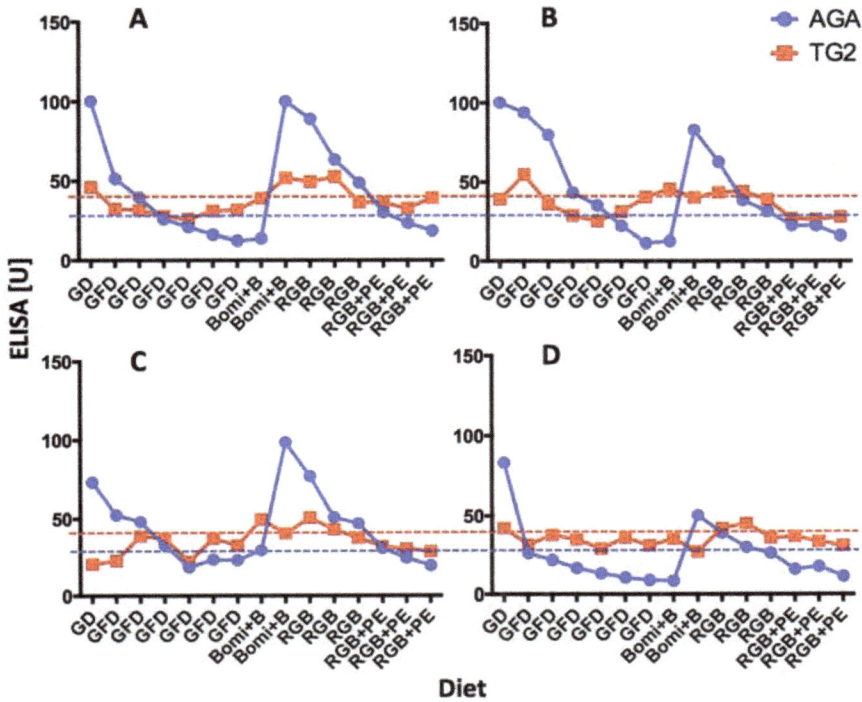

Figure 1. Anti-gliadin antibodies (AGA) and anti-intestinal tissue transglutaminase (TG2) plasma antibodies in four gluten-sensitive (GS) rhesus macaques (**A–D**). Gluten-modified diets (GD, GFD, Bomi + B, RGB and RGB + PE) that were used to feed the macaques are indicated. Individual time points represent two-week intervals. Blue dashed line represents AGA baseline, i.e., 25 ELISA units while red dashed line represents TG2 antibody baseline, i.e., 40 units. Values elevated above these lines were significantly greater ($p < 0.05$) than values generated with plasmas from healthy, normal macaques.

Notably, decrease in AGA and TG2 antibodies continued after the introduction of PE into RGB diet (RGB + PE). Only upon RGB + PE diet administration did the AGA and TG2 antibodies decline below or close to baseline levels. There were noticeable similarities in the dynamics of AGA and TG2 antibody formation in studied GS macaques but also differences in magnitude of these responses, likely attributed to heterogeneous *Mamu* II backgrounds of the GS macaques used. As previously reported, none of the healthy controls used in phase one of this study developed any AGA or TG2 antibody serum responses [7].

3.2. Clinical Diarrhea Scores

Clinical diarrhea scores (Figure 2) reflected plasma AGA and to a lesser extent TG2 antibody levels following the administration of the four experimental diets (Figures 1 and 2). Despite the fact that the Bomi + B diet was fed for no longer than one month, re-introduction of barley- and wheat-derived gluten in this diet caused clinical diarrhea in GS macaques. The significantly ($p < 0.05$) elevated clinical diarrhea scores of Bomi + B diet fed macaques above those of GFD fed macaques were suggestive of progression towards more severe diarrhea in the scenario where Bomi + B diet would not be replaced by RGB diet (Figure 2). Once Bomi + B diet was replaced by RGB and later followed by RGB + PE diets, clinical diarrhea scores returned to normal, healthy animal levels within two months.

Clinical Diarrhea Scores

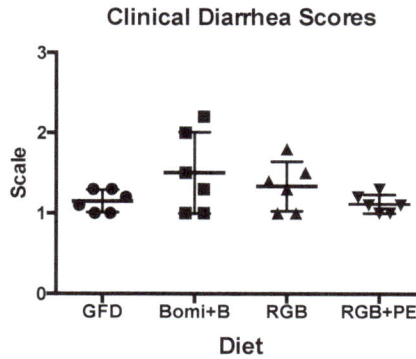

Figure 2. Clinical diarrhea scores generated with GS macaques fed gluten-modified diets (GFD, Bomi + B, RGB and RGB + PE) are shown.

3.3. Rhesus Macaque Small Intestinal Tissue Architecture

H & E staining of small intestinal biopsy tissues from juvenile GS macaques while on GFD revealed normal tissue architecture, without villous atrophy or extensive lymphocytic infiltrations of lamina propria (Figure 3A), unlike the considerable GSE that is seen in GS macaques on a long-term GD [14,16].

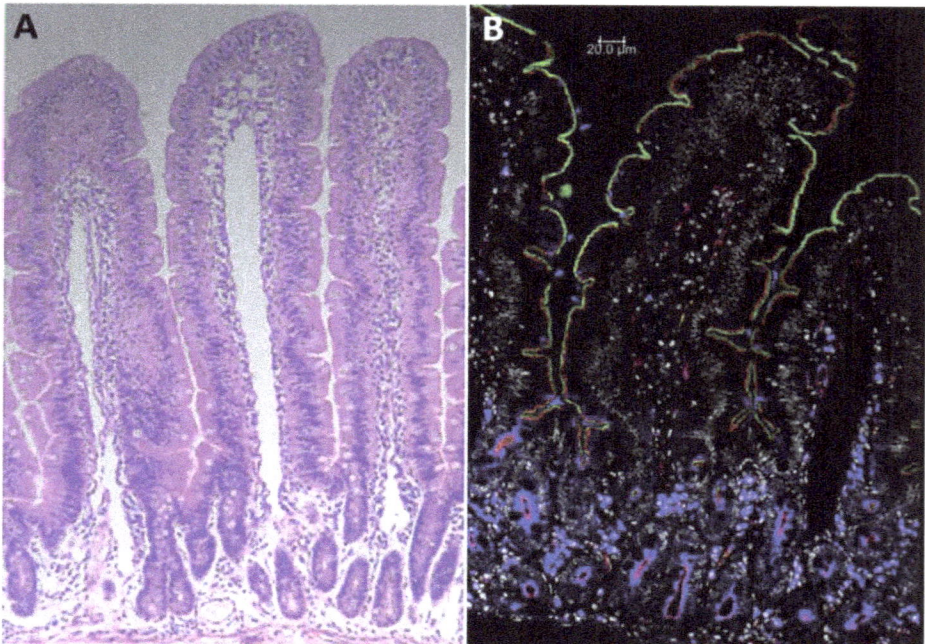

Figure 3. H & E staining of jejunum from a GS macaque while on GFD reveals normal-range intestinal architecture, magnification 10× (**A**); Four-color confocal microscopy of jejunum from another animal on GFD (**B**) shows undisrupted continuity of villin (**green**) and tight junction protein ZO-1 staining (**red**). Abundant IgA-positive B cells are seen in the subepithelium (**blue**). Gray = nuclear DNA.

Typically, an advanced GSE is in macaques accompanied with discontinuous expression of tight junction proteins such as ZO-1, resulting in a compromised epithelial barrier function [15,17] but this was not seen in juvenile macaques fed Bomi + B diet. The IgA-positive B cells were observed in lamina propria of GS macaques regardless of GFD treatment (Figure 3B).

3.4. Gluten Diet-Dependent Apoptotic Changes in Small Intestine

In order to study histopathological changes on a cellular level, confocal microscopy of small intestinal biopsies was used (Figure 4). Epithelial and subepithelial (lamina propria, i.e., LP) cells that were positive for active caspase were designated as "apoptotic" and their proportions (%) from total epithelial and LP cells were recorded. The highest proportions of apoptotic cells were found in historical GSE controls, i.e., adult rhesus macaques with CD-like symptoms that were not part of this study except for use as comparisons. Both epithelial and LP apoptotic cell counts from GSE controls were significantly higher ($p < 0.001$) than those generated with juvenile GS macaques, regardless of the GFD, RGB + G, or Bomi + B diets (Figure 4A–E). The highest proportions of apoptotic cells in juvenile GS macaques were found in biopsies taken while animals were fed Bomi + B diet. After the switch from Bomi + B to RGB diets, the numbers of apoptotic cells started to decline. After one month on RGB diet, followed by one month on RGB + PE diet, apoptotic cell counts decreased to levels comparable with those ascribed to GFD (Figure 4D,E).

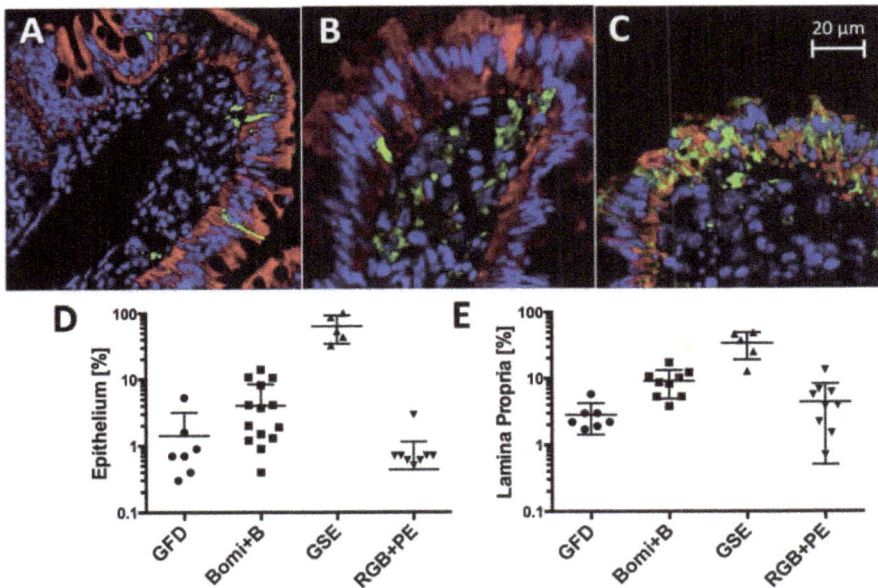

Figure 4. The combination of cytokeratin 1 (**red** = epithelial cells), active caspase (**green** = cells undergoing apoptosis) and diamino-2-phenylindole (DAPI, **blue** = nuclear DNA) antibodies was used to examine the diet-induced changes within intestinal mucosa. Jejunum from juvenile GS macaques on gluten-free diet (GFD) shows prominent red staining corresponding to epithelial cells with very few of the green cells (**A**); Jejunum from macaque on Bomi + B diet shows an increased number of green/apoptotic cells positive for active caspase inside the lamina propria (LP) (**B**); Control jejunum tissue from an adult macaque with gluten-sensitive enteropathy (GSE) exhibits high % of epithelial apoptotic cells (**C**); Charts reflecting the proportions (%) of apoptotic cells inside the epithelium (**D**) and LP (**E**) of GS macaques fed dietary gluten-modified diets in this study plus the control GSE macaques fed regular monkey (gluten-containing) chow are shown.

It is important to emphasize that differences between counts of apoptotic cells ascribed to Bomi + B vs. RGB + PE diets were significant ($p < 0.05$) for both epithelial and LP counts although not as robust as those observed with GSE controls ($p < 0.001$, Figure 4D,E). In summary, it was observed that after being placed on RGB + PE diet, juvenile GS macaques lowered their numbers of apoptotic enterocytes to levels similar to those associated with a GFD.

3.5. IL-15 Expression in Small Intestine

Due to emerging evidence regarding the key role of IL-15 in NKT-cell-mediated pathogenesis of CD/GSE [18–20], selected jejunum biopsies from three GS and one healthy control macaques fed Bomi + B diets were evaluated for the presence of IL-15. Biopsies from GS macaques showed prominent IL-15 staining (Figure 5A,B) while lower intensity (but not completely negative) of such signal was detected also in tissues stained with unrelated, isotype-matched antibodies as well as healthy control jejunum (Figure 5C,D).

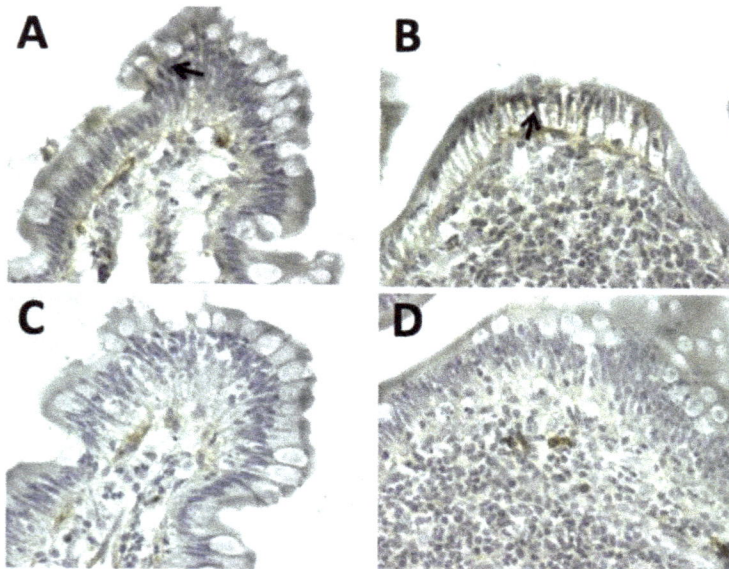

Figure 5. Jejunum biopsies collected from GS macaques on Bomi + B diet show an increased IL-15 staining, indicated by arrows (**A,B**) while lower intensity of such signal was detected in tissues stained with unrelated, isotype-matched antibodies or in healthy control biopsies (**C,D**), magnification 40×.

3.6. Expression of Pro- and Anti-Inflammatory Mediators by PBMCs

Proportions of IFN-γ, TNF and CTLA-4 inflammation-regulatory molecules—expressed by peripheral blood lymphocytes—were measured by multi-color FACS. Significant and consistent increases in expression of IFN-γ by CD3 + CD8 + T cells and TNF by CD20 + B cells were found in Bomi + B diet-fed GS macaques (Figure 6A,B). Only a non-significant trend for increased expression of TNF by CD3 + CD4 + T cells was detected following the administration of Bomi + B diet (Figure 6C and Supplementary Materials Figure S3).

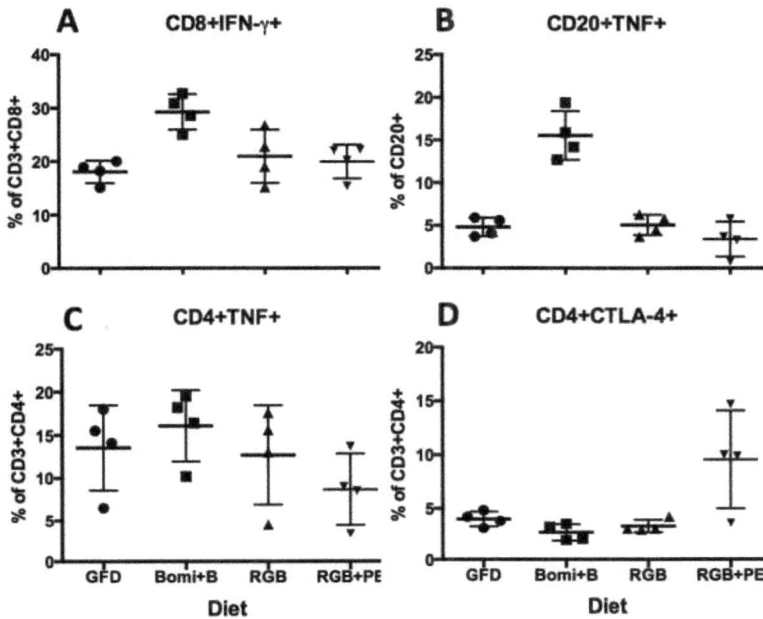

Figure 6. Proportions of pro- and anti-inflammatory mediator expressions by peripheral blood mononuclear cells (PBMCs) following the administration of gluten-modified diets are shown. Significant differences in IFN-γ production between the GFD vs. Bomi + B fed macaques ($p = 0.006$) were found (**A**). Bomi + B vs. RGB or RGB + PE fed macaques also differed significantly ($p < 0.05$) in IFN-γ production (**A**); A similar but more robust difference ($p < 0.0001$) between the Bomi + B fed macaques and other diets was found in the case of TNF production by CD20 + B cells (**B**); Non-significant trends for differences were found in the case of TNF production by CD4 + T cells (**C**) while an increase in expression of anti-inflammatory CTLA-4 (CD152) by CD4 + T cells ($p < 0.05$) was observed after the macaques were placed on RGB + PE diet (**D**). Time intervals between indicated measurements correspond to four weeks.

An increase ($p < 0.05$) in expression of anti-inflammatory CTLA-4 (CD152) molecule by CD3 + CD4 + T cells was revealed upon introduction of RGB + PE regimen (Figure 6D). Taken together, these findings suggest that several pro-inflammatory changes take place in GS juvenile macaques upon introduction of dietary gluten. Notably, these changes can be reversed upon introduction of RGB + PE diet—the effects of which are comparable with the effects of a GFD.

4. Discussion

In order to extend the findings from our recently completed phase one study and to evaluate if inclusion of oral glutenase (*Aspergillus niger*-derived prolyl endopeptidase, i.e., PE) into a reduced-gluten RGB diet will further ameliorate symptoms of GS in juvenile macaques, we conducted this (phase two) study. In accord with phase one, despite its beneficial effects, RGB diet alone was not sufficient to eliminate symptoms of GS in macaques, most likely due to residual quantities of dietary gluten (200 ppm) in RGB chow [7]. Consumption of RGB diet alone in GS macaques is characterized by intermediate levels of TNF and IFN-γ production by peripheral lymphocytes, low-grade intestinal inflammation, and border-line AGA (IgG) plasma levels. Our hypothesis was that these effects would further be abrogated upon inclusion of PE oral glutenase supplement.

Past attempts to utilize PE as oral therapy in celiac patients yielded promising results. The initial report that suggested the applicability of a PE in treatment of CD dates back to 2002 [8]. Since then, several studies—including clinical trials—have been conducted, which have focused on the ability of PEs to proteolytically degrade gluten, which comprises peptides with hard-to-digest, immunotoxic sequences featuring a high proline content [1–3]. Some unanswered questions still remain regarding the delivery of oral PE supplement can avoid the proteolytic degradation during gastric passage while ensuring the optimal dosing in small intestine [3,10]. Regardless, PE remains the only digestive supplement capable of degrading most of the gluten-derived immunotoxic epitopes [11]. Due to their biological similarities with human celiac patients, GS rhesus macaques were used to evaluate combined effects of PE and barley-derived, reduced-gluten diet. Juvenile GS macaques that did not yet have the fully-developed form of the disease (GSE) were used to assure the prompt and effective response upon administration of RGB + PE diet and treatment, as opposed to some adult rhesus macaques with severe GSE where dietary gluten withdrawal and treatment takes a much longer time to have an effect [16]. Variable levels of villous atrophy and lymphocytic infiltration of lamina propria were observed in juvenile macaques consuming Bomi + B diet [7]. In contrast to the severe GSE that develops as a consequence of life-long dietary gluten consumption in some—but not all—GS adult rhesus macaques [14,16], one month's administration of Bomi + B diet to juvenile GS macaques did not result in morphologically distinguishable, severe GSE but only mild enteritis. A commercially available form of PE was used (Tolerase G®, DSM, Heerlen, The Netherlands), following the manufacturer's recommended dose and route of administration to ameliorate the symptoms of GS.

In addition to established hallmarks of GS in macaques such as AGA and TG2 serum antibodies, chronic diarrhea, enteritis, compromised epithelial integrity (measured by ZO-1 tight junction protein expression), and/or GSE, as well as increased expression of IFN-γ by peripheral and/or intestinal lymphocytes, the following measurements were examined in this study: (1) Quantitative analysis of enteric (small intestine) apoptosis; and (2) Qualitative evaluation of IL-15 production in small intestine. It was demonstrated that apoptosis plays a role in CD and diabetes mellitus patients in enterocyte destruction, preceding the development of villous atrophy (VA) [21–23]. It was found that cytokeratin 18 caspase-cleaved fragment, granzyme B, and other factors play roles in this process. It has also been reported that down-regulation of apoptotic inhibitors in patients with refractory CD induces further pro-apoptotic effects [22]. Although severe VA can develop in adult rhesus macaques with GS, it was not yet fully evident in this study's juvenile animals. Therefore, a morphometric evaluation of enteric mucosa was conducted, hypothesizing that reduced-gluten diets and PE treatment would have an impact on epithelial enterocytes' apoptosis. A high resolution, multi-laser Leica confocal microscope equipped with Volocity cell imaging software was used for this purpose. Interestingly, apoptosis not only took place in intestinal epithelium upon introduction of dietary gluten (Bomi + B diet) but its extent was significantly different between GS macaques fed Bomi + B and RGB + PE diets. This result alone represents the most significant finding from our study. It illustrates that enteropathy-associated changes that occur in intestinal mucosa prior to development of severe GSE are reversible, and can be achieved not only upon administration of GFD but also by RGB + PE diet. These findings provide guidance for further research involving gluten-modified diets and also illustrate the usefulness of the GS rhesus model in preclinical research.

Evaluation of IL-15 production within the small intestine of GS macaques confirmed the anticipated increased presence of this key regulator of CD immunopathology [20]. Clearly, IL-15 production represents an entirely different (NKT-cell mediated epithelial cell destruction) mechanism of GSE pathogenesis than that linked with intestinal apoptosis. Nonetheless, elevated levels of IL-15 in GS macaques corroborate the overall validity of the GS macaque model and suggest that more than one mechanism contributes to GSE pathogenesis. An unanticipated increase in CTLA-4 expression by peripheral CD4 + T cells following the supplementation of RGB diet with PE was also observed (Figure 6D). Considering the beneficial role CTLA-4 was suggested to play in down-regulation of autoimmune diseases including CD [24,25], this result deserves further examination. Intestinal apoptosis, IL-15, and CTL-4 traits of CD pathogenesis should be investigated on a molecular level in future studies. The rhesus GS model is a "natural-disease model" that closely resembles the biology and pathogenesis of human CD and does not require genetic manipulation of its host. Future studies might also be conducted with inhibitors of intestinal apoptosis and/or NKT-cell mediated autoimmunity as alternative treatments of CD.

As our study was underway, a publication appeared [26] indicating that additional gluten-reducing mutations had been combined with the *lys3a* mutant present in the RGB used in the present study to produce an ultra-low gluten barley (ULGB). This ULGB has been used to brew beer that can be classified as gluten-free (containing less than 20 ppm gluten). Presumably at this low level of gluten, beer made with ULGB may be safe for celiac patients, although this remains to be rigorously evaluated. Treatments such as the glutenase Tolerase® G would likely provide an additional margin of safety. Efforts to produce an analogous ultra-low gluten wheat are less likely to be successful both because of the more complex genetics of tetraploid pasta and hexaploid bread wheat and because of the constraints imposed by the required functional properties of the wheat, in which the gluten proteins play a major role.

5. Conclusions

Our recently reported results suggest that partial improvement but not complete remission of gluten-induced disease can be accomplished by 100-fold reduction of dietary gluten—by replacement of conventional dietary sources with barley-derived, reduced gluten (*lys3a* barley) source. The main focus of this study was to determine if the inflammatory effects of leftover gluten in the RGB grain could be further reduced by oral supplementation with PE. Our results show that PE supplementation of RGB diet induces more complete immunological, histopathological, and clinical remission than RGB diet alone. The beneficial effects of the RGB + PE treatment on GS juvenile macaques were comparable with those of the GFD. These findings provide guidance for further research involving gluten-modified diet alternatives.

Supplementary Materials: The following are available online at http://www.mdpi.com/2072-6643/8/7/401/s1, Figure S1: Confocal microscopy of paraffin-fixed tissue sections labeled with fluorescein-conjugated antibodies to active caspase (apoptotic cells = green), cytokeratin 1 (epithelial cells = red) and nuclear DNA (blue) was used in conjunction with 6.3 Volocity 3D cell imaging software (PerkinElmer) to enumerate the apoptotic cells on a software-generated grid; Figure S2: Negative mock (A) and positive control, human and rhesus IL-15 transfected Expi 293F cells, were used to optimize the IL-15 staining; Figure S3: Peripheral blood populations of CD3 + T and CD20 + B lymphocytes (A) were evaluated for the production of regulatory and inflammatory cytokines including IFN-γ and TNF. CD3 + T lymphocytes were subdivided into CD4 + and CD8 + cells (B).

Acknowledgments: The authors wish to thank Carol Coyne, Julie Bruhn, Calvin Lanclos, Cecily Conerly, William J. Austill, Cate McGuire, Paul Gallawa and Meir Gadisman for their excellent technical support. For assistance with milling the barley grain we are grateful to Craig Morris and his staff at the ARS Western Wheat Quality Lab in Pullman, WA. We are grateful to DSM Nutritional Products Ltd. for donating Tolerase® G. Tolerase G® is not intended to treat or prevent celiac disease. For guidance with the oral supplementation of the primate diet with PE we are grateful to Maaike Bruins of DSM Biotechnology Center, Delft, The Netherlands and Marc Plaum of DSM Nutritional Products, Kaiseraugst, Switzerland. The authors thank Harold Bockelman at the USDA National Small Grains Collection in Aberdeen, ID for samples of Bomi and *lys3a* barley (Risø 1508). This work was funded by the National Institute of Diabetes and Digestive and Kidney Diseases of the National Institutes of Health under Award Number R42DK097976. The authors alone are responsible for the content of this article and this work does not necessarily represent the views of the National Institutes of Health. The study was completed as part of the collaboration between Arcadia Biosciences, PreCliniTria, LLC. and Tulane University.

Author Contributions: Karol Sestak wrote the manuscript, coordinated the overall work, participated in work related to multi-color flow cytometry and analyzed the data. Hazel Thwin processed and distributed samples from rhesus macaques and participated in execution of laboratory immunoassays. Jason Dufour provided veterinary care, executed surgical procedures and helped with coordination of dietary regimens. Xavier Alvarez directed immunohistochemistry and confocal microscopy work. David X. Liu was responsible for H & E evaluation of intestinal biopsies. David Laine, Adam Clarke and Anthony Doyle were responsible for IL-15-related work. Pyone P. Aye and James Blanchard helped with preparation and coordination of animal studies. Charles P. Moehs was responsible for growth and characterization of the barley varieties, preparation of the experimental diets as well as for the study's overall coordination and manuscript preparation.

Conflicts of Interest: The authors declare no conflict of interests.

References

1. Piper, J.L.; Gray, G.M.; Khosla, C. Effect of prolyl endopeptidase on digestive-resistant gliadin peptides in vivo. *J. Pharmacol. Exp. Ther.* **2004**, *311*, 213–219. [CrossRef] [PubMed]
2. Mitea, C.; Havenaar, R.; Drijfhout, J.W.; Edens, L.; Dekking, L.; Koning, F. Efficient degradation of gluten by a prolyl endoprotease in a gastrointestinal model: Implications for coeliac disease. *Gut* **2008**, *57*, 25–32. [CrossRef] [PubMed]
3. Tack, G.J.; van de Water, J.M.; Bruins, M.J.; Kooy-Winkelaar, E.M.; van Bergen, J.; Bonnet, P.; Vreugdenhil, A.C.; Korponay-Szabo, I.; Edens, L.; von Blomberg, B.M.; et al. Consumption of gluten with gluten-degrading enzyme by celiac patients: A pilot study. *World J. Gastroenterol.* **2013**, *19*, 5837–5847. [CrossRef] [PubMed]
4. Tanner, G.; Howitt, C.; Forrester, R.; Campbell, P.; Tye-Din, J.; Anderson, R. Dissecting the T-cell response to hordeins in coeliac disease can develop barley with reduced immunotoxicity. *Aliment. Pharmacol. Ther.* **2010**, *32*, 1184–1191. [CrossRef] [PubMed]
5. Wen, S.; Wen, N.; Pang, J.; Langen, G.; Brew-Appiah, R.A.; Mejias, J.H.; Osorio, C.; Yang, M.; Gemini, R.; Moehs, C.P.; et al. Structural genes of wheat and barley 5-methylcytosine DNA glycosylases and their potential applications for human health. *Proc. Natl. Acad. Sci. USA* **2012**, *109*, 20543–20548. [CrossRef] [PubMed]
6. Gil-Humanes, J.; Piston, F.; Altamirano-Fortoul, R.; Real, A.; Comino, I.; Sousa, C.; Rosell, C.M.; Barro, F. Reduced-gliadin wheat bread: An alternative to the gluten-free diet for consumers suffering gluten-related pathologies. *PLoS ONE* **2014**, *9*, e90898. [CrossRef] [PubMed]
7. Sestak, K.; Thwin, H.; Dufour, J.; Aye, P.P.; Liu, D.X.; Moehs, C.P. The effects of reduced gluten barley diet on humoral and cell-mediated systemic immune responses of gluten-sensitive rhesus macaques. *Nutrients* **2015**, *7*, 1657–1671. [CrossRef] [PubMed]
8. Shan, L.; Molberg, O.; Parrot, I.; Hausch, F.; Filiz, F.; Gray, G.M.; Sollid, L.M.; Khosla, C. Structural basis for gluten intolerance in celiac sprue. *Science* **2002**, *297*, 2275–2279. [CrossRef] [PubMed]
9. Ehren, J.; Govindarajan, S.; Moron, B.; Minshull, J.; Khosla, C. Protein engineering of improved prolyl endopeptidases for celiac sprue therapy. *Protein Eng. Des. Sel.* **2008**, *21*, 699–707. [CrossRef] [PubMed]
10. Alvarez-Sieiro, P.; Martin, M.C.; Redruello, B.; Del Rio, B.; Ladero, V.; Palanski, B.A.; Khosla, C.; Fernandez, M.; Alvarez, M.A. Generation of food-grade recombinant *Lactobacillus casei* delivering *Myxococcus xanthus* prolyl endopeptidase. *Appl. Microbiol. Biotechnol.* **2014**, *98*, 6689–6700. [CrossRef] [PubMed]
11. Janssen, G.; Christis, C.; Kooy-Winkelaar, Y.; Edens, L.; Smith, D.; van Veelen, P.; Koning, F. Ineffective degradation of immunogenic gluten epitopes by currently available digestive enzyme supplements. *PLoS ONE* **2015**, *10*, e0128065. [CrossRef] [PubMed]
12. Salden, B.N.; Monserrat, V.; Troost, F.J.; Bruins, M.J.; Edens, L.; Bartholome, R.; Haenen, G.R.; Winkens, B.; Koning, F.; Masclee, A.A. Randomised clinical study: *Aspergillus niger*-derived enzyme digests gluten in the stomach of healthy volunteers. *Aliment. Pharmacol. Ther.* **2015**, *42*, 273–285. [CrossRef] [PubMed]
13. Sestak, K.; Merritt, C.K.; Borda, J.; Saylor, E.; Schwamberger, S.R.; Cogswell, F.; Didier, E.S.; Didier, P.J.; Plauche, G.; Bohm, R.P.; et al. Infectious agent and immune response characteristics of chronic enterocolitis in captive rhesus macaques. *Infect. Immun.* **2003**, *71*, 4079–4086. [CrossRef] [PubMed]
14. Xu, H.; Feely, S.L.; Wang, X.; Liu, D.X.; Borda, J.T.; Dufour, J.; Li, W.; Aye, P.P.; Doxiadis, G.G.; Khosla, C.; et al. Gluten-sensitive enteropathy coincides with decreased capability of intestinal T cells to secrete IL-17 and IL-22 in a macaque model for celiac disease. *Clin. Immunol.* **2013**, *147*, 40–49. [CrossRef] [PubMed]
15. Mazumdar, K.; Alvarez, X.; Borda, J.T.; Dufour, J.; Martin, E.; Bethune, M.T.; Khosla, C.; Sestak, K. Visualization of transepithelial passage of the immunogenic 33-residue peptide from α-2 gliadin in gluten-sensitive macaques. *PLoS ONE* **2010**, *5*, e10228. [CrossRef] [PubMed]
16. Bethune, M.T.; Borda, J.T.; Ribka, E.; Liu, M.X.; Phillipi-Falkenstein, K.; Jandacek, R.J.; Doxiadis, G.G.M.; Gray, G.M.; Khosla, C.; Sestak, K. A non-human primate model for gluten sensitivity. *PLoS ONE* **2008**, *3*, e1614. [CrossRef] [PubMed]
17. Bethune, M.T.; Ribka, E.; Khosla, C.; Sestak, K. Transepithelial transport and enzymatic detoxification of gluten in gluten-sensitive rhesus macaques. *PLoS ONE* **2008**, *3*, e1857. [CrossRef] [PubMed]

18. Pagliari, D.; Cianci, R.; Frosali, S.; Landolfi, R.; Cammarota, G.; Newton, E.E.; Pandolfi, F. The role of IL-15 in gastrointestinal diseases: A bridge between innate and adaptive immune response. *Cytokine Growth Factor Rev.* **2013**, *24*, 455–466. [CrossRef] [PubMed]

19. Abadie, V.; Jabri, B. IL-15: A central regulator of celiac disease immunopathology. *Immunol. Rev.* **2014**, *260*, 221–234. [CrossRef] [PubMed]

20. Van Bergen, J.; Mulder, C.J.; Mearin, M.L.; Koning, F. Local communication among mucosal immune cells in patients with celiac disease. *Gastroenterology* **2015**, *148*, 1187–1194. [CrossRef] [PubMed]

21. Pohjanen, V.M.; Kokkonen, T.S.; Arvonen, M.; Augustin, M.A.; Patankar, M.; Turunen, S.; Vahasalo, P.; Karttunen, T.J. Decreased expression of protease inhibitor 9, a granzyme B inhibitor, in celiac disease: A potential mechanism in enterocyte destruction and villous atrophy. *Int. J. Immunopathol. Pharmacol.* **2013**, *26*, 897–905. [PubMed]

22. Shalimar, D.M.; Prasenjit, D.; Vishnubhatla, S.; Siddhartha, D.G.; Subrat, K.P.; Makharia, G.K. Mechanism of villous atrophy in celiac disease—Role of apoptosis and epithelial regeneration. *Arch. Pathol. Lab. Med.* **2013**, *137*, 1262–1269. [CrossRef] [PubMed]

23. Hoffmanova, I.; Sanchez, D.; Habova, V.; Andel, M.; Tuckova, L.; Tlaskalova-Hogenova, H. Serological markers of enterocyte damage and apoptosis in patients with celiac disease, autoimmune diabetes mellitus and diabetes mellitus type 2. *Physiol. Res.* **2015**, *64*, 537–546. [PubMed]

24. Tavares, N.A.; Santos, M.M.; Moura, R.; Araujo, J.; Guimaraes, R.L.; Crovella, S.; Brandao, L.A. Association of TNF-α, CTLA-4, and PTPN22 polymorphisms with type 1 diabetes and other autoimmune diseases in Brazil. *Genet. Mol. Res.* **2015**, *14*, 18936–18944. [CrossRef] [PubMed]

25. Simone, R.; Brizzolara, R.; Chiappori, A.; Milintenda-Floriani, F.; Natale, C.; Greco, L.; Schiavo, M.; Bagnasco, M.; Pesce, G.; Saverino, D. A functional soluble form of CTLA-4 is present in the serum of celiac patients and correlates with mucosal injury. *Int. Immunol.* **2009**, *9*, 1037–1045. [CrossRef] [PubMed]

26. Tanner, G.J.; Blundell, M.J.; Colgrave, M.L.; Howitt, C.A. Creation of the first ultra-low gluten barley (*Hordeum vulgare* L.) for coeliac and gluten-intolerant populations. *Plant Biotechnol.* **2016**, *4*, 1139–1150. [CrossRef] [PubMed]

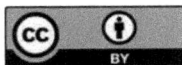

nutrients

MDPI

Article

Gastrointestinal Symptoms in Celiac Disease Patients on a Long-Term Gluten-Free Diet

Pilvi Laurikka [1], Teea Salmi [1,2], Pekka Collin [1,3], Heini Huhtala [4], Markku Mäki [5], Katri Kaukinen [1,6] and Kalle Kurppa [5,*]

[1] School of Medicine, University of Tampere, Tampere 33014, Finland; laurikka.pilvi.l@student.uta.fi (P.L.); teea.salmi@uta.fi (T.S.); pekka.collin@uta.fi (P.C.); markku.maki@uta.fi (K.K.)
[2] Department of Dermatology, Tampere University Hospital, Tampere 33014, Finland
[3] Department of Gastroenterology and Alimentary Tract Surgery, Tampere University Hospital, University of Tampere, Tampere 33014, Finland
[4] Tampere School of Health Sciences, University of Tampere, Tampere 33014, Finland; heini.huhtala@staff.uta.fi
[5] Centre for Child Health Research, University of Tampere and Tampere University Hospital, Tampere 33014, Finland; markku.maki@uta.fi
[6] Department of Internal Medicine, Tampere University Hospital, Tampere 33014, Finland
* Correspondence: kalle.kurppa@uta.fi; Tel.: +358-3-3551-8403

Received: 17 May 2016; Accepted: 11 July 2016; Published: 14 July 2016

Abstract: Experience suggests that many celiac patients suffer from persistent symptoms despite a long-term gluten-free diet (GFD). We investigated the prevalence and severity of these symptoms in patients with variable duration of GFD. Altogether, 856 patients were classified into untreated (n = 128), short-term GFD (1–2 years, n = 93) and long-term GFD ($\geqslant$3 years, n = 635) groups. Analyses were made of clinical and histological data and dietary adherence. Symptoms were evaluated by the validated GSRS questionnaire. One-hundred-sixty healthy subjects comprised the control group. Further, the severity of symptoms was compared with that in peptic ulcer, reflux disease, inflammatory bowel disease (IBD) and irritable bowel syndrome (IBS). Altogether, 93% of the short-term and 94% of the long-term treated patients had a strict GFD and recovered mucosa. Untreated patients had more diarrhea, indigestion and abdominal pain than those on GFD and controls. There were no differences in symptoms between the short- and long-term GFD groups, but both yielded poorer GSRS total score than controls (p = 0.03 and p = 0.05, respectively). Furthermore, patients treated 1–2 years had more diarrhea (p = 0.03) and those treated >10 years more reflux (p = 0.04) than controls. Long-term treated celiac patients showed relatively mild symptoms compared with other gastrointestinal diseases. Based on our results, good response to GFD sustained in long-term follow-up, but not all patients reach the level of healthy individuals.

Keywords: celiac disease; gastrointestinal diseases; symptoms; gluten-free diet

1. Introduction

The only current treatment for celiac disease is a life-long gluten-free diet. Commencement of a strict diet usually results in prompt relief of clinical symptoms, while recovery of small-bowel mucosal damage may take even years [1,2]. Although mucosal healing is the ultimate goal of the dietary treatment [3], from the patient's perspective alleviation of self-perceived clinical symptoms is usually the most rewarding outcome. A good clinical response in the early stages of dietary treatment further motivates to maintain a strict diet, which consequently facilitates mucosal recovery. There is some evidence that after the initial enthusiasm has faded, many patients experience ongoing symptoms while maintaining an apparently strict gluten-free diet [4–7]. Such persistence of symptoms despite burdensome dietary restriction is frustrating and may even predispose to poor dietary adherence and thus further worsen the situation. Hitherto, however, neither the prevalence nor the severity of the persistent symptoms in celiac disease patients on a gluten-free diet has been well characterized, let alone their impact on patients' daily life. Data on these aspects would be necessary in order to optimize the follow-up of patients and, in the future, to develop interventions on top of the gluten-free diet.

The aim of the present nationwide study was to define the prevalence and severity of gastrointestinal symptoms in a large cohort of long-term dietary treated adult celiac disease patients and to compare these with those seen in untreated and short-term treated patients and in healthy controls. Further, symptom severity was compared with other common gastrointestinal diseases based on a literature search.

2. Materials and Methods

2.1. Study Design and Participants

The large cross-sectional study was carried out at Tampere University Hospital and the University of Tampere. The celiac disease patients were collected from our prospectively maintained research database, in which the patients have been recruited via newspaper advertisements and via local and national celiac disease associations from different parts of Finland. Exclusion criteria for the present study were age under 15 years and uncertain diagnosis of celiac disease (not based on biopsy). The final study cohort comprised 856 consecutive subjects with confirmed celiac disease. All celiac disease patients had received professional dietary counseling and were placed on a strict gluten-free diet soon after the diagnosis was confirmed.

Clinical data were collected systematically from the medical records. Further, all study subjects were interviewed by an experienced physician or a study nurse in the study clinic and asked about demographics, clinical presentation of the disease at the time of diagnosis, family history of celiac disease, duration of gluten-free diet, and adherence to dietary treatment. The main mode of presentation of celiac disease at diagnosis was further classified into gastrointestinal symptoms (e.g., indigestion, diarrhea and signs of malabsorption), extraintestinal symptoms (e.g., dermatitis herpetiformis, dental enamel defects and neurological symptoms) and patients detected by screening at-risk groups (celiac disease in family, type I diabetes, thyroid disease, Sjögren's syndrome, Addison's disease and IgA nephropathy). The results of serum endomysial antibody (EmA) measurements and small-bowel mucosal biopsy sampling were collected systematically.

In order to compare differences in the presence and severity of persistent gastrointestinal symptoms between subjects dieting for different periods of gluten-free diet the celiac disease patients were further divided into three groups based on the duration of the gluten-free diet as follows: (i) newly diagnosed patients (no diet); (ii) patients with short-term treatment (diet 1–2 years) and (iii) patients with long-term treatment (diet $\geqslant$ 3 years). For a more detailed analysis the long-term treatment group was further divided into subjects who had been on a gluten-free diet either 3–5 years, 6–10 years or > 10 years.

One-hundred-and-sixty healthy individuals (72% females, median age 55 (range 23–87) years) with no first-degree relatives with celiac disease served as a control group in the comparison of gastrointestinal symptoms.

The Regional Ethics Committee of the Tampere University Hospital District approved the study protocol and all participants gave written informed consent.

2.2. Celiac Disease Serology and Small-Bowel Mucosal Histology

Serum IgA class EmA were measured by an indirect immunofluorescence method with human umbilical cord as substrate [8], and a dilution of 1: $\geqslant$5 was considered positive. Positive samples were further diluted up to 1:4000 until negative. In cases of selective IgA deficiency, the corresponding IgG class antibodies were measured. Serum transglutaminase 2 antibodies had also been measured in most of the patients, but since test methods and reference values had varied during the study period these readings were not used here. The degree of small-bowel mucosal damage was systematically measured from several well-orientated duodenal biopsy samples and reported by quantitative villous height crypt depth ratio (VH/CrD) as previously described [9]. Here VH/CrD < 2.0 was considered to indicate active celiac disease [9].

2.3. Gastrointestinal Symptoms

For the systematic evaluation of current gastrointestinal symptoms, participants in each group filled a self-administered, structured Gastrointestinal Symptom Rating Scale (GSRS) questionnaire. This is a validated questionnaire used widely in research on celiac disease and other gastrointestinal disorders [10–15]. The questionnaire measures five sub-dimensions of gastrointestinal symptoms: Indigestion, diarrhea, abdominal pain, reflux and constipation. It comprises altogether 15 separate items. Values for each of the five sub-dimension scores were calculated as a mean of the respective items and the total GSRS score as a mean of all 15 items. The scoring is based on a Likert scale from 1 to 7 points, where 1 point signifies minimal gastrointestinal symptoms and 7 points the most severe symptoms.

To further identify patients with persistent gastrointestinal symptoms, a cut-off for significantly worsened symptoms was set in the GSRS total and sub-dimension scores. This was the case when the subject's GSRS total score or subscore was higher than 1 standard deviation (SD) compared with the corresponding mean score or subscore of the healthy controls [4,16–18].

Besides between study groups, the GSRS scores in untreated and long-term treated celiac disease patients were compared with those seen in subjects with common gastrointestinal disorders, namely peptic ulcer, gastro-esophageal reflux disease (GER), inflammatory bowel disease (IBD) and irritable bowel syndrome (IBS) as established by literature search [11,13–15]. In all diseases the GSRS scores were from untreated patients at diagnosis except for IBD, where the subjects were on treatment.

2.4. Adherence to the Gluten-Free Diet

Based on dietary interview, a subject was considered to be adherent to the gluten-free diet in the case of minor inadvertent gluten intake a few times a year or less. In addition, an objective estimation of dietary adherence was carried out by measuring the percentage of EmA-positive subjects in each treatment group. Positivity for EmA was considered to represent non-adherence when detected after two years on a gluten-free diet [19].

2.5. Statistics

Categorical data were described using percentages and quantitative data using either medians with range or means with 95% confidence intervals. Cross-tabulation with Pearson's χ2 test was used to analyze differences between categorical variables. To compare means between study groups, one-way ANOVA with Bonferroni post hoc analysis was used in normally distributed variables and Kruskal-Wallis test in non-parametric variables. To investigate correlation between variables, correlation coefficient (r) was calculated using Spearman's correlation. To take account of the effect of age, a covariance analysis was used. Analyses were made with the whole study cohort and also separately for males and females. A *p*-value < 0.05 was considered statistically significant. All data were analyzed by SPSS (Statistical Package for the Social Sciences) Statistics Version 21 (IBM Corporation, Armonk, NY, USA).

3. Results

The median age of all 856 celiac disease patients was 54 years (range 15–85 years) and 75% were females. In 64% the reasons for celiac disease suspicion were gastrointestinal symptoms and in 18% extraintestinal symptoms; 18% were detected by screening. There were no significant differences between the celiac disease groups in either gender, median age at time of study, clinical presentation at diagnosis or celiac disease in the family (Table 1). Among patients on a gluten-free diet the long-term treated cohort contained lower percentage of EmA-positive subjects than the short-term treated, while there were no differences in self-reported dietary adherence or VH/CrD.

Table 1. Demographic characteristics and selected celiac disease-associated data on untreated, short-term (1–2 years) treated and long-term (≥3 years) treated celiac patients and healthy controls.

	Celiac Patients on a GFD *n* = 728			Non-Celiac Controls *n* = 160
	Untreated Patients *n* = 128	Short Treatment *n* = 93	Long Treatment *n* = 635	
Females, %	76	72	75	72
Current age, median (range)	47 (15–72)	51 (16–80)	55 (17–85)	55 (23–87)
GFD, median (range), years.	0	1 (1–2)	12 (3–48)	0
Mode of presentation at diagnosis, %				
Gastrointestinal	66	63	64	0
Extraintestinal [a]	12	16	19	0
Screen-detected [b]	23	20	17	0
Celiac disease in family, %	47	54	61	0
Self-reported strictness of GFD, (%)				
Strict diet	0	93	94	0
Occasional gluten	0	7	6	0
No diet	100	0	0	100
Positive EMA, %	93	8 [c]	3 [c,d]	0 [e]
VH/CrD, mean (95% CI)	0.5 (0.4–0.6)	2.7 (2.5–2.9) [c,f]	2.8 (2.6–2.9) [c,g]	3.2 (3.0–3.3) [h]

[a] Dermatitis herpetiformis, aphtous ulcerations, enamel defects, elevated liver enzymes, neurological and musculoskeletal symptoms, psychiatric symptoms, infertility or early menopause; [b] Family history of celiac disease, type I diabetes, thyroidal disease, Sjögren's syndrome, Addison's disease, IgA nephropathy; [c] $p < 0.001$ compared with untreated patients; [d] $p = 0.028$ compared with short treatment group; [e–h] Data available on [e] 50 subjects, [f] 20 subjects, [g] 191 subjects and [h] 35 subjects. GFD, gluten-free diet; EMA, endomysial antibodies; VH/CrD, small-bowel mucosal villous height crypt depth ratio; CI, confidence interval.

Untreated celiac patients had significantly higher (more symptoms) GSRS scores on indigestion, diarrhea, abdominal pain and total scores than those on a gluten-free diet and healthy controls, whereas there was no difference in any of the scores between long-term and short-term treated patients (Figure 1). Long-term treated patients yielded higher GSRS reflux scores, and short-term treated higher diarrhea and total scores compared with the healthy controls. In more detailed analysis reflux was seen particularly in patients treated >10 years (data not shown). None of the gastrointestinal symptoms correlated with VH/CrD levels either in the whole cohort (r varying between −0.013 and −0.220) or in the different durations of gluten-free diet (r varying between −0.146 and 0.142).

When analyzing the occurrence of significantly increased (by definition, GSRS score > 1 SD compared with healthy controls) gastrointestinal symptoms, the untreated celiac disease patients again showed significant overrepresentation in all GSRS scores except constipation compared with the other study groups (Table 2). In addition, both long- and short-term treatment groups evinced more reflux and total gastrointestinal symptoms than controls; the short-term treated patients also reported more diarrhea (Table 2). In treatment groups the mean VH/CrD levels did not differ between patients with and without increased symptoms in any of the GSRS sub-groups (data not shown). In separate analysis, long-term treated women had higher GSRS total scores (2.0 vs. 1.8, $p = 0.001$) and indigestion scores (2.5 vs. 2.3, $p = 0.034$) than men, whereas short-term treated men had higher diarrhea scores (2.4 vs. 1.7, $p = 0.003$). The overrepresentation of increased (>1 SD) reflux and total scores seen in the long-term treatment group in both genders combined remained significant in women ($p = 0.002$ and $p = 0.015$, respectively) but not in men. The GSRS diarrhea scores were also increased in short-term treated men and long-term treated women compared with healthy controls (2.4 vs. 1.5, $p < 0.001$ and 1.7 vs. 1.5, $p = 0.042$, respectively).

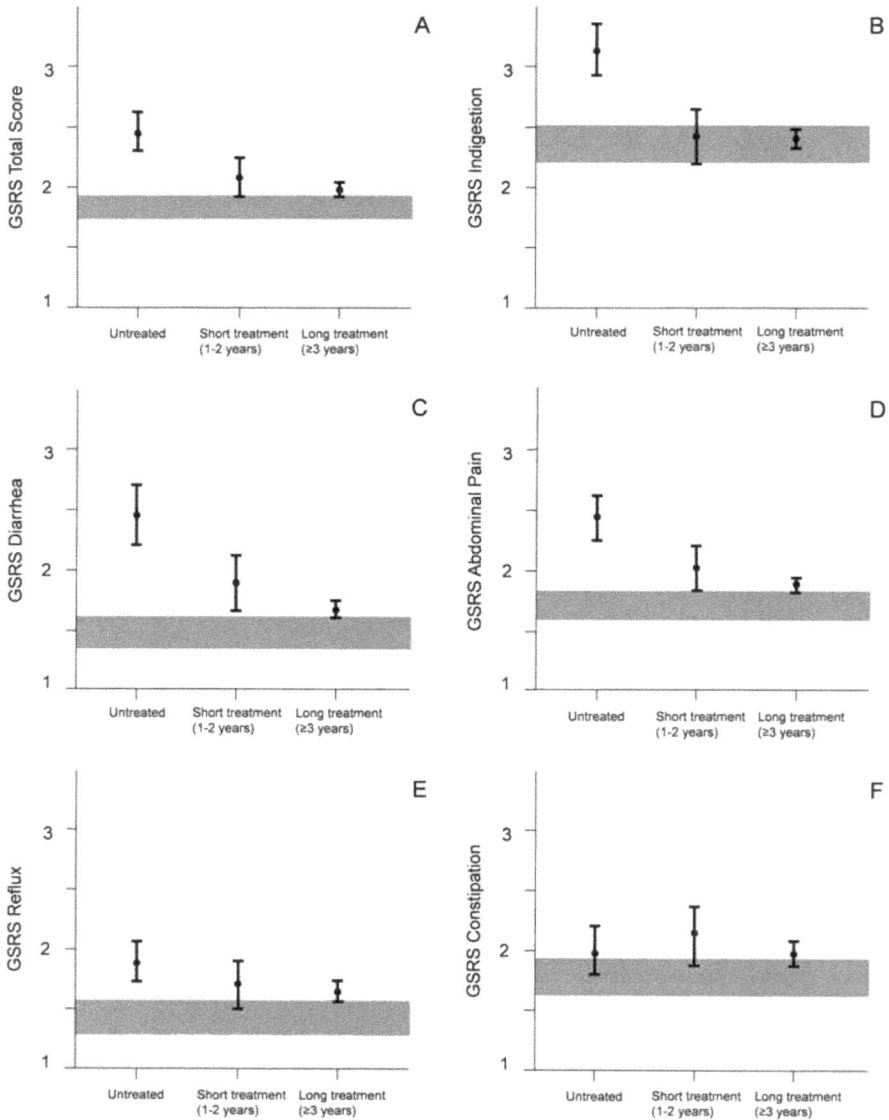

Figure 1. Gastrointestinal Symptom Rating Scale (GSRS) total (**A**) and sub-dimension (**B**–**F**) scores in untreated, short-term treated and long-term treated patients compared with healthy controls. Values are expressed as means with 95% confidence intervals (CI) and gray bars denote 95% CIs of controls. There were significant differences between the groups as follows: (**A**) Untreated patients and all other groups ($p < 0.001$), and short-term treated patients and healthy controls ($p = 0.03$); (**B**) Untreated and all other groups ($p < 0.001$); (**C**) Untreated and short-term treated ($p = 0.015$) and long-term treated ($p < 0.001$) patients, and short-term treated patients and healthy controls ($p = 0.010$); (**D**) Untreated patients and all other groups ($p < 0.001$); (**E**) Healthy controls and untreated ($p < 0.001$) and long-term treated ($p = 0.013$) patients.

Table 2. Presence (%) of increased gastrointestinal symptoms[a] in untreated, short-term (GFD 1–2 years) treated and long-term (GFD $\geqslant$ 3 years) treated celiac disease patients and in healthy controls.

GSRS Score	Celiac Patients on a GFD *n* = 728			
	Untreated Patients *n* = 128	Short Treatment *n* = 93	Long Treatment *n* = 635	Non-Celiac Controls *n* = 160
Total score	48 [b]	27 [c]	23 [c]	16
Indigestion	41 [b]	18	17	14
Diarrhea	47 [b]	32 [c,d]	21	15
Abdominal pain	43 [b]	20	18	14
Reflux	34 [b]	20 [c]	19 [c]	11
Constipation	16	18	18	16

GSRS, Gastrointestinal Symptom Rating Scale; GFD, gluten-free diet. [a] Defined as GSRS scores > 1 SD compared to mean values of healthy controls; [b] $p < 0.05$ compared with short and long treatment groups and with controls; [c] $p < 0.05$ compared with healthy controls; [d] $p < 0.05$ compared with long treatment group.

Comparisons of GSRS scores between celiac disease patients in the present study (untreated and long-term treated) and those with other gastrointestinal disorders can be seen in Figure 2. In general, untreated celiac patients suffered from a wider spectrum of symptoms compared with other gastrointestinal disease groups, the most severe being indigestion, diarrhea and abdominal pain (Figure 2). However, in long-term treated patients the gastrointestinal symptoms were clearly milder.

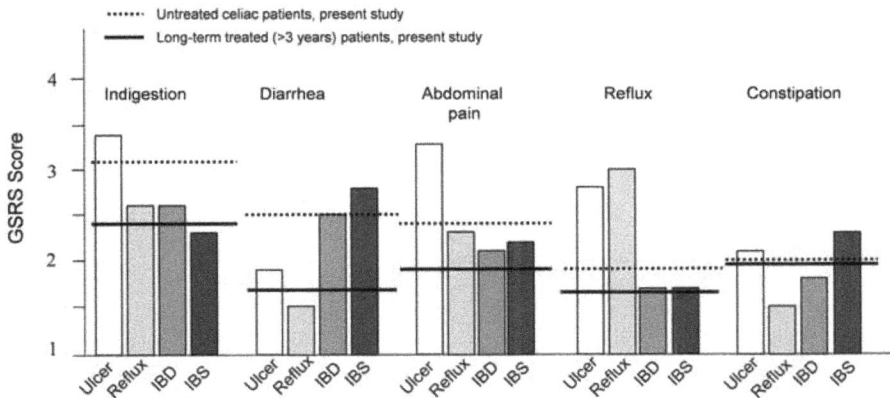

Figure 2. The mean Gastrointestinal Symptom Rating Scale (GSRS) sub-dimension scores of untreated and long-term treated patients (present study) compared with other gastrointestinal diseases [11,13–15]. Ulcer, peptic ulcer disease; Reflux, gastroesophageal reflux disease; IBD, inflammatory bowel disease; IBS, irritable bowel syndrome.

4. Discussion

The main finding in the present study was that both short-term and long-term dietary treated celiac disease patients have more symptoms than non-celiac controls. However, although the majority of gastrointestinal symptoms are alleviated well on a strict gluten-free diet, not all patients reach the level of the general population even in long-term follow-up.

Here, the majority of the celiac disease patients showed rapid relief of symptoms during the first year on a gluten-free diet. This is in accord with previous studies investigating short-term responses, where the diet has also alleviated typical gastrointestinal symptoms within the first few months after diagnosis [20–22]. The only exception here was diarrhea, which, although alleviated on a long-term diet, remained fairly common in short-term-treated patients. This raises the question whether the alleviation of diarrhea requires more complete histological recovery than other symptoms. However, in a recent study we observed no differences in symptoms or quality of life between patients evincing full histological recovery and those with ongoing mucosal damage after one year [22]. Hence, incomplete mucosal recovery would not appear to explain slow recovery from diarrhea in our patients. The few previous studies investigating this issue have obtained somewhat contradictory results. In accord with our observations, Pulido and colleagues showed very slow resolution of diarrhea on treatment within five or more years [7], whereas a group under Murray observed improvement of diarrhea already within six months [20]. The reason for these considerable variations between the studies remains unclear, but might for example involve differences in interpretation and definition of symptoms. Obviously different study designs and populations may also have an effect, as we had demographic characteristics and design similar to those of Pulido and colleagues [7], whereas Murray and group [20] investigated mainly short-term responses to a gluten-free diet in one well-defined geographical region.

In contrast to the well-documented short-term outcome [2], the long-term response to a gluten-free diet has thus far been poorly investigated. Judging from our results, in most patients with good adherence and recovered villi the good initial response to the diet remains after several years, demonstrating that it is not only based on a short-term "honeymoon" effect. Notwithstanding this long-lasting positive effect, we found even long-term dietary treated patients to have more symptoms than healthy controls. Such ongoing symptoms may in the long run discourage patients from adhering to what is a socially restrictive and expensive treatment mode if they consider it ineffective. In such cases, it is particularly important for physicians to urge patients to persist with a strict gluten-free diet in order to prevent disease-associated complications [2]. In addition to the increased GSRS total score, particularly reflux symptoms showed a tendency to persist for several years. Gastroesophageal reflux is common in general populations [23] and in earlier studies it has appeared to be approximately as common in celiac patients [24]. Then again, initiation of a gluten-free diet has often reduced reflux symptoms rapidly [25–27], and the response has also persisted in the long term [27]. In some studies reflux symptoms have been suggested to be more common in aged people [28], but this is controversial and did not explain the difference in the present study. Altogether, the reason for the increase in reflux symptoms in long-term treated celiac disease remains unclear and needs to be clarified in future studies.

We observed long-term treated celiac disease women to experience more symptoms than men. Previously Hallert and associates has reported similar findings in Swedish women [6,29,30], and Pulido and colleagues observed more symptoms in both undiagnosed Canadian women and those on dietary treatment [7]. One plausible explanation for the gender difference might be the higher prevalence of concomitant functional gastrointestinal disorders in women, which have also been shown to be exacerbated by psychological distress such as that involved in following a burdensome dietary treatment [31–33]. Women may also find the inevitable social restrictions caused by the gluten-free diet harder to cope with [29]. Other possible reasons could be differences in fiber intake and the symptom-modifying effect of gonadal hormones [34–36]. In any case, physicians should acknowledge the higher risk of persistent symptoms in women and provide adequate support if needed.

In comparison with the other common gastrointestinal disorders as reported in the literature [11,13–15], we observed that untreated celiac patients evince a fairly wide range of symptoms. In line with this, other recent studies have reported that nowadays only a minority of patients present with classical symptoms, such as diarrhea and malabsorption, but, instead, suffer from a plethora of "atypical" symptoms or have no symptoms at all [4,19,37]. As well as in the diagnostic workout, this heterogeneous clinical presentation also needs to be taken into account when evaluating the long-term dietary response. In particular, although the specific GSRS scores here were mostly fairly low, physicians should remember that suffering from multiple, even if moderate, symptoms simultaneously may constitute a substantial burden in individual patients.

The most common reason for the persistence of symptoms in celiac disease has been ongoing gluten consumption [5,38]. However, in agreement with our previous studies [19,39,40], more than 90% of the patients here were strictly adherent and even in the few who reported lapses these were only occasional. This conception was further confirmed by the well-recovered histology and low EmA-positivity among patients on the diet. Thus, although gluten intake should always be excluded [41], other explanations for persistent symptoms must be sought in patients with proven strict adherence. These include for example small-intestinal bacterial overgrowth or some other concomitant disorder such as IBD and microscopic colitis, and refractory celiac disease [5,41]. An interesting new research topic related to this issue is dysbiosis of the intestinal microbiota [42]. We have recently shown that celiac patients suffering from persistent symptoms on a gluten-free diet had an altered balance and reduced richness of duodenal microbiota [43]. The intestinal microbiota affects the complex gut-brain axis along with the enteric nervous system, immune system and external environment, and alterations in this axis may predispose to chronic pain in functional gastrointestinal disorders and perhaps also in celiac disease [44]. A deeper understanding of these mechanisms would be important in order to make the development of new pharmacological interventions possible.

Several novel adjunct therapies to improve the treatment of celiac disease are currently under development [45]. In these circumstances evaluating long-term symptoms in treated celiac disease patients becomes more and more important. For now, gluten-free diet remains the gold standard treatment for celiac disease and thus every new therapeutic approach needs to be compared with the response to the diet. The present study provides solid information of the response of celiac individuals to gluten-free diet and could thus be used as baseline to the future pharmacological trials.

Strengths of the present study were the large and nationwide cohort of clinically representative celiac disease patients and the use of well-validated and structured symptom questionnaire. A major limitation was the retrospective cross-sectional study design, this, however, being offset by the fact that patients with different durations of gluten-free diet were comparable regarding most of the clinical and demographic parameters and were diagnosed and treated similarly according to nationwide guidelines. Another limitation was that the majority of the participants were recruited via celiac disease associations, which may cause some selection bias. Finally, celiac disease was not excluded among all healthy controls, a few of whom might have been suffering unrecognized.

5. Conclusions

In conclusion, we showed that the good initial clinical response to a gluten-free diet is sustained also in the long run. However, it is important for physicians to realize that one year might not be long enough for all symptoms to abate, and that some patients may continue to have mild or moderate gastrointestinal symptoms despite long-term and strict dietary treatment. A fuller understanding of the factors behind persistent symptoms in celiac disease would provide new treatment possibilities in the future.

Acknowledgments: The study was supported by the Academy of Finland, the Sigrid Juselius Foundation, the Competitive State Research Financing of the Expert Area of Tampere University Hospital (grants 9R034, 9R018, 9T023 and 9T058) and Seinäjoki Central Hospital (VTR16), Kaarina Savolainen's Fund Allocated for the Development of Cancer Treatment, the Finnish Medical Foundation, the Mary and Georg Ehrnrooth Foundation, and the Foundation for Pediatric Research.

Author Contributions: Pilvi Laurikka, Teea Salmi, Pekka Collin, Heini Huhtala, Markku Mäki, Katri Kaukinen and Kalle Kurppa conceived and designed the study; Pekka Collin and Markku Mäki contributed to the acquisition of data; Pilvi Laurikka, Heini Huhtala, Katri Kaukinen and Kalle Kurppa analyzed the data; Pilvi Laurikka and Kalle Kurppa drafted the manuscript and Teea Salmi, Pekka Collin, Heini Huhtala, Markku Mäki and Katri Kaukinen revised the manuscript for important intellectual content.

Conflicts of Interest: The authors declare no conflict of interest. The sponsors had no role in the study design; in the collection, analyses, or interpretation of data; in the writing of the manuscript, and in the decision to publish the results.

References

1. Wahab, P.J.; Meijer, J.W.; Mulder, C.J. Histologic follow-up of people with celiac disease on a gluten-free diet: Slow and incomplete recovery. *Am. J. Clin. Pathol.* **2002**, *118*, 459–463. [CrossRef] [PubMed]
2. See, J.A.; Kaukinen, K.; Makharia, G.K.; Gibson, P.R.; Murray, J.A. Practical insights into gluten-free diets. *Nat. Rev. Gastroenterol. Hepatol.* **2015**, *12*, 580–591. [CrossRef] [PubMed]
3. Haines, M.L.; Anderson, R.P.; Gibson, P.R. Systematic review: The evidence base for long-term management of coeliac disease. *Aliment. Pharmacol. Ther.* **2008**, *28*, 1042–1066. [CrossRef] [PubMed]
4. Paarlahti, P.; Kurppa, K.; Ukkola, A.; Collin, P.; Huhtala, H.; Maki, M.; Kaukinen, K. Predictors of persistent symptoms and reduced quality of life in treated coeliac disease patients: A large cross-sectional study. *BMC Gastroenterol.* **2013**, *13*, 75. [CrossRef] [PubMed]
5. Dewar, D.H.; Donnelly, S.C.; McLaughlin, S.D.; Johnson, M.W.; Ellis, H.J.; Ciclitira, P.J. Celiac disease: Management of persistent symptoms in patients on a gluten-free diet. *World J. Gastroenterol.* **2012**, *18*, 1348–1356. [CrossRef] [PubMed]
6. Midhagen, G.; Hallert, C. High rate of gastrointestinal symptoms in celiac patients living on a gluten-free diet: Controlled study. *Am. J. Gastroenterol.* **2003**, *98*, 2023–2026. [CrossRef] [PubMed]
7. Pulido, O.; Zarkadas, M.; Dubois, S.; Macisaac, K.; Cantin, I.; La Vieille, S.; Godefroy, S.; Rashid, M. Clinical features and symptom recovery on a gluten-free diet in Canadian adults with celiac disease. *Can. J. Gastroenterol.* **2013**, *27*, 449–453. [CrossRef] [PubMed]
8. Sulkanen, S.; Collin, P.; Laurila, K.; Mäki, M. IgA- and IgG-class antihuman umbilical cord antibody tests in adult coeliac disease. *Scand. J. Gastroenterol.* **1998**, *33*, 251–254. [PubMed]
9. Taavela, J.; Koskinen, O.; Huhtala, H.; Lahdeaho, M.L.; Popp, A.; Laurila, K.; Collin, P.; Kaukinen, K.; Kurppa, K.; Mäki, M. Validation of morphometric analyses of small-intestinal biopsy readouts in celiac disease. *PLoS ONE* **2013**, *8*, e76163. [CrossRef] [PubMed]
10. Hopman, E.G.; Koopman, H.M.; Wit, J.M.; Mearin, M.L. Dietary compliance and health-related quality of life in patients with coeliac disease. *Eur. J. Gastroenterol. Hepatol.* **2009**, *21*, 1056–1061. [CrossRef] [PubMed]
11. Simren, M.; Axelsson, J.; Gillberg, R.; Abrahamsson, H.; Svedlund, J.; Björnsson, E.S. Quality of life in inflammatory bowel disease in remission: The impact of IBS-like symptoms and associated psychological factors. *Am. J. Gastroenterol.* **2002**, *97*, 389–396. [CrossRef] [PubMed]
12. Svedlund, J.; Sjödin, I.; Dotevall, G. GSRS—A clinical rating scale for gastrointestinal symptoms in patients with irritable bowel syndrome and peptic ulcer disease. *Dig. Dis. Sci.* **1988**, *33*, 129–134. [CrossRef] [PubMed]
13. Olafsson, S.; Hatlebakk, J.G.; Berstad, A. Patients with endoscopic gastritis and/or duodenitis improve markedly following eradication of Helicobacter pylori, although less so than patients with ulcers. *Scand. J. Gastroenterol.* **2002**, *37*, 1386–1394. [CrossRef] [PubMed]
14. Hori, K.; Matsumoto, T.; Miwa, H. Analysis of the gastrointestinal symptoms of uninvestigated dyspepsia and irritable bowel syndrome. *Gut Liver* **2009**, *3*, 192–196. [CrossRef] [PubMed]
15. Dimenäs, E.; Carlsson, G.; Glise, H.; Israelsson, B.; Wiklund, I. Relevance of norm values as part of the documentation of quality of life instruments for use in upper gastrointestinal disease. *Scand. J. Gastroenterol. Suppl.* **1996**, *221*, 8–13.
16. Häuser, W.; Stallmach, A.; Caspary, W.F.; Stein, J. Predictors of reduced health-related quality of life in adults with coeliac disease. *Aliment. Pharmacol. Ther.* **2007**, *25*, 569–578.
17. Zeltzer, L.K.; Lu, Q.; Leisenring, W.; Tsao, J.C.; Recklitis, C.; Armstrong, G.; Mertens, A.C.; Robison, L.L.; Ness, K.K. Psychosocial outcomes and health-related quality of life in adult childhood cancer survivors: A report from the childhood cancer survivor study. *Cancer Epidemiol. Biomark. Prev.* **2008**, *17*, 435–446. [CrossRef] [PubMed]
18. Wilt, T.J.; Rubins, H.B.; Collins, D.; O'Connor, T.Z.; Rutan, G.H.; Robins, S.J. Correlates and consequences of diffuse atherosclerosis in men with coronary heart disease. *Arch. Intern. Med.* **1996**, *156*, 1181–1188. [CrossRef] [PubMed]
19. Kurppa, K.; Lauronen, O.; Collin, P.; Ukkola, A.; Laurila, K.; Huhtala, H.; Maki, M.; Kaukinen, K. Factors associated with dietary adherence in celiac disease: A nationwide study. *Digestion* **2012**, *86*, 309–314. [CrossRef] [PubMed]
20. Murray, J.A.; Watson, T.; Clearman, B.; Mitros, F. Effect of a gluten-free diet on gastrointestinal symptoms in celiac disease. *Am. J. Clin. Nutr.* **2004**, *79*, 669–673. [PubMed]

21. Zarkadas, M.; Cranney, A.; Case, S.; Molloy, M.; Switzer, C.; Graham, I.D.; Butzner, J.D.; Rashid, M.; Warren, R.E.; Burrows, V. The impact of a gluten-free diet on adults with coeliac disease: Results of a national survey. *J. Hum. Nutr. Diet.* **2006**, *19*, 41–49. [CrossRef] [PubMed]

22. Pekki, H.; Kurppa, K.; Mäki, M.; Huhtala, H.; Sievänen, H.; Laurila, K.; Collin, P.; Kaukinen, K. Predictors and Significance of Incomplete Mucosal Recovery in Celiac Disease After 1 Year on a Gluten-Free Diet. *Am. J. Gastroenterol.* **2015**, *110*, 1078–1085. [CrossRef] [PubMed]

23. Rasmussen, S.; Jensen, T.H.; Henriksen, S.L.; Haastrup, P.F.; Larsen, P.V.; Söndergaard, J.; Jarbol, D.E. Overlap of symptoms of gastroesophageal reflux disease, dyspepsia and irritable bowel syndrome in the general population. *Scand. J. Gastroenterol.* **2015**, *50*, 162–169. [CrossRef] [PubMed]

24. Mooney, P.D.; Evans, K.E.; Kurien, M.; Hopper, A.D.; Sanders, D.S. Gastro-oesophageal reflux symptoms and coeliac disease: No role for routine duodenal biopsy. *Eur. J. Gastroenterol. Hepatol.* **2015**, *27*, 692–697. [CrossRef] [PubMed]

25. Cuomo, A.; Romano, M.; Rocco, A.; Budillon, G.; Del Vecchio, B.C.; Nardone, G. Reflux oesophagitis in adult coeliac disease: Beneficial effect of a gluten free diet. *Gut* **2003**, *52*, 514–517. [CrossRef] [PubMed]

26. Collin, P.; Mustalahti, K.; Kyrönpalo, S.; Rasmussen, M.; Pehkonen, E.; Kaukinen, K. Should we screen reflux oesophagitis patients for coeliac disease? *Eur. J. Gastroenterol. Hepatol.* **2004**, *16*, 917–920. [CrossRef] [PubMed]

27. Nachman, F.; Vazquez, H.; Gonzalez, A.; Andrenacci, P.; Compagni, L.; Reyes, H.; Sugai, E.; Moreno, M.L.; Smecuol, E.; Hwang, H.J.; et al. Gastroesophageal reflux symptoms in patients with celiac disease and the effects of a gluten-free diet. *Clin. Gastroenterol. Hepatol.* **2011**, *9*, 214–219. [CrossRef] [PubMed]

28. Diaz-Rubio, M.; Moreno-Elola-Olaso, C.; Rey, E.; Locke, G.R., III; Rodriguez-Artalejo, F. Symptoms of gastro-oesophageal reflux: Prevalence, severity, duration and associated factors in a Spanish population. *Aliment. Pharmacol. Ther.* **2004**, *19*, 95–105. [CrossRef] [PubMed]

29. Hallert, C.; Grännö, C.; Hulten, S.; Midhagen, G.; Ström, M.; Svensson, H.; Valdimarsson, T. Living with coeliac disease: Controlled study of the burden of illness. *Scand. J. Gastroenterol.* **2002**, *37*, 39–42. [CrossRef] [PubMed]

30. Hallert, C.; Grännö, C.; Grant, C.; Hulten, S.; Midhagen, G.; Ström, M.; Svensson, H.; Valdimarsson, T.; Wickström, T. Quality of life of adult coeliac patients treated for 10 years. *Scand. J. Gastroenterol.* **1998**, *33*, 933–938. [CrossRef] [PubMed]

31. Chang, L.; Heitkemper, M.M. Gender differences in irritable bowel syndrome. *Gastroenterology* **2002**, *123*, 1686–1701. [CrossRef] [PubMed]

32. Flier, S.N.; Rose, S. Is functional dyspepsia of particular concern in women? A review of gender differences in epidemiology, pathophysiologic mechanisms, clinical presentation, and management. *Am. J. Gastroenterol.* **2006**, *101*, S644–S653. [CrossRef] [PubMed]

33. Koloski, N.A.; Talley, N.J.; Boyce, P.M. Does psychological distress modulate functional gastrointestinal symptoms and health care seeking? A prospective, community Cohort study. *Am. J. Gastroenterol.* **2003**, *98*, 789–797. [CrossRef] [PubMed]

34. Storey, M.; Anderson, P. Income and race/ethnicity influence dietary fiber intake and vegetable consumption. *Nutr. Res.* **2014**, *34*, 844–850. [CrossRef] [PubMed]

35. Kuba, T.; Quinones-Jenab, V. The role of female gonadal hormones in behavioral sex differences in persistent and chronic pain: Clinical versus preclinical studies. *Brain Res. Bull.* **2005**, *66*, 179–188. [CrossRef] [PubMed]

36. Mulak, A.; Taché, Y. Sex difference in irritable bowel syndrome: Do gonadal hormones play a role? *Gastroenterol. Polska* **2010**, *17*, 89–97.

37. Leffler, D.A.; Green, P.H.R.; Fasano, A. Extraintestinal manifestations of coeliac disease. *Nat. Rev. Gastroenterol. Hepatol.* **2015**, *12*, 561–571. [CrossRef] [PubMed]

38. Abdulkarim, A.S.; Burgart, L.J.; See, J.; Murray, J.A. Etiology of nonresponsive celiac disease: Results of a systematic approach. *Am. J. Gastroenterol.* **2002**, *97*, 2016–2021. [CrossRef] [PubMed]

39. Viljamaa, M.; Collin, P.; Huhtala, H.; Sievänen, H.; Mäki, M.; Kaukinen, K. Is coeliac disease screening in risk groups justified? A fourteen-year follow-up with special focus on compliance and quality of life. *Aliment. Pharmacol. Ther.* **2005**, *22*, 317–324. [CrossRef] [PubMed]

40. Ukkola, A.; Mäki, M.; Kurppa, K.; Collin, P.; Huhtala, H.; Kekkonen, L.; Kaukinen, K. Patients' experiences and perceptions of living with coeliac disease—Implications for optimizing care. *J. Gastrointest. Liver Dis.* **2012**, *21*, 17–22.

41. Leffler, D.A.; Dennis, M.; Hyett, B.; Kelly, E.; Schuppan, D.; Kelly, C.P. Etiologies and predictors of diagnosis in nonresponsive celiac disease. *Clin. Gastroenterol. Hepatol.* **2007**, *5*, 445–450. [CrossRef] [PubMed]

42. Verdu, E.F.; Galipeau, H.J.; Jabri, B. Novel players in coeliac disease pathogenesis: Role of the gut microbiota. *Nat. Rev. Gastroenterol. Hepatol.* **2015**, *12*, 497–506. [CrossRef] [PubMed]

43. Wacklin, P.; Laurikka, P.; Lindfors, K.; Collin, P.; Salmi, T.; Lähdeaho, M.L.; Saavalainen, P.; Mäki, M.; Mättö, J.; Kurppa, K.; Kaukinen, K. Altered duodenal microbiota composition in celiac disease patients suffering from persistent symptoms on a long-term gluten-free diet. *Am. J. Gastroenterol.* **2014**, *109*, 1933–1941. [CrossRef] [PubMed]

44. Mayer, E.A.; Labus, J.S.; Tillisch, K.; Cole, S.W.; Baldi, P. Towards a systems view of IBS. *Nat. Rev. Gastroenterol. Hepatol.* **2015**, *12*, 592–605. [CrossRef] [PubMed]

45. Kurppa, K.; Hietikko, M.; Sulic, A.M.; Kaukinen, K.; Lindfors, K. Current status of drugs in development for celiac disease. *Expert Opin. Investig. Drugs* **2014**, *23*, 1079–1091. [CrossRef] [PubMed]

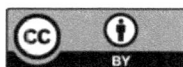

nutrients

MDPI

Article

Persistent Intraepithelial Lymphocytosis in Celiac Patients Adhering to Gluten-Free Diet Is Not Abolished Despite a Gluten Contamination Elimination Diet

Barbara Zanini [1,*], Monica Marullo [1], Vincenzo Villanacci [2], Marianna Salemme [2], Francesco Lanzarotto [1], Chiara Ricci [1] and Alberto Lanzini [1]

1   Gastroenterology Unit, University and Spedali Civili of Brescia, Piazzale Spedali Civili, Brescia I-25123, Italy; mon.ya@live.it (M.M.); francesco.lanzarotto@asst-spedalicivili.it (F.L.); chiara.ricci@unibs.it (C.R.); alberto.lanzini@unibs.it (A.L.)
2   Histopathology Unit, University and Spedali Civili of Brescia, Piazzale Spedali Civili, Brescia I-25123, Italy; villanac@alice.it (V.V.); mariannasalemme@alice.it (M.S.)
*   Correspondence: barbara.zanini@unibs.it; Tel.: +39-303-399-2541; Fax: +39-030-399-5817

Received: 8 July 2016; Accepted: 16 August 2016; Published: 26 August 2016

Abstract: The gluten-free diet (GFD) is the only validated treatment for celiac disease (CD), but despite strict adherence, complete mucosal recovery is rarely obtained. The aim of our study was to assess whether complete restitutio ad integrum could be achieved by adopting a restrictive diet (Gluten Contamination Elimination Diet, GCED) or may depend on time of exposure to GFD. Two cohorts of CD patients, with persisting Marsh II/Grade A lesion at duodenal biopsy after 12–18 months of GFD (early control) were identified. Patients in Cohort A were re-biopsied after a three-month GCED (GCED control) and patients in Cohort B were re-biopsied after a minimum of two years on a standard GFD subsequent to early control (late control). Ten patients in Cohort A and 19 in Cohort B completed the study protocol. There was no change in the classification of duodenal biopsies in both cohorts. The number of intraepithelial lymphocytes, TCRγδ+ (T-Cell Receptor gamma delta) T cell and eosinophils significantly decreased at GCED control (Cohort A) and at late control (Cohort B), compared to early control. Duodenal intraepithelial lymphocytosis persisting in CD patients during GFD is not eliminated by a GCED and is independent of the length of GFD. [NCT 02711696]

Keywords: gluten free diet; celiac disease; mucosal recovery; gluten contamination

1. Introduction

Celiac disease is a systemic autoimmune disorder triggered by the ingestion of gluten, a complex of proteins contained in wheat, barley and rye, in genetically predisposed patients. The autoimmune process is responsible for alterations in the duodenal mucosa graded according to Marsh and the New Classification as Marsh I/Grade A (intraepithelial lymphocytosis), Marsh II/Grade A (+ glandular hyperplasia) and Marsh III (+ IIIa partial, IIIb subtotal or IIIc total villous atrophy)/Grade B (B1 low-moderate or B2 severe atrophy) [1–5].

The only treatment for celiac disease is exclusion of gluten from the diet; however, despite strict dietary compliance, complete restitutio ad integrum of the duodenal mucosa is rarely achieved. In most cases, a variable degree of inflammation persists characterized by persistent intraepithelial lymphocytosis without or with associated glandular hyperplasia (Marsh I-II/Grade A) at control biopsy usually performed after 6–18 months of gluten-free diet (GFD) [6–10]. In our experience on

463 cases, complete normalization to Marsh 0 stage was observed in 8% of patients, with Marsh I and II lesions persisting in 65% of patients with duodenal atrophy at baseline [7].

The cause of persistence of this inflammation, even in patients fully adherent to GFD, poses a "million-dollar question" [11]. It is well known that there is a high degree of variability in individual response to gluten, with some patients' worsening of duodenal histology on exposure to very small amounts of gluten [12–14]. This observation suggests that contamination with gluten from commercially available processed food and/or small amounts of gluten present in products labeled "gluten-free" (up to 20 ppm) may prevent complete mucosal recovery. This explanation is indirectly supported in a study by Hollon and colleagues [15] showing that persistence of gastrointestinal symptoms in celiac patients on a GFD is eliminated in 81% of cases by adopting a diet based exclusively on naturally gluten-free products, and on removal from the diet of commercially available processed food and products labeled "gluten free" (Gluten Contamination Elimination Diet, GCED). Unfortunately, information on the effects of this diet on duodenal histology was largely incomplete. Another explanation to gluten contamination is that complete mucosal recovery during GFD may go undetected, as the time of follow-up biopsies at 12–18 months may be too short.

The aim of our study was to assess whether complete recovery of duodenal mucosa in patients with persistent Marsh I-II/Grade A lesion after one year of GFD: (i) can be achieved by adopting a GCED; and/or (ii) may depend on the time of exposure to GFD. To achieve this aim, we studied two cohorts of patients with Marsh I-II/Grade A lesion after one year of GFD: cohort A was re-biopsied after three months on GCED, and cohort B after a minimum of two years subsequent to the first follow-up biopsy at 6–18 months.

2. Materials and methods

This study is a prospective, open label, interventional study involving celiac patients on regular follow up at our Celiac Disease Clinic during GFD. We identified 2 cohorts of patients.

2.1. Recruitment

Cohort A consisted of patients from the Clinic with persistent Marsh II/Grade A lesion at follow-up duodenal biopsy performed on GFD (early control), who were instructed to adopt a GCED for three months, before repeating biopsy. Cohort B consisted of patients on long-term follow-up, who accepted to repeat biopsy at least 60 months after the early control biopsy on GFD (late control). In both cohorts, patient selection criteria included: (i) Marsh II/Grade A lesion at duodenal biopsy performed at 12–18 months after starting GFD; (ii) negative CD related serology on GFD; (iii) strict adherence to GFD without digression; (iv) absence of gastrointestinal or extra intestinal symptoms; and (v) absence of *Helicobacter pylori* infection and no history of chronic NSAIDs (NonSteroidal Anti-Inflammatory Drugs) use.

Patients in cohort A were informed of the rationale for adopting a GCED and of the characteristics of the diet by a physician and a professional dietitian expert on CD and with the help of leaflets (AL and MM). Patients were seen monthly at the Clinic by the physician and the dietician to ensure adherence to the diet and to boost compliance with the protocol. The GCED was designed as indicated by Hollon et al. [15] and patients were required to stay on the GCED for a minimum of 3 months or more if well tolerated. Patients were given 2 kg of rice macaroni (Riso Viazzo, Crova, VC, Italy), 2 kg of rice (Riso Viazzo, Crova, VC, Italy) and 2 kg of corn flour (Molino Bresciano, Azzano Mella, Bs, Italy) free of charge for each month of the study. Before and after the GCED patients were asked to fill in a questionnaire on gastrointestinal symptoms using the Gastrointestinal Symptom Rating Scale (GSRS) questionnaire [16,17] that includes 15 items related to gastrointestinal symptoms grouped into 5 dimensions: abdominal pain, reflux, indigestion, diarrhea and constipation, and scored according to a 7-point Likert scale graded 1 (no discomfort at all) to 7 (very severe discomfort) referring to the previous week.

Patients in cohort B were assessed by the dietitian for adherence to GFD and invited to a repeated duodenal biopsy after long-term GFD (late control). Adherence to GFD was assessed by the dietician using 4 point Likert scale (1 = no digression; 4 = no adherence at all) as previously described [18].

2.2. Serology

IgA t-TG antibodies were measured on the same day as duodenal biopsy with the enzyme-linked immunosorbent assay procedure employing the human recombinant t-Tg antigen (Eu t-Tg$^{®}$Eurospital, Trieste, Italy), and anti-endomysial antibodies (EMA) were detected by indirect immunofluorescence using monkey esophagus tissue as substrate (Antiendomysium$^{®}$, Eurospital, Trieste, Italy). HLA genotype was assessed with commercial kits [7].

2.3. Histology

According to our Institutional protocol [7], a minimum of 4 endoscopic biopsies were obtained from the duodenum and specimens were oriented mucosal-up on cellulose filter. Duodenal histology was classified according to Marsh [1] and to the New Classification [3–5]. For pathology assessment two serials of 4-micron-thick were cut from each biopsy, one serial stained with H&E (Haematoxylin and Eosin) and one serial routinely used for CD 3 identification by immunohistochemistry using rabbit monoclonal antihuman antibodies 1:250 (Neomarker, Fremont, CA, USA). Intraepithelial lymphocytes (IEL) were counted on the H&E stained sections and on the corresponding CD 3 immuno-stained sections after counting at least 300 epithelial cells on both sides of five villous bodies. A cut-off value of 25 IEL/100 epithelial cells was used.

TCRγδ+ T cells were identified using a commercially available method suitable for formalin fixed paraffin embedded (FFPE) small bowel biopsies [19]. Serial cut sections (4 μm thick) of FFPE were stained using anti TCRCγM1 (Thermo Scientific, Fremont, CA, USA). After the appropriate antigen retrieval, the reaction was revealed using EnVisio (Dako, Glostrrup, Denmark) and Novolink polymer (Novocastra, Newcastle upon Tyne, UK). Diamonobenzidine was used as chromogen and Meyer's hematoxylin as counterstaining. Sections were digitalized with Aperio Scanscope CS (Nikon) and a mean of the count was obtained with a cut off value of 4/100 epithelial cells. Eosinophils have also been counted with a cut off value of 2/100 epithelial cells. For Villous Height-Crypt Depth ratio (VH:CD), a cut-off value of 2 was considered to categorize patients as having active celiac disease (VH:CD <2) or not (VH:CD ≥2) [20]. All endoscopic biopsies were reviewed by experienced pathologists (V.V. and M.S.).

2.4. Statistics

Results were expressed as mean ± SD, and differences were tested for statistical significance using paired t test or Wilcoxon matched pairs test as appropriate, after testing normality with D'Agostino and Pearson omnibus normality test. A p value of <0.05 was used to reject the null hypothesis. The GraphPad Prism 5 statistical package (GraphPad Software, La Jolla, CA, USA) was used for statistical analysis and graphs.

2.5. Ethics

Our Institutional ethical committee approved of the study protocol on 10 February 2014. ClinicaTrials.gov identifier was NCT02711696.

3. Results

3.1. Patients' Characteristics

Cohort A consisted of 13 patients (F 69%, mean age 38 ± 14 years) and cohort B of 19 patients (F 79%, mean age 34 ± 10 years). A flow chart of the study design and the main baseline characteristics in both cohorts reported in Figure 1 and Table 1, respectively.

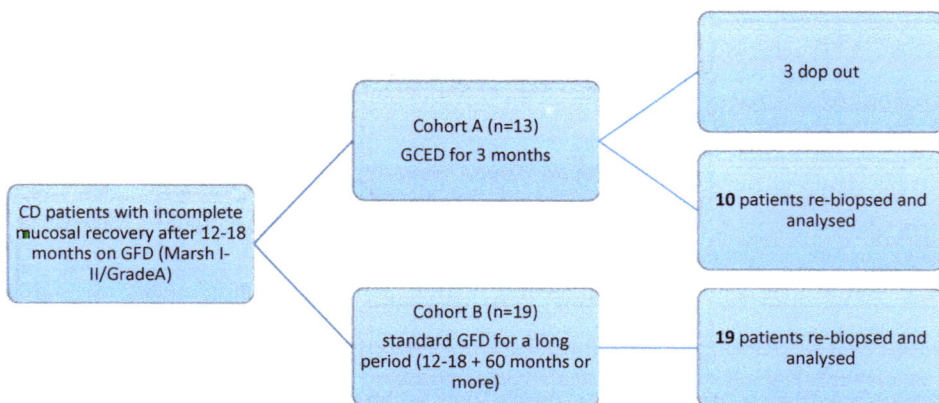

Figure 1. Study design flow-chart and patients assignment in the two cohorts.

Table 1. Main characteristics of Cohorts A and B at the time of diagnosis of Celiac Disease.

Cohort A					Cohort B				
n	Gender	Age	Marsh	NC	*n*	Gender	Age	Marsh	NC
1	M	23	3a	B1	1	F	38	3c	B2
2	M	30	3c	B2	2	F	34	3c	B2
3	F	22	3c	B2	3	M	38	3c	B2
4	F	30	3a	B1	4	M	46	3c	B2
5	F	30	3a	B1	5	F	45	3c	B2
6	F	43	3b	B1	6	F	22	3a	B1
7	F	47	3b	B1	7	F	46	3a	B1
8	F	49	3c	B2	8	F	19	3	B1
9	F	26	3a	B1	9	F	25	3c	B2
10	F	68	3b	B1	10	F	42	3b	B1
11	M	44	3a	B1	11	F	20	3b	B1
12	F	29	3c	B2	12	F	44	2	A
13	M	58	2	A	13	M	32	3b	B1
					14	M	29	3b	B1
					15	F	26	3c	B2
					16	F	30	3c	B2
					17	F	26	3c	B2
					18	F	52	3b	B1
					19	F	38	3c	B2

NC: New Classification [3–5].

3.2. Effect of GCED: Cohort A

Ten of the 13 patients enrolled in cohort A completed the trial. Two patients withdrew immediately after starting, and one patient after two months because of difficulties in adherence to GCED (patients 3 and 6, and 8 in Table 2, respectively).

As for selection criteria patients were virtually asymptomatic at control biopsy, and during GCED, GSRS dimension scores remained virtually unchanged for abdominal pain (2.40 ± 0.54 vs. 1.97 ± 0.81, $p = 0.0954$), reflux (1.7 ± 0.67 vs. 1.5 ± 0.85, $p = 0.4962$), diarrhea (2.23 ± 1.51 vs. 1.70 ± 0.97, $p = 0.5736$), constipation (2.03 ± 1.20 vs. 1.23 ± 0.35, $p = 0.0502$) and statistically improved for indigestion (2.93 ± 1.22 vs. 1.93 ± 0.83, $p = 0.0183$). All patients reported improvement in general wellbeing. There was no significant change in body weight with a tendency in patients to gain BMI (22.5 ± 5.2 vs. 23.0 ± 4.9, $p = 0.5625$).

Table 2. Effect of Gluten Contamination Elimination Diet (GCED) on histological characteristics of duodenal biopsies.

n	Time of Diagnosis							Early Control (after 1 Year GFD)								GCED Control (after 3 Months of Restricted Diet)							
	BMI	Ttg	VH/CD	IEL	γδ	Eos	Months	BMI	Ttg	Marsh	NC	VH/CD	IEL	γδ	Eos	Days	BMI	Marsh	NC	VH/CD	IEL	γδ	Eos
1	19.3	>100/16	<2	35	8	3	13	19.0	13/16	2	A	≥2	30	7	2	95	18.5	2	A	≥2	29	6	1
2	38.0	>100/16	<2	50	10	4	13	36.3	5.1/16	2	A	≥2	41	8	2	109	32.4	2	A	≥2	35	5	1
3	19.7	>100/16	<2	50	10	4	13	19.7	8.2/16	2	A	≥2	41	8	2	d.o.	-	-	-	-	-	-	-
4	18.6	7.5/7	<2	48	8	3	14	19.0	3.4/16	2	A	≥2	40	5	2	92	18.4	2	A	≥2	35	4	1
5	21.1	>100/16	<2	50	13	5	14	23.5	4.2/16	2	A	≥2	40	11	3	79	23.0	2	A	≥2	36	10	2
6	19.4	8.1/7	<2	50	13	5	16	20.0	5./16	2	A	≥2	40	11	3	d.o.	-	-	-	-	-	-	-
7	28.3	>100/16	<2	50	8	2	13	31.4	7.7/16	2	A	≥2	42	5	1	85	29.2	2	A	≥2	35	3	1
8	19.8	18/16	<2	50	8	2	15	19.2	5./16	2	A	≥2	42	5	1	d.o.	-	-	-	-	-	-	-
9	25.0	11.6/16	<2	45	10	5	15	24.6	3.2/16	2	A	≥2	35	8	3	109	24.1	2	A	≥2	30	6	2
10	20.0	29/16	<2	45	7	5	13	20.5	3.0/16	2	A	≥2	35	6	3	92	20.9	2	A	≥2	31	5	2
11	22.7	80/16	<2	50	8	4	14	22.3	4./16	2	A	≥2	40	6	2	95	21.7	2	A	≥2	30	5	1
12	19.3	>100/16	<2	50	7	4	15	19.7	7.9/16	2	A	≥2	40	6	1	99	20.4	2	A	≥2	35	4	1
13	22.9	8.8/16	<2	50	7	4	29	22.9	5.9/16	2	A	≥2	35	9	5	95	20.9	2	A	≥2	30	8	4

BMI: Body Mass Index; Ttg: Tissue Transglutaminases; NC: New Classification [3–5]; VH/CD: Villous Height/Crypt depth ratio; IEL: IntraEpithelial Lymphocytes; Eos: Eosinophils; d.o.: Drop Out.

There was no change in the classification of duodenal biopsies and in VH:CD category at the end of GECD compared with results of the early control biopsies taken after a mean 15 ± 4 months of GFD. In all patients, biopsies were classified as Marsh II/Grade A with VH:CD ≥ 2 on both occasions (Table 2). The number of intraepithelial lymphocytes decreased from 47.9 ± 4.3 at the time of CD diagnosis to 38.5 ± 3.6 at early control biopsies ($p = 0.0015$) with further decrease to 32.6 ± 2.8 after GCED ($p = 0.0056$). The number of TCR$\gamma\delta+$ T cells decreased from 9.0 ± 2.1 at the time of CD diagnosis to 7.3 ± 2.1 at early control biopsies ($p = 0.0006$) with further decrease to 5.6 ± 2.1 after GCED ($p < 0.0001$). The number of eosinophils decreased from 3.8 ± 1.1 at the time of CD diagnosis to 2.3 ± 1.1 at early control biopsies ($p < 0.0001$) with further decrease to 1.6 ± 1.0 after GCED ($p = 0.006$) (Figure 2).

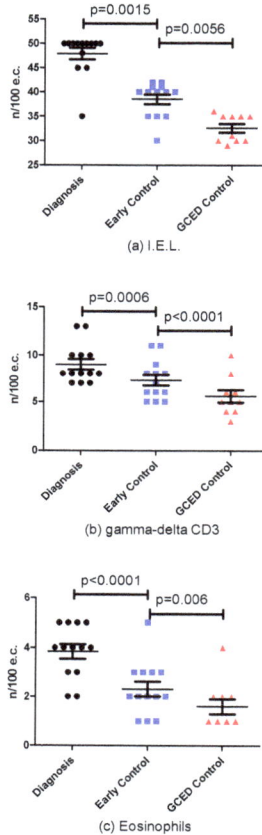

(a) I.E.L.

(b) gamma-delta CD3

(c) Eosinophils

Figure 2. Histologic Changes at the time of diagnosis, at early control and during Gluten Elimination Contamination Diet (GCED) in the number of: IntraEpithelial Lymphocytes (IEL) (**a**); gamma-delta CD3 (**b**); and eosinophils (**c**).

3.3. Effect of Long Term GFD

Nineteen patients enrolled in cohort B had repeated biopsies 96 ± 47 months (range 54–216) after the first control biopsy taken 16 ± 7 months (range 12–36) after starting GFD (Table 3). There was no change in classification of duodenal biopsies and in VH:CD category after long-term GFD compared with results obtained at the early control biopsy. In all patients, biopsies were classified as Marsh II/Grade A with VH:CD ≥ 2 on both occasions (Table 3) and in no case revealed compete normalization. The number of intraepithelial lymphocytes decreased from 45.1 ± 7.3 at the time of CD diagnosis to 41.9 ± 3.3 at the early control biopsy (p = 0.0071) with a further decrease to 34.5 ± 5.1 after long-term GFD (p = 0.0012). The number of TCRγδ+ T cells decreased from 13.0 ± 2.0 at the time of CD diagnosis to 10.5 ± 1.8 at early control biopsy (p < 0.0001) with further decrease to 9.1 ± 1.5 after long-term GFD (p < 0.0001). The number of eosinophils decreased from 4.0 ± 0.7 at the time of CD diagnosis to 2.4 ± 0.8 at early control biopsies (p < 0.0001) with further decrease to 1.4 ± 0.7 after long-term GFD (p = 0.0012) (Figure 3).

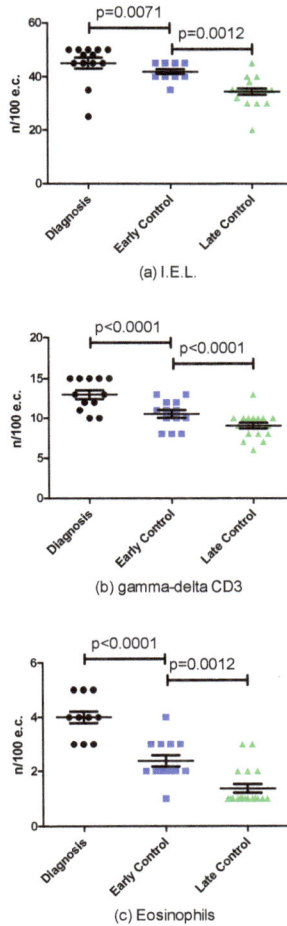

(a) I.E.L.

(b) gamma-delta CD3

(c) Eosinophils

Figure 3. Histologic Changes at the time of diagnosis, at early and late control during Gluten Free Diet (GFD) in the number of: IntraEpithelial Lymphocytes (IEL (**a**); gamma-delta CD3 (**b**); and eosinophils (**c**).

Table 3. Effect of time on histological characteristics of duodenal biopsies.

n	Time of Diagnosis				Early Control (after 1 Year GFD)							Late Control (after Longer Period of GFD)						
	VH/CD	IEL	γδ	Eos	Months	Marsh	NC	VH/CD	IEL	γδ	Eos	Months	Marsh	NC	VH/CD	IEL	γδ	Eos
1	<2	45	10	3	13	2	A	≥2	40	8	2	103	2	A	≥2	35	6	1
2	<2	50	15	4	12	2	A	≥2	45	12	3	54	2	A	≥2	35	10	2
3	<2	48	12	4	13	2	A	≥2	45	10	2	102	2	A	≥2	40	8	1
4	<2	48	13	5	16	2	A	≥2	45	11	3	78	2	A	≥2	40	10	1
5	<2	45	10	3	14	2	A	≥2	40	8	2	67	2	A	≥2	38	7	1
6	n.a	>25	n.a	n.a	12	2	A	n.a	>25	n.a	n.a	204	2	A	≥2	35	10	3
7	n.a	>25	n.a	n.a	12	2	A	≥2	45	10	4	54	1	A	≥2	35	8	1
8	<2	50	15	4	12	2	A	n.a	>25	n.a	n.a	216	2	A	≥2	45	13	1
9	<2	50	15	4	12	2	A	≥2	45	13	3	48	1	A	≥2	20	8	1
10	n.a	>25	n.a	n.a	12	2	A	≥2	40	11	2	63	2	A	≥2	35	9	1
11	n.a	>25	n.a	n.a	24	2	A	≥2	40	8	1	85	2	A	≥2	35	7	1
12	≥2	35	11	5	15	2	A	n.a	>25	n.a	n.a	80	2	A	≥2	32	9	3
13	n.a	>25	n.a	n.a	12	2	A	n.a	>25	n.a	n.a	60	2	A	≥2	35	9	2
14	<2	45	15	4	12	1	A	n.a	>25	n.a	n.a	63	2	A	≥2	30	10	1
15	<2	50	13	3	16	2	A	≥2	45	11	2	90	2	A	≥2	35	10	1
16	<2	50	12	5	13	2	A	≥2	40	10	3	116	2	A	≥2	35	9	2
17	n.a	>25	n.a	n.a	36	2	A	n.a	n.a	n.a	n.a	137	2	A	≥2	30	9	1
18	n.a	>25	n.a	n.a	22	2	A	≥2	35	13	2	85	2	A	≥2	30	10	1
19	<2	45	15	4	19	2	A	≥2	40	12	2	113	0	A	≥2	35	10	1

NC: New Classification [3–5]; VH/CD: Villous Height/Crypt Depth ratio; IEL: IntraEpithelial Lymphocytes; Eos: Eosinophils; n.a.: not available.

4. Discussion

Our study shows that duodenal intraepithelial lymphocytosis persisting in celiac patients during GFD is not completely eliminated despite a GCED, and is independent of the time of adherence to GFD. Although the number of patients studied is limited, in none of the 10 patients completing the three-month GCED trial, there was a regression in the histological stage from Marsh II/Grade A to Marsh 0. Our finding, obtained in a prospective way, at predetermined time of histological assessment extends the similar retrospective observations obtained in four out of five patients studied by Hollon et al. [15]. Given these results, we felt it unethical to enroll more patients mainly because of the alarmed reaction elicited by the proposal of a trial dealing with "incomplete mucosal recovery", and because adherence to the very restrictive GCED was very difficult, despite an improvement in wellbeing, mainly for social and psychological reasons, especially in asymptomatic patients.

The reason why GCED did not result in mucosal recovery is unclear. One possible explanation is that gluten contamination is unavoidable in our gluten-rich environment where the risk of contamination is high even in inherently gluten free food [21]. A Significant increase of IEL is an early event in the kinetics of histological response to gluten challenge in celiacs [22] thus acting as a sensitive marker of ongoing gluten ingestion. In our study, we did not allow for cereals except for rice and maize obtained by producers that exclusively process these two cereals. Besides contamination, a potential for maize prolamins to induce a gluten-like cellular immune response has been hypothesized [23] and this may contribute to persistent intraepithelial lymphocytosis at least in some patients.

A further possible explanation is that a three months of GCED is too short to achieve complete mucosal recovery and switching off the immunological process that characterizes CD. We have chosen a three-month period, because it proved sufficient in improving symptoms in 81% of the patients studied by Hollon et al. [15]. The study by Hollon et al. focused on the identification of refractory celiac disease (RCD) in non-responsive CD (biopsy-proven with persistence of symptoms and/or villous atrophy on strict GFD for at least 12 months) and on the proposal of a new algorithm to identify CD patients with RCD type 1 or type 2. Beside these differences in the study design, we felt it unethical to ask our patients (asymptomatic and without villous atrophy on GFD) for a longer period of GCED.

A third possibility is that persistence of intraepithelial lymphocytosis during GFD and the more restricted GCED may be speculatively attributable to characteristics of intestinal microbiota. Intestinal microbiota has a well-recognized role in the shaping of the intestinal immune system [24,25] and research is focusing on its potential role in the pathogenesis of celiac disease as a key factor in association with genetic predisposition and gluten [26]. Many factors known to influence intestinal microbiota have been identified as risk factors for CD. These include caesarean delivery [27] and breast feeding practices [28], although evidence is conflicting [29–31], history of infection and antibiotics use [31]. Furthermore quantitative and qualitative differences of intestinal and fecal microbiota have been identified between CD patients and controls [32–35], and composition of duodenal microbiota appears to be in relation to clinical manifestations of CD [35]. An intestinal disbiosis also persists during GFD even after reconstitution of the villous structure [32,36,37] and is different in patients with persisting symptoms and those who are asymptomatic [38]. Small intestinal microbiota respond metabolically to dietary changes [37] and it is reasonable to hypothesize that dietary components of GFD and GCED may cause pro-inflammatory changes in the intestinal mucosa thus preventing the mucosa from progress beyond reconstitution of the villous structure. This hypothesis is supported in a recent study by Tjellstrom et al. [39] in children with CD showing that challenge with strictly gluten free oats caused an increase of in fecal SCFA, acetic acid and n-butyric acid consistent with changes in the gut microflora and resulting in increased "fermentation index", a pro-inflammatory index.

Our study also confirms no further progression of intraepithelial lymphocytosis to normal limits after eight years of GFD compared with results obtained after 1–2 years [7,40]. Tuire et al. [40] reported a progressive reduction of in the prevalence of intraepithelial lymphocytosis from 85% at two years to 48% after 20 years of strict GFD and conclude that intraepithelial lymphocytosis may not disappear in treated CD over time. The reason for this persistence, besides common causes other than CD [41] that were excluded in our study and that of Tuire et al. [40] may, as in the case of lack of improvement with GCED, be related to gluten contamination or changes in microbiota during GFD.

Despite persistence of Marsh II/Grade A lesion, both patients treated with GCED and those on long-term GFD exhibited a slight although statistically significant reduction of IEL-CD3, Delta-gamma and eosinophils. This slight amelioration of the duodenal histology can be explained increased strictness in the GFD, that was inherent to the GCED, and the well established phenomenon of stricter adherence to dietary recommendations for patients enrolled in a clinical trial.

5. Conclusions

In conclusion, our study shows that residual duodenal inflammatory changes persist during GFD despite adherence to a diet based on products that are in nature gluten-free and despite long-term adherence to GFD. This incomplete mucosal recovery has, however, marginal clinical relevance and is unlikely to affect long-term prognosis [42].

Acknowledgments: We thank Mirna De Gregorio for her valuable help and kind assistance. We are grateful to Nurse Elvira Spreafichi and to Mrs Anna Tomasini for their assistance in clinical practice. Rice and corn flour were kindly provided by Riso Viazzo, Crova, VC, Italy and Molino Bresciano; Azzano Mella, BS, Italy, respectively.

Author Contributions: B.Z. jointly had the original idea for the study, and was involved in its design, acquisition and interpretation of data, and in the drafting of the manuscript. M.M. provided dietetic support, assisted in the acquisition and interpretation of data. V.V. reviewed all duodenal biopsies and assisted in interpretation of data. M.S. reviewed all duodenal biopsies and assisted in interpretation of data. F.L. assisted in the acquisition and interpretation of data. C.R. assisted in the acquisition and interpretation of data. A.L. jointly had the original idea of the study, and was involved in the interpretation of data and revision of the manuscript. All authors read and approved the final manuscript.

Conflicts of Interest: The authors declare no conflict of interest.

References

1. Marsh, M.N. Gluten, major histocompatibility complex and the small intestine. A molecular and immunobiologic approach to the spectrum of gluten sensitivity (celiac sprue). *Gastroenterology* **1992**, *102*, 330–354. [CrossRef]

2. Oberhuber, G.; Granditsch, G.; Volgelsang, H. The histopathology of celiac disease: Time for a standardized report scheme for pathologists. *Eur. J. Gastroenterol. Hepatol.* **1999**, *11*, 1185–1194. [CrossRef] [PubMed]

3. Corazza, G.R.; Villanacci, V. Coeliac Disease. Some considerations on the histological classification. *J. Clin. Pathol.* **2005**, *58*, 573–574. [CrossRef] [PubMed]

4. Corazza, G.R.; Villanacci, V.; Zambelli, C.; Milione, M.; Luinetti, O.; Vindigni, C.; Chioda, C.; Albarello, L.; Bartolini, D.; Donato, F. Comparison of the interobserver reproducibility with different histologic criteria used in celiac disease. *Clin. Gastroenterol. Hepatol.* **2007**, *5*, 838–843. [CrossRef] [PubMed]

5. Villanacci, V.; Ceppa, P.; Tavani, E.; Vindigni, C.; Volta, U.; Gruppo Italiano Patologi Apparato Digerente (GIPAD); Società Italiana di Anatomia Patologica e Citopatologia Diagnostica/International Academy of Pathology, Italian division (SIAPEC/IAP). Coeliac disease: The histology report. *Dig. Liver. Dis.* **2011**, *43*, S385–S395. [CrossRef]

6. Wahab, P.J.; Meijer, J.W.; Mulder, C.J. Histologic follow-up of people with celiac disease on a gluten free diet: Slow and incomplete recovery. *Am. J. Clin. Pathol.* **2002**, *118*, 459–463. [CrossRef] [PubMed]

7. Lanzini, A.; Lanzarotto, F.; Villanacci, V.; Mora, A.; Bertolazzi, S.; Turini, D.; Carella, G.; Malagoli, A.; Ferrante, G.; Cesana, B.M.; et al. Complete recovery of intestinal mucosa occurs very rarely in adult celiac patients despite adherence to gluten free diet. *Aliment. Pharmacol. Ther.* **2009**, *29*, 1299–1308. [CrossRef] [PubMed]

8. Ciacci, C.; Cirillo, M.; Cavallaro, R.; Mazzacca, G. Long term follow-up of celiac adults on gluten-free diet: Prevalence and correlates of intestinal damage. *Digestion* **2002**, *66*, 178–185. [CrossRef] [PubMed]

9. Lee, S.K.; Lo, W.; Memeo, L.; Rotterdam, H.; Green, P.H. Duodenal histology in patients with celiac disease after treatment with a gluten-free diet. *Gastrointest Endosc.* **2003**, *57*, 187–191. [CrossRef] [PubMed]

10. Bardella, M.T.; Velio, P.; Cesana, B.M.; Prampolini, L.; Casella, G.; Di Bella, C.; Lanzini, A.; Gambarotti, M.; Bassotti, G.; Villanacci, V. Coelic disease: A histological follow-up study. *Histopathology* **2007**, *50*, 465–471. [CrossRef] [PubMed]

11. Koning, F.; Mol, M.; Mearin, M.L. The million-dollar question: Is gluten-free food safe for patients with celiac disease? *Am. J. Clin. Nutr.* **2013**, *97*, 3–4. [CrossRef] [PubMed]

12. Catassi, C.; Fabiani, E.; Iacono, G.; D'Agate, C.; Francavilla, K.; Biagi, F.; Volta, U.; Accomando, S.; Picarelli, A.; De Vitis, I.; et al. A prospective, double-blind, placebo-controlled trial to estabilish a safe gluten threshold for patients with celiac disease. *Am. J. Clin. Nutr.* **2007**, *85*, 160–166. [PubMed]

13. Biagi, F.; Campanella, J.; Martucci, S.; Pezzimenti, D.; Ciclitira, P.J.; Ellis, H.J.; Corazza, G.R. A milligram of gluten a day keeps the mucosal recovery away: A case report. *Nutr. Rev.* **2004**, *62*, 360–363. [CrossRef] [PubMed]

14. Akobneg, A.K.; Thomas, A.G. Systematic review: Tolerable amount of gluten for people with celiac disease. *Aliment. Pharmacol. Ther.* **2008**, *27*, 1044–1052. [CrossRef] [PubMed]

15. Hollon, J.R.; Cureton, P.A.; Martin, M.L.; Puppa, E.L.; Fasano, A. Trace gluten contamination may play a role in mucosal and clinical recovery in a subgroup of diet-adherent non-responsive celiac disease patients. *BMC Gastroenterol.* **2013**. [CrossRef] [PubMed]

16. Svedlund, J.; Sjödin, I.; Dotevall, G. GSRS-A clinical rating scale for gastrointestinal symptoms in patients with irritable bowel syndrome and peptic ulcer disease. *Dig. Dis. Sci.* **1988**, *33*, 129–134. [CrossRef] [PubMed]

17. Zanini, B.; Ricci, C.; Bandera, F.; Caselani, F.; Magni, A.; Laronga, A.M.; Lanzini, A. Incidence of post-infectious irritable bowel syndrome and functional intestinal disorders following a water-borne viral gastroenteritis outbreak. *Am. J. Gastroenterol.* **2012**, *107*, 891–899. [CrossRef] [PubMed]

18. Zanini, B.; Lanzarotto, F.; Mora, A.; Bertolazzi, F.; Turini, D.; Cesana, B.; Donato, F.; Ricci, C.; Lonati, F.; Vassallo, F.; et al. Five years time course of celiac disease serology during gluten free diet: Results of a community based "CD.Watch" program. *Dig. Liv. Dis.* **2010**, *42*, 865–870. [CrossRef] [PubMed]

19. Lonardi, S.; Villanacci, V.; Lorenzi, L.; Lanzini, A.; Lanzarotto, F.; Carabellese, N.; Volta, U.; Facchetti, F. Anti-TCR gamma antibody in celiac disease. The value of count on formalin-fixed paraffin-embedded biopsies. *Virchows Arch.* **2013**, *463*, 409–413. [CrossRef] [PubMed]

20. Saukkonen, J.; Kaikinen, K.; Koivisto, A.M.; Maki, M.; Laurila, K.; Sievänen, H.; Collin, P.; Kurppa, K. Clinical characteristics and the dietary response in celiac disease patients presenting with or without anemia. *J. Clin. Gastroenterol.* **2016**, in press. [CrossRef] [PubMed]

21. Thompson, T.; Lee, A.R.; Grace, T. Gluten contamination of grains, seeds, and flours in the United States: A pilot study. *J. Am. Diet. Assoc.* **2010**, *110*, 937–940. [CrossRef] [PubMed]

22. Leffler, D.; Schuppan, D.; Pallav, K.; Najarian, R.; Goldsmith, J.D.; Hansen, J.; Kabbani, T.; Dennis, M.; Kelly, C.P. Kinetics of the histological, serological and symptomatic responses to gluten challenge in adults with coeliac disease. *Gut* **2013**, *62*, 996–1004. [CrossRef] [PubMed]

23. Ortiz-Sanchez, J.P.; Cabrera-Chavez, F.; de la Barca, A.M. Maize prolamins could induce a gluten-like cellular immune response in some celiac disease patients. *Nutrients* **2013**, *5*, 4174–4183. [CrossRef] [PubMed]

24. Galipeau, H.J.; McCarville, J.L.; Huebener, S.; Litwin, O.; Meisel, M.; Jabri, B.; Sanz, Y.; Murray, J.A.; Jordana, M.; Alaedini, A.; et al. Intestinal microbiota modulates gluten-induced immunopathology in humanized mice. *Am. J. Pathol.* **2015**, *185*, 2969–2982. [CrossRef] [PubMed]

25. Mowat, A.M.; Agace, W.W. Regional specialization within the intestinal immune system. *Nat. Rev. Immunol.* **2014**, *14*, 667–685. [CrossRef] [PubMed]

26. Verdu, E.F.; Galipeau, H.J.; Jabri, B. Novel players in coeliac disease pathogenesis: Role of the gut microbiota. *Nat. Rev. Gastroenterol. Hepatol.* **2015**, *12*, 497–506. [CrossRef] [PubMed]

27. Decker, E.; Hornef, M.; Stockinger, S. Cesarean delivery is associated with celiac disease but not inflammatory bowel disease in children. *Gut Microb.* **2011**, *2*, 91–98. [CrossRef] [PubMed]

28. Ivarsson, A.; Persson, L.A.; Nystrom, L.; Ascher, H.; Cavell, B.; Danielsson, L.; Dannaeus, A.; Lindberg, T.; Lindquist, B.; Stenhammar, L.; et al. Epidemic of coeliac disease in Swedish children. *Acta. Paediatr.* **2000**, *89*, 165–171. [CrossRef] [PubMed]

29. Emilsson, L.; Magnus, M.C.; Stordal, K. Perinatal risk factors for development of celiac disease in children, based on the prospective Norwegian Mother and Child Cohort Study. *Clin. Gastroenterol. Hepatol.* **2015**, *13*, 921–922. [CrossRef] [PubMed]

30. Lionetti, E.; Castellaneta, S.; Francavilla, R.; Pulvirenti, A.; Tonutti, E.; Amarri, S.; Barbato, M.; Barbera, C.; Barera, G.; Bellantoni, A.; et al. Introduction of gluten, HLA status, and the risk of celiac disease in children. *N. Engl. J. Med.* **2014**, *371*, 1295–1303. [CrossRef] [PubMed]

31. Vriezinga, S.L.; Auricchio, R.; Bravi, E.; Castillejo, G.; Chmielewska, A.; Crespo, E.P.; Kolacek, S.; Koletzko, S.; Korponay-Szabo, I.R.; Mummert, E.; et al. Randomized feeding intervention in infants at high risk for celiac disease. *N. Engl. J. Med.* **2014**, *371*, 1304–1315. [CrossRef] [PubMed]

32. Collado, M.C.; Donat, E.; Ribes-Koninckx, C.; Calabuig, M.; Sanz, Y. Specific duodenal and faecal bacterial groups associated with paediatric coeliac disease. *J. Clin. Pathol.* **2009**, *62*, 264–269. [CrossRef] [PubMed]

33. Nadal, I.; Donat, E.; Ribes-Koninckx, C.; Calabuig, M.; Sanz, Y. Imbalance in the composition of the duodenal microbiota of children with coeliac disease. *J. Med. Microbiol.* **2007**, *56*, 1669–1674. [CrossRef] [PubMed]

34. Sanchez, E.; Donat, E.; Ribes-Koninckx, C.; Fernandez-Murga, M.L.; Sanz, Y. Duodenal-mucosal bacteria associated with celiac disease in children. *Appl. Environ. Microbiol.* **2013**, *79*, 5472–5479. [CrossRef] [PubMed]

35. Wacklin, P.; Kaukinen, K.; Tuovinen, E.; Collin, P.; Lindfors, K.; Partanen, J.; Maki, M.; Matto, J. The duodenal microbiota composition of adult celiac disease patients is associated with the clinical manifestation of the disease. *Inflamm. Bowel. Dis.* **2013**, *19*, 934–941. [CrossRef] [PubMed]

36. Nistal, E.; Caminero, A.; Herran, A.R.; Arias, L.; Vivas, S.; de Morales, J.M.; Calleja, S.; de Miera, L.E.; Arroyo, P.; Casqueiro, J. Differences of small intestinal bacteria populations in adults and children with/without celiac disease: Effect of age, gluten diet, and disease. *Inflamm. Bowel. Dis.* **2012**, *18*, 649–656. [CrossRef] [PubMed]

37 Zoetendal, E.G.; Raes, J.; van den Bogert, B.; Arumugam, M.; Booijink, C.C.; Troost, F.J.; Bork, P.; Wels, M.; de Vos, W.M.; Kleerebezem, M. The human small intestinal microbiota is driven by rapid uptake and conversion of simple carbohydrates. *ISME J.* **2012**, *6*, 1415–1426. [CrossRef] [PubMed]

38 Wacklin, P.; Laurikka, P.; Lindfors, K.; Collin, P.; Salmi, T.; Lahdeaho, M.L.; Saavalainen, P.; Maki, M.; Matto, J.; Kurppa, K.; et al. Altered duodenal microbiota composition in celiac disease patients suffering from persistent symptoms on a long-term gluten-free diet. *Am. J. Gastroenterol.* **2014**, *109*, 1933–1941. [CrossRef] [PubMed]

39. Tjellstrom, B.; Stenhammar, L.; Sundqvist, T.; Falth-Magnusson, K.; Hollen, E.; Magnusson, K.E.; Norin, E.; Midtvedt, T.; Hogberg, L. The effects of oats on the function of gut microflora in children with coeliac disease. *Aliment. Pharmacol. Ther.* **2014**, *39*, 1156–1160. [CrossRef] [PubMed]

40. Tuire, I.; Marja-Leena, L.; Teea, S.; Katri, H.; Jukka, P.; Päivi, S.; Heini, H.; Markku, M.; Pekka, C.; Katri, K. Persistent duodenal intraepithelial lymphocytosis despite a long-term strict gluten-free diet in celiac disease. *Am. J. Gastroenterol.* **2012**, *107*, 1563–1569. [CrossRef] [PubMed]

41. Aziz, I.; Evans, K.E.; Hopper, A.D.; Smillie, D.M.; Sanders, D.S. A prospective study into the aetiology of lymphocytic duodenosis. *Aliment. Pharmacol. Ther.* **2010**, *32*, 1392–1397. [CrossRef] [PubMed]

42. Pekki, H.; Kurppa, K.; Maki, M.; Huhtala, H.; Sievanen, H.; Laurila, K.; Collin, P.; Kaukinen, K. Predictors and significance of incomplete mucosal recovery in celiac disease after 1 year on a Gluten-Free diet. *Am. J. Gastroenterol.* **2015**, *110*, 1078–1085. [CrossRef] [PubMed]

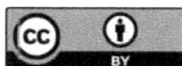

nutrients

Article

Properties of Gluten Intolerance: Gluten Structure, Evolution, Pathogenicity and Detoxification Capabilities

Anastasia V. Balakireva [1] and Andrey A. Zamyatnin Jr. [1,2,*]

[1] Institute of Molecular Medicine, Sechenov First Moscow State Medical University, Moscow 119991, Russia; balakireva.anastacia@gmail.com

[2] Belozersky Institute of Physico-Chemical Biology, Lomonosov Moscow State University, Moscow 119992, Russia

* Correspondence: zamyat@belozersky.msu.ru; Tel.: +7-495-609-1400 (ext. 3028)

Received: 28 August 2016; Accepted: 11 October 2016; Published: 18 October 2016

Abstract: Theterm gluten intolerance may refer to three types of human disorders: autoimmune celiac disease (CD), allergy to wheat and non-celiac gluten sensitivity (NCGS). Gluten is a mixture of prolamin proteins present mostly in wheat, but also in barley, rye and oat. Gluten can be subdivided into three major groups: S-rich, S-poor and high molecular weight proteins. Prolamins within the groups possess similar structures and properties. All gluten proteins are evolutionarily connected and share the same ancestral origin. Gluten proteins are highly resistant to hydrolysis mediated by proteases of the human gastrointestinal tract. It results in emergence of pathogenic peptides, which cause CD and allergy in genetically predisposed people. There is a hierarchy of peptide toxicity and peptide recognition by T cells. Nowadays, there are several ways to detoxify gluten peptides: the most common is gluten-free diet (GFD), which has proved its effectiveness; prevention programs, enzymatic therapy, correction of gluten pathogenicity pathways and genetically modified grains with reduced immunotoxicity. A deep understanding of gluten intolerance underlying mechanisms and detailed knowledge of gluten properties may lead to the emergence of novel effective approaches for treatment of gluten-related disorders.

Keywords: gluten; celiac disease; NCGS; wheat allergy; gluten intolerance; gliadin; glutenin; hordein; secalin; avenin

1. Introduction

Gluten intolerance is an umbrella term integrating three major types of gluten-related disorders: autoimmune celiac disease (CD), allergy to wheat and non-celiac gluten sensitivity (NCGS) [1–3]. Although these disorders possess similar symptoms, which include bloating, vomiting and diarrhea, a number of principle differences of their pathogenesis are remarkable (Table 1).

Celiac disease is an autoimmune enteropathy caused by genetic and environmental factors, with an estimated worldwide prevalence of about 1%. The huge prevalence of CD in the Saharawi people (5.6%) probably indicates that events linked to wheat domestication 10,000 years ago were a 'founder effect' related to the positive selection of HLA-DQ2 haplotype [4].

CD is usually diagnosed by serological examination [5]. Duodenal biopsy is not necessary for the diagnosis of CD but is necessary for the treatment [6]. Disease is induced by gluten-containing food in people carrying HLA-DQ2 or DQ8 haplotype (human leukocyte antigen Class II with DQ2 and/or DQ8 molecules on antigen-presenting cells). CD is not only characterized by gastrointestinal symptoms but also by extraintestinal manifestations, some of which are a direct consequence of autoimmunity responses—for example, dermatitis herpetiformis or gluten ataxia—while others are an indirect consequence of anaemia, such as osteoporosis, short stature and delayed puberty [7].

After gluten enters into the digestive system, glutamine and proline-rich gluten composing proteins are partially hydrolyzed by proteases presented in the gastrointestinal tract [8] (Figure 1). The upregulation of intestinal peptide zonulin, involved in tight junction regulation, appears to be partly responsible for the increased permeability characteristic of the gut [9]. As a result, generated gluten-derived peptides reach the lamina propria (mucosa) by transcellular or paracellular transport where they are modified by tissue transglutaminase (tTG) enhancing their affinity to MHC II molecules, and thereby making them toxic and immunogenic in HLA-DQ2 or DQ8 containing patients [10]. The repetitive presence of glutamine and proline residues determines the gluten-derived peptides as a preferred substrate for tTG. tTG-mediated modifications occur in two ways: deamidation (cleavage of the ε-amino group of a glutamine side chain) or more frequently transamidation (cross-linking of a glutamine residue from the gliadin peptide to a lysine residue of tTG). Further peptides presentation by HLA-DQ2/DQ8 protein subunits in the surface of dendritic cells to gluten-specific T cells induces two levels of immune response: the innate response and the adaptive (T-helper cell mediated) response with the production of interferon-γ and IL-15. As a result, it causes immune-mediated enteropathy, intestinal inflammation, followed by the atrophy of villi, crypt hyperplasia and increased infiltration by intraepithelial lymphocytes [11]. It also produces weight loss and chronic diarrhea. Although the causative agent is a dietary protein, the disease has marked autoimmune features, which are indicated by the presence of autoantibodies against tTG. Cross-linking between gliadin and tTG is covalent resulting in the formation of new epitopes, which trigger the primary immune response, and by which the autoantibodies against tTG are developed [12].

Table 1. Comparative major characteristics of gluten intolerance manifestations.

	Celiac Disease	Allergy	NCGS
Underlying cause	Genetic: HLA-DQ2 or/and –DQ8 haplotype	Atopy (100%)	Probably, genetic: DQ2 and/or DQ8 (up to 50% of patients)
Laboratory markers	IgA (IgG) anti-tTG, IgA(IgG) anti-endomysium (anti-EMA), anti-deamidated gliadin peptides antibodies	Specific IgE for wheat, specific IgE for ω-5 gliadin, specific IgE for non-specific lipid transfer proteins	IgG antigliadin antibodies (in only a part of the patients)
Histopathological intestine symptoms	Atrophy of villi, crypt hyperplasia, increased infiltration by intraepithelial lymphocytes	Any mucosal damage or increased infiltration by intraepithelial lymphocytes or atrophy of villi and crypt hyperplasia	Any mucosal damage or increased infiltration by intraepithelial lymphocytes

Allergy to wheat is represented by a food IgE-mediated allergy, which is most frequently based on the sensitization to wheat protein allergens. It has been shown that wheat ω5-gliadin is the main allergen of gluten, inducing wheat-dependent exercise-induced anaphylaxis [13]. Furthermore, some data suggest that α- and γ-gliadins are IgE-binding proteins [14]. Allergy occurs within a few hours and causes no permanent gastrointestinal or other organ damage.

One more gluten-related disorder has recently been proposed—NCGS—and its pathogenesis is still not clear. Gluten ataxia (GA) is one of a number of different neurological manifestations attributed to CD, but Rodrigo et al. have suggested that it is related to NCGS [15]. Recently, special criteria aimed at optimizing the clinical care in clarifying the core of NCGS have been accepted [3].

Gluten triggers all kinds of gluten related disorders and represent proteins of wheat, barley, rye and, probably, oat. The gluten proteins of different species are the major subject of this present review along with the currently used proposed gluten detoxification strategies and the development of effective prevention and treatment of gluten related disorders.

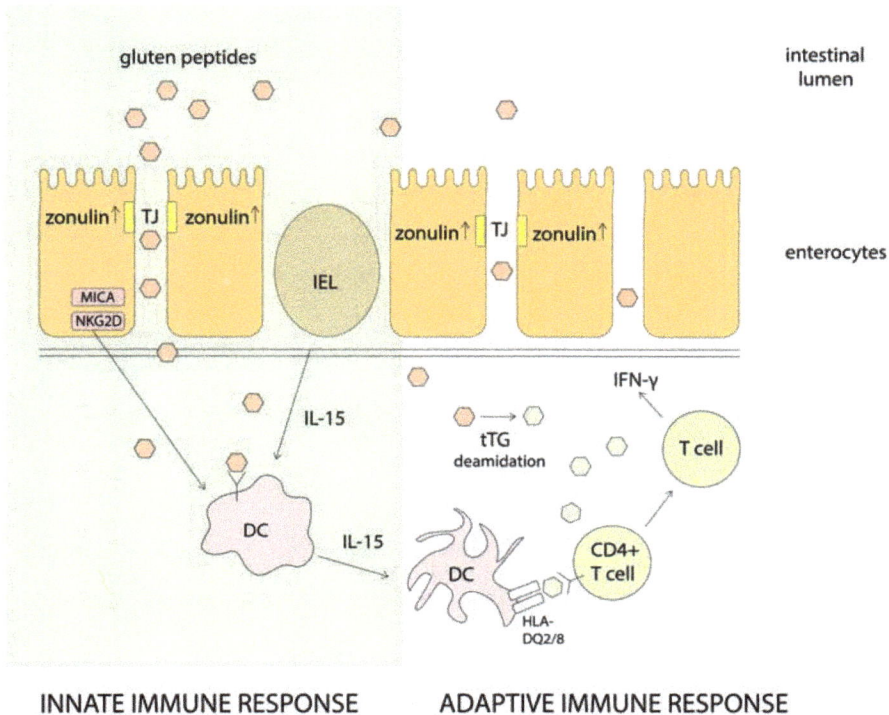

Figure 1. Schematic representation of major pathways in celiac disease (CD) pathogenesis. MICA, NKG2D—stress molecules on enterocytes, IEL—intraepithelial lymphocyte, DC—dendritic cell.

2. Classification and Structure of Gluten Proteins

Gluten is a mixture of seed storage proteins found in grains such as wheat, rye, barley and oat. Wheat, rye and barley are closely related members of the *Triticeae* tribe. They contain kindred groups of proteins. Rye (*Secale cereal* L., genome composition RR) and barley (*Hordeum vulgare* L.) are diploid, while wheat is represented by the most widely studied hexaploid bread wheat (*Triticum aestivum* L., genome composition AABBDD), tetraploid pasta wheat (*Triticum durum* L., genome composition AABB) and diploid wheat (*Triticum monococcum* L., genome composition AA). Oat (*Avena sativa* L.) is the most closely related cereal to the *Triticeae* and belongs to a separate *Aveneae* tribe within the same sub-family (*Festucoideae*).

Gluten proteins appear to be prolamins due to the significant amount of glutamine and proline amino acid residues present in their primary structures. Prolamins are the major endosperm storage proteins in grains. Prolamin genes are present in the A, B and D genomes of wheat, and, consequently, hexaploid and tetraploid wheat prolamin fractions consist of more individual components than in barley and rye. There is also a difference in the number and properties of prolamin polypeptides. Despite these variations, all prolamins are related and, usually referred to as three broad groups: sulphur-rich (S-rich), sulphur-poor (S-poor) and high molecular weight (HMW) prolamins (Table 2) [16]. They comprise the Prolamin Superfamily, along with the prolamins of oat, maize and rice, (Figure 2).

The proteins and polypeptides within these groups possess similar structures: signal peptide for translocation into cellular compartments, a non-repetitive *N*-terminal region, a non-repetitive *C*-terminal region and a long repetitive central region (Figure 3). The central region contains glutamine-rich and proline-rich repeat units unique to each group. It has been shown that the motifs in central region of S-rich and S-poor groups are clearly related and the cysteine positions in HMW proteins and S-rich group prolamins are highly conserved. Thus, the conclusion was that all these groups have a common evolutionary origin [17]. Now, we will discuss every prolamin group in detail.

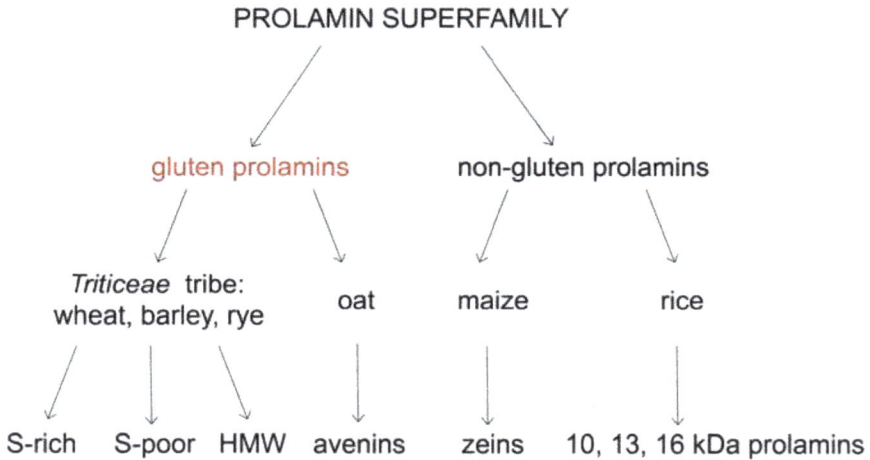

Figure 2. Prolamin Superfamily composition.

Table 2. Classification of gluten prolamins.

Grain Species	Components	Molecular Weight (% Total)	Polymers or Monomers
HMW Prolamins			
Wheat	HMW subunits of glutenin	65–90 kDa (6%–10%)	Polymers
Barley	D-hordeins	>100 kDa (2%–4%)	Polymers
Rye	HMW secalins	>100 kDa (2%)	Polymers
S-rich prolamins			
	γ-gliadins		Monomers
Wheat	α-gliadins	30–45 kDa (70%–80%)	Monomers
	B- and C-type LMW subunits of glutenin		Polymers
Barley	B-hordeins and γ-hordeins	32–45 kDa (80%)	Aggregated type, monomers or single chain polypeptide
Rye	γ-secalins	40–75 kDa (80%)	Polymers
S-poor prolamins			
Wheat	ω-gliadins	30–75 kDa (10%–20%)	Monomers
	D-type LMW subunits of glutenin		Aggregated type, polymers
Barley	C-hordeins	40–72 kDa (10%–15%)	Monomers
Rye	ω-secalins	48–55 kDa (10%–15%)	Monomers
Other gluten prolamins			
Oat	avenins	18.5–23.5 kDa (10%)	Monomers

2.1. Wheat

Wheat prolamins appear to be the first identified gluten proteins. According to their solubility they are usually divided into two classes: alcohol-soluble fraction named gliadins (monomeric) and insoluble—glutenins (polymeric, soluble in dilute acids and bases) [18]. It has been shown that gliadins contribute to the cohesiveness and extensibility of the gluten, whereas glutenins play a role in the maintenance of the elasticity and strength of the gluten [18]. Integrally, these proteins represent 80%–85% of gluten proteins and define viscoelastic properties of dough.

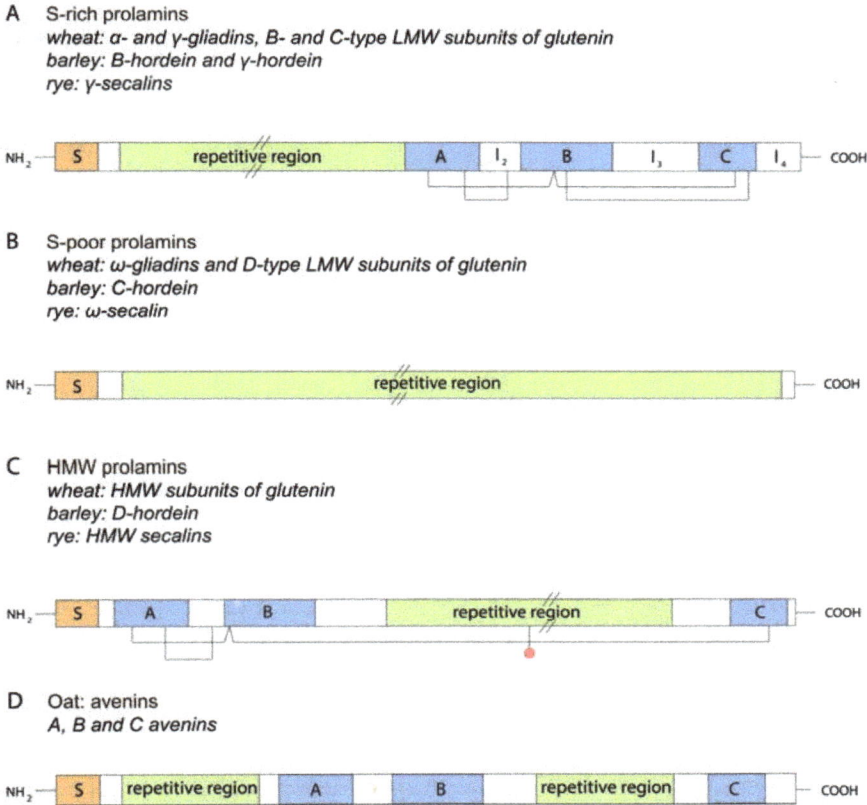

A S-rich prolamins
wheat: α- and γ-gliadins, B- and C-type LMW subunits of glutenin
barley: B-hordein and γ-hordein
rye: γ-secalins

B S-poor prolamins
wheat: ω-gliadins and D-type LMW subunits of glutenin
barley: C-hordein
rye: ω-secalin

C HMW prolamins
wheat: HMW subunits of glutenin
barley: D-hordein
rye: HMW secalins

D Oat: avenins
A, B and C avenins

Figure 3. Schematic representation of typical structure of prolamin group members: S-rich, S-poor, HMW and avenins. S—signal peptide; A, B, C—conserved regions, lines—disulfide bonds, red circles—unpaired cysteine residue, I_2–I_4—variant regions; parallel lines—contracted repetitive region. (**A**) Typical structure of S-rich prolamin. It contains conservative domains, repetitive region and is able to form intrachain disulfide bonds; (**B**) Typical structure of S-poor prolamin. It lacks conservative domains and cysteine residues, and is therefore not able to form any disulfide bonds; (**C**) Typical structure of HMW prolamin. It contains conservative domains, repetitive region and is able to form intra- and interchain disulfide bonds; (**D**) Typical structure of avenin. It contains conservative domains, repetitive regions and is able to form interchain disulfide bonds only.

This difference in solubility largely reflects the ability of these proteins to form inter- or intramolecular disulfide bonds. Gliadins are monomeric proteins and are connected to each other through intrachain disulfide bonds (α/β-, and γ-gliadins), or not connected at all (ω-gliadins) [19]. It has been reported that C and D groups of LMW glutenin subunits (LMW-GS) are mainly composed of α-, β-, γ-, and ω-gliadins but mutated in cysteine residues. It means that LMW-GS can act as chain extenders depending on how many bonds it may form, and gliadins may serve as chain terminators [20]. The polymeric form contributes to the strength of gluten and improves dough quality.

(1) Gliadins

Gliadins are represented as single chain polypeptides, and it is accepted that gliadins are divided into four major groups (from fastest mobility to slowest): α-, β-, γ-, and ω-gliadins, according to their electrophoretic mobility in SDS-PAGE at low pH [18]. Precisely, ω-, α/β-, and γ-gliadins exist. Proteins from α- and β-groups are similar, so this group is referred to as α-gliadins [21]. ω-gliadins can be arranged into three types, which will be discussed further.

Genes encoding gliadin proteins are located on the short arms of Groups 1 and 6 chromosomes at three homologous loci—*Gli-A1*, *Gli-B1*, and *Gli-D1* (Group 1) and—*Gli-A2*, *Gli-B2*, and *Gli-D2* (Group 6) [22]. Some of the α- and γ-gliadins are encoded by *Gli-2* genes. The estimated copy number of α-gliadins in hexaploid wheat is between 25 and 150 copies. *Gli-1* contains genes encoding not only γ- and ω-gliadins but also LMW-GS, so there is a tight linkage between them [23].

Gliadins of different types bear distinct secondary structure. Thus, ω-gliadins contain randomly coiled β-turns without α-helices or β-sheets. In contrast, α/β- and γ-gliadins possess α-helices and β-sheets, which, in turn, allow these proteins to not only stabilize by disulfide bonds but also by the support of hydrogen bonds within their helices and sheets [24].

Gliadins are monomers but they are able to form intramolecular disulfide bonds. Free SH groups of glutenin, generated by β-elimination from cysteine, initiate SH–SS interchain reaction between gliadin and glutenin. This mechanism was proposed by Schofield et al. [25], which postulates that these SH–SS interchange reactions cause transformation from intra- to intermolecular SS bonds of gliadins [26]. Even the addition of free SH groups, such as cysteine, starts gliadin polymerization according to first-order reaction kinetics [27]. Such polymers are used as biodegradable films.

Gliadins are transported via the Golgi to the protein storage vacuole, whereas others, principally glutenins, are retained within the ER [16]. The precise mechanism determining the transportation of prolamins is not clear. There are no classical signal peptides targeting proteins neither to ER nor to vacuole.

(1.1) α- and γ-gliadins

α- and γ-gliadins are very similar in their amino acid sequences. These types of proteins belong to S-rich group of prolamins and have similar structures (Figure 3). α- and γ-gliadins contain a relatively high composition of cysteine and methionine, but few glutamine, proline and phenylalanine residues. Eight cysteine residues allow the formation of intrachain disulphide bonds responsible for its folding (Figure 3) [28]. α- and γ-gliadins are able to form three and four intramolecular disulfide bonds, respectively. Their folded structures determine further non-covalent interactions, including hydrogen bonds and hydrophobic interactions [29].

N-terminal domain of α-gliadins consists of five residues and the central domain is about 113–134 amino acid residues. Central domain contains proline- and glutamine-rich heptapeptide PQPQPFP and pentapeptide PQQPY. This domain contains the most characteristic immunogenic fragment: 33-mer peptide comprising six overlapping epitopes significant for CD pathogenesis. Based on the differences in epitopes comprising 33-mer peptide, α-gliadins can be divided into six types. Only Type 1 encompasses proteins including 33-mer peptide (from hexaploid wheat), whereas other types do not [30].

C-terminal segment of α- and γ-gliadins is about 150 residues. In α-gliadins, almost all the glutamic acid and aspartic acid residues are present in amide forms [31]. γ-gliadins contain a 12 residues signal peptide and have more cysteine residues in their primary structure than α-gliadins. All these cysteine residues are involved in intrachain disulfide bonds formation (Figure 3).

Recently, a conformational equilibrium toward a beta-parallel structure was reported in the case of 33-mer peptide of α/β-gliadins under physiological conditions [32]. Gliadin nanoparticles formation was reported in distilled water (probably at pH 6–7) [33]. Then, self-organization capabilities of 33-mer peptide were investigated under gastrointestinal environment [34]. The spontaneous self-organization at pH 3.0 leads to the formation of aggregates such as micelles of amphiphilic molecules. Then, on increasing the pH to 7.0, gliadin nanostructures repulsion decreases due to proximity to the isoelectric point.

(1.2)   ω-gliadins

This group differs from other groups of gliadins. It is related to S-poor group of proteins lacking methionine or cysteine residues in their primary structure. Thus, ω-gliadins are incapable of disulfide bonds formation (Figure 3). As a result, no compact structure exists for these proteins. Proline, glutamine and phenylalanine residues comprise the majority of amino acids (80%) in ω-gliadins. They are more polar than α- and γ-gliadins [35].

On the basis of the *N*-terminal sequences, three different types of ω-gliadins have been distinguished from wheat proteins and related proteins from other species such as C-hordeins and ω-secalins: ARQ-, KEL-, and SRL-types depending on the first three amino acids [36]. The KEL-type differs from the ARQ-type by the absence of the first eight residues in its structure.

(2)   Glutenins

Glutenins consist of subunits and are usually divided into two classes according to their molecular weight defined by SDS-PAGE: high molecular weight glutenin subunits (HMW-GS) and low molecular weight glutenin subunits (LMW-GS) (Table 2) [37]. They are encoded by *Glu-1* loci on the long arms of 1A, 1B, 1D chromosomes of wheat.

Each HMW-GS locus contains two tightly linked genes encoding larger x-type (82–90 kDa) and smaller y-type (60–80 kDa) subunits, respectively [38]. Both types of subunits have similar structures (Figure 3). Repetitive central region is the cause of the difference between HMW-GS and LMW-GS. It may have various lengths provided by three types of repeat units: tripeptides (GQQ), hexapeptides (PGQGQQ), and nonapeptides (GYYPTSLQQ), and it is worth mentioning that the tripeptide units only exist in the x-type subunits, and both x- and y-type subunits possess hexapeptide and nonapeptide units [39]. The y-type glutenin subunits possess more cysteine residues than x-type subunits, and, are therefore capable of more inter- and intramolecular disulfide bonds formation, which mediates the aggregation of HMW-GSs with the involvement of LMW-GSs and results in an improved dough quality [16].

LMW-GS are classically subdivided into B, C, and D-type on the basis of their SDS-PAGE mobility and pI (Table 2) [40]. The B-type is the major group of LMW-GS. It represents the most numerous of LMW proteins. C-type proteins are the fastest moving type and the later discovered proteins comprise the D-type group. The B- and C-type subunits are encoded by genes located in the *Gli-3*, *Gli-1* and *Gli-2* loci on the short arm of homologous Groups 1 and 6 chromosomes. Genes at the *Gli-1* loci encode D subunits [41].

LMW-GS can be divided into two groups: one of which contains subunits with methionine as *N*-terminal amino acid (LMW-m) in their amino acid sequences, whereas the other group contains serine as *N*-terminal amino acid (LMW-s). In B- and C-types of LMW, there are both m- and s-types. D-type subunits are the less abundant group of LMW-GS. It has been shown that they could be formed by the mutation in one or more genes encoding ω-gliadins, resulting in the appearance of a single cysteine and allowing for the formation of an additional interchain disulfide bond in the glutenin macropolymer [42].

2.2. Barley

Hordeins are the major storage proteins in barley, and these proteins, like gliadins, are also alcohol-soluble prolamins and appear to be rich in glutamine and proline residues but poor in charged amino acids. Hordein polypeptides are not glycosylated. Two-dimensional polyacrylamide gel electrophoresis (with immobilized pH gradients in first dimension) of barley seed proteins reveal the occurrence of A, B, γ, C and D hordeins depending on their molecular mass and amino acid composition [43]. The A hordeins are of low molecular weight and do not seem to be true storage proteins. B and γ-hordeins are rich in sulfur and account for about 80% of the total hordein amount. They belong to S-rich prolamin group (Table 2, Figure 3); the C hordeins belong to S-poor group, and the D hordeins to HMW protein group. B and C hordeins collectively account for over 95% of barley seed storage proteins and are encoded by linked loci *Hor 2* (B hordein) and *Hor 1* (C hordein) located on the short arm of the chromosome 5 [44]. D hordeins and γ-hordeins are encoded by structural loci *Hor 3* and *Hor 5* located on the long arm of chromosome 5.

It has been suggested that B and C hordeins belong to common evolutionary origin due to the shared short tandem repeats [45]. The occurrence of two distinct domains in B hordein (one is related to C hordein and one is not) suggests that an unusual evolutionary pathway links these two groups of prolamin storage proteins.

The structural features of hordein proteins are similar to those of wheat proteins and are indicated in Figure 3. Three conserved regions (A, B, C) are present in all hordeins, except C hordein. These three regions also show a homology with each other, and contain cysteine residues that may be conserved within the groups or between the different groups of proteins. Shewry at al. concluded that S-poor prolamins originated from S-rich group because they have similar glutamine- and proline-rich motifs and evolved by the further amplification of repeat units and deletion on conserved regions A, B, and C [36].

(1)   B and γ-hordein

B hordeins are the orthologous prolamin family to wheat LMW-GS group [17]. It has been estimated that B hordeins are represented by 11 different proteins and are now divided into closely related subgroups: SDS-PAGE revealed two major bands of B1 and B3 hordeins, and minor band with intermediate mass called B2. Three pseudogenes of B hordein have been identified [46]. Most of the B hordein are present in monomeric form or as single polypeptide subunits within the globules of low electron density of endosperm cells along with C, γ 1-, γ 2- and possibly γ 3-hordein polypeptides [47].

B hordeins can form a wedge or tadpole-shaped structure stabilized with interchain disulphide bonds formed between unpaired cysteine residues in the *N*- and *C*-terminal domains [48].

γ-hordein is homologues to γ-gliadin of wheat. γ-hordein is presented in γ1-, γ2-, γ3-types. Analysis of primary sequences revealed a distant relation between γ3-hordein to γ2- and B hordein, while γ2-hordein is very close to γ-gliadin and γ-secalin (Figure 4) [47]. In addition, γ1- and γ2-types have identical *N*-terminal sequences. Signal peptides allow γ1-, γ2-hordeins to be co-translationally transported into the rough endoplasmic reticulum. They present in small aggregates (hordein polypeptides) soluble in 55% isopropanol. γ1- and γ2-hordein can form intermolecular disulfide bridges but γ3-hordein exists as a monomer only.

(2)   C hordein

C hordein is a group of homologous proteins that have molecular weights of about 50 kDa. C1 and C2 types of C hordein were identified [49]. They are homologous to wheat ω-gliadin. C hordeins lack cysteine residues and always present in monomeric form due to their inability to form disulfide bonds. Their primary sequences are rich in glutamine, proline and phenylalanine residues. They possess short *N*- and *C*-terminal (unique sequence of 6 amino acid residues) domains and central domain containing P/LQQPY and PQQPFPQQ repetitive motifs (Figure 3) [45]. Structural studies of C hordein showed that these proteins have a conserved but unusual secondary structure—repetitive β-turns [50]. Further analysis performed by l'Anson e al. indicates that such primary structure results in a similarly conserved supersecondary structure called "worm-like" chain. This is a loose spiral based on elements of P-turn and poly-L-proline II helix [51]. C hordeins are located within the globules of low electron density along with γ-hordein and B hordein [47]. These globules merge with each other in cytoplasm.

(3) D hordein

D hordein is homologous to HMW glutenins of wheat. They have been studied in detail due to their importance in the quality and strength of dough. D hordein and polymeric B hordein are present in polymeric form as aggregates of polypeptide subunits linked by interchain disulfide bonds. It is always deposited in the vacuole [52]. D hordein possesses a similar amino acid composition as HMW-GSs of wheat. It has repeat units such as tripeptides (GQQ), hexapeptides (PGQGQQ), and nonapeptides (GYYPTSLQQ). These subunits form spiral supersecondary structure provided by repeating β-turns [53]. Nevertheless, it has unique tetrapeptide present in C-terminal part of repetitive domain. D hordein has an extended rod-like structure. In addition, D hordein differs from HMW-GS in terms of the number and distribution of cysteine residues.

2.3. Rye

Rye is one of the major cereal species along with wheat and barley. Prolamins of rye are called secalins and are divided into three classes: HMW secalins, γ-secalins and ω-secalins (Table 2) [17].

(1) HMW secalin subunits (HMW-SS)

These high molecular weight proteins are encoded by two genes of *Sec-3 (Glu-R1)* locus located at the long arm of 1R rye chromosome [54]. As HMW glutenins are subdivided into x- and y-types, *Sec-3* also consists of two paralogous alleles (*Glu-R1x* and *Glu-R1y*) of duplication origin. They encode x-(more abundant) and y-types of subunits [55]. HMW-SS are always present as one or two individual subunits similar to D hordeins and in contrast to five to six subunits of wheat HMW-GS.

HMW-SS are homologous to HMW-GS but there is a significant difference in the properties and structural parameters determining gluten formation (see below, Triticale).

Repetitive domain of HMW-SS contains tripeptide, nonapeptide and hexapeptide consensus motifs discussed in Section (2) Glutenin section. Scanning tunnelling microscopy of a purified HMW secalin subunit demonstrated aligned rods with a diameter of about 1.9 nm containing diagonal striations (presumably corresponding to turns of the spiral) and having a pitch of about 1.5 nm [56].

(2) γ-secalins

γ-secalins are encoded by five to 10 genes of *Sec-1* and *Sec-2* loci at 1R and 2R chromosomes of rye, respectively. The structures of γ-secalin and other γ-type prolamins are alike (Figure 3). It has eight cysteine residues involved in intramolecular disulfide bonds formation and unpaired cysteine residue involved in intermolecular bonds formation. Rye also encodes 75 kDa γ-secalins that have no analogues in other cereals. It amounts to about 50% of total seed proteins in rye and is sometimes separated from other secalins into distinct types.

(3) ω-secalins

Sec-1 locus is a gene region of ω-secalins located at the short arm of chromosome 1RS. This arm contains *Sec-1* disease resistant genes tightly linked to leaf, stem and stripe rusts and powdery mildew [57]. This linkage results in some dough quality defects such as marked stickiness, reduced strength and intolerance to overmixing. Clarke et al. reported that the *Sec-1* locus of rye consists of approximately 145 kb of DNA containing a tandem gene array of 15 ω-secalin gene units [58]. FISH analysis shows that the sizes of the *Sec-1* region range from 131 to 164 kb on the DNA fiber specimen [59]. Rye genome contains not only ω-secalin genes with ORFs but also pseudogenes, which may be the subject of a reduced selection pressure [60].

ω-secalins are related to S-poor group of prolamins and possess a typical structure for this group. These proteins are monomers and cannot form interchain disulfide bonds like the other proteins in this group: C-hordeins and ω-gliadins. This was discussed earlier for C hordein, ω-secalin has no A, B or C conservative domains. Repetitive domain of ω-secalin is flanked by short unique sequences of *N*-terminal 12 amino acid residues and four amino acids on its *C*-terminus. Repetitive region of ω-secalin also has an unusual supersecondary structure similar to that in C hordein of barley.

2.4. Triticale

Hybrid species triticale (X *Triticosecale Wittmack*) also contains gluten, and originates from species durum wheat (*Triticum durum* L., AABB genome) and rye (*Secale cereal* L., RR genome). The hexaploid triticale genome (AABBRR) encodes three sets of HMW glutenins (1A and 1B chromosomes), HMW secalins (1R), 75K γ-secalins (2R) of rye and LMW glutenins (1A and 1B). This complex was named "secaloglutenin", while "secalogluten" refers to the hydrated network of secaloglutenin with some monomers [61]. This network is weak and incohesive and the dough strength is between the dough strength of *Triticum durum* L. and *Secale cereale* L. and requires less mixing time. Currently, many papers focus on the elucidation of possible methods for the improvement of triticale dough.

2.5. Oat

Prolamins in oat (*Avena sativa* L.) are represented by avenins. Oat avenins differ from other grain prolamins in the lower amount of proline. Furthermore, oats contains a relatively low content of storage proteins; approximately 10% only of the total grain protein amount compared with 40%–50% in wheat, barley, and rye [62]. This is a cause of the inability to divide oat prolamins into HMW proteins, S-rich and S-poor groups in a manner of *Triticeae* tribe. Avenins were shown to be homologous to α,′ β-gliadin and γ-gliadin of wheat, B-hordein of barley and γ-secalin of rye (S-rich group) [63].

Avenins can be well analyzed with HPLC technique, and contain insoluble and soluble fractions. Insoluble in alcohol but soluble in reducing solution fraction named "glutelin fraction" [64]. The molecular weight of avenins is about 18.5–23.5 kDa and contain two blocks of glutamine- and proline-rich repeated sequences, whose length varies from six to 11 residues (Figure 3). Avenins are monomers and only contain interchain disulfide bonds [62].

Although avenins are very similar [65], only differing by point mutations, they are subdivided into A, B and C groups according to the neighbor-joining phylogeny method [66]. Avenin sequences belonging to B and C groups possess eight cysteine residues, whereas sequences from A group bear 9. Thus, avenins from group A are capable of interchain disulfide bonds formation and a polymer in a wheat glutenin manner with a use of unpaired nineth cysteine. Generated polymer may consist of only A avenins or from other prolamins resulting in heteropolymer formation. It has been proposed that A avenins are LMW-GS-like (glutelin fraction). B and C avenins show up to be α- and γ-gliadins-like proteins. The expression levels of avenins of different groups have not yet been well studied, but it is clear that α- and γ-gliadins-like proteins (group C and B) expression is greater than that of LMW-GS-like avenins from group A [66]. Avenins are synthesized and assembled into vacuolar protein bodies in developing endosperm tissue along with globulin storage proteins. Immunogold staining of this tissue demonstrated that prolamins were located in the light-staining regions. These proteins appear to aggregate within the rough ER, while most of the globulin appear to aggregate in the vacuole [67].

3. Gluten Evolution

Although the prolamin superfamily seems to be a relatively unique group of proteins, there is evidence of a relationship between these proteins and other seed protein groups. First, proteins within one group (S-rich, S-poor or HMW) have a similar structure. For example, comparison of prolamin C-terminal domain sequences from S-rich group of proteins (wheat, barley and rye) including oat avenins showed significant similarity. Particularly, three conserved regions of length about 30 residues were identified and called A, B and C (Figure 3) [17]. They include a conserved number and position of cysteine residues. It is interesting that these regions share some similarity indicating the probable triplication of a short ancestral sequence (Figure 4) [62]. Moreover, such short similar sequences were found not only in gluten prolamins but also in other seed and non-seed proteins.

Comparison of regions of A, B and C conserved domains (Figure 3, see I_2–I_4) identified subgroups within S-rich group: α-type and γ-type, B hordein [68]. γ-type is considered to be the most ancient among the gluten proteins. It is worth mentioning that regions A, B and C are also present in the HMW prolamins, although in this case regions A and B are located within the *N*-terminal domain while region C is within the *C*-terminal domain indicating that proteins of S-rich and HMW groups arose from a single ancestor by insertion of I_2–I_4 blocks and repeated sequences. It has been shown that α- and γ-gliadins are both related to LMW-GS. Moreover, it has been suggested that C and D groups of glutenins are mainly composed of α-, β-, γ-, and ω-gliadins but mutated in cysteine residues [20].

Proteins of S-poor group of prolamins do not contain conserved regions. It is also clear that repeated sequences of S-poor prolamins (ω-type, C hordein) are related to repeated sequences in S-rich prolamins indicating that S-poor group of proteins originated from S-rich group through amplification of repeats and deletion of *C*-terminal domain. The evolutionary events leading to emergence of prolamin superfamily are summarized in Figure 4.

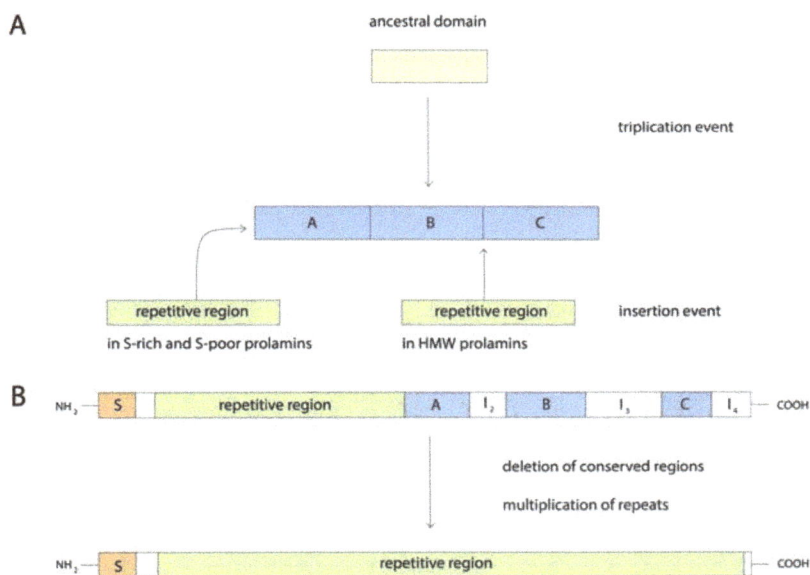

Figure 4. Summary of evolutionary events that probably contributed to the divergence of Prolamin Superfamily proteins. A, B, C—conserved regions, S—signal peptide, I_2–I_4—variant regions. (**A**) Conservative domains A, B and C of prolamins are thought to originate from the ancestral domain by triplication. S-rich and HMW prolamins emerged after insertions of repetitive regions in a manner showed on a Figure; (**B**) S-poor prolamins are suggested to originate from S-rich prolamins by deletion of conserved A, B and C regions, and by multiplication of repeated sequences.

4. Gluten Intolerance Pathogenesis

4.1. Cross-Reactivity between Gluten Proteins

Primarily, gluten is a source of flour and, consequently, bread and flour products. Consumption of gluten-containing food makes such food an immune system target. Digested gluten is a reason for the emergence of different antigens and immunogens. Cross-reactivity implies the reaction between an antibody and an antigen that differs from the immunogen, and it has been shown in glutenin-specific and gliadin-specific T-cells. Such T-cells could respond to gliadin and glutenin and vice versa due to their directivity to repetitive sequence highly homologous in these proteins [69]. Such cross-reactivity contributes to the development and spread of T-cell response and inflammation. It is also known that CD is characterized not only by inflammation and small intestine tissue remodeling but also by neurologic defects such as axonal neuropathy and cerebellar ataxia [70,71]. It has been shown that such neurological implications may occur partly due to the cross-reactivity between antigliadin antibody and synapsin I protein [72]. This protein is a cytosolic phosphoprotein found in most neurons of the central and peripheral nervous systems. Although gliadins are not homologous to synapsin I, there is a glutamine- and proline-rich-region in C-terminal sequence of synapsin I, which includes PQP and PQQP motifs similar to those in gliadin.

Evidence of the cross-reactivity of prolamin proteins was also reported in the course of allergy. ω5-gliadin is the major wheat allergen. It was shown that anti-ω5-gliadin antibodies bind to rye γ70-secalin, rye γ35-secalin and barley γ3-hordein [73]. In about 90% of patients with wheat-dependent exercise-induced anaphylaxis, IgE antibodies against these proteins were found. Rye γ70- and γ35-secalin and barley γ3-hordein cross-react with ω5-gliadin. This probably happens due to the fact that IgE antibodies bind to structurally similar epitopes; found proteins are related to the same evolutionary group of γ-type prolamins.

Even though there is no cross-reactivity between allergens in oat and other gluten species, avenins show immunological cross-reactivity to γ-secalin due to their considerable homology [74]. First immunogenic peptides in hordein, secalin and avenin were revealed on the basis of T-cell cross-reactivity against wheat gluten proteins [75]. Epitopes defined in hordein and secalin were recognized by α-gliadin-reactive T-cell lines in vitro while avenin epitopes were not. That explains why rye and barley were considered to be pathogenic for CD patients, whereas oat was included in the "gluten-free" group of food.

Later, it was shown that oat consumption is safe for the majority of CD patients [76], even for children [77]. It is well known that the greater the proline residues in storage protein the more pathogenic this protein is for CD patients [78]. Low proline content may be the reason why oat avenins are less immunogenic compared to wheat prolamins but may still be toxic in large quantities. However, there was no direct (in vivo) evidence of the activation of gluten-reactive T-cells following ingestion of oats. Hardy et al. provided in vivo evidence that ingestion of oats activates avenin-specific T-cells in 10% of CD patients [79]. Moreover, they showed T-cells to be cross-reactive against hordein and avenin. After oral challenge with barley (and not wheat or rye) the majority of HLA-DQ2.5 CD patients harbor T-cells capable of being activated by avenin peptides ex vivo, but the ingestion of oats itself provides rather weak antigenic stimulation for this population of T-cells. Avenins are probably less stimulatory because they do not contain proteolytically resistant peptides longer that 10 amino acid residues. They have reduced binding stability to HLA-DQ2.5 compared to hordein peptides. This means that avenin-reactive T-cells are activated by the consumption of barley rather than oat.

4.2. Celiac Disease

As described in the introduction, gluten is impregnable by the gastric, pancreatic and intestinal digestive proteases of people carrying HLA-DQ2 or/and DQ8 haplotype. HLA-DQ is a part of the MHC class II antigen-presenting receptor system and distinguishes its own and foreign cells. HLA-DQ protein consists of two subunits, which are encoded by the HLA-DQA1 and HLA-DQB1 genes located on the short arm of the 6 chromosome. Mainly, people with celiac disease have DQ2 or DQ8 isoforms because these receptors bind to gliadin peptides more tightly than other forms.

However, there are multiple DQ2 haplotypes. The most associated with celiac disease (95% of patients) is the two-gene HLA-DQ2 haplotype referred to as DQ2.5. This haplotype is composed of subunits α^5 and β^2 encoded by two adjacent gene alleles DQA1*0501 and DQB1*0201 (Figure 5). Four percent of CD patients have the DQ2.2 isoform (DQA1*0201:DQB1*0202) and the remaining have DQ8 (encoded by the haplotype DQA1*03:DQB1*0302).

After the gluten enters into the digestive system, prolamin proteins are not fully hydrolyzed by proteases, which results in the emergence of gluten peptides. They are deamidated by tTG enhancing their affinity to MHC II molecules. Deamidated peptide is then recognized by DQ molecule on the surface of a dendritic cell and is presented to T cells inducing immune response. It is interesting that both DQ2 and DQ8 lack canonical aspartic acid residue at DQβ57. It results in the compensation of this negative charge by negatively charged residues either in the T cell receptor or in the deamidated peptide. Absence of aspartic acid residue leads to cross-reactive and stronger responses by T cells [80].

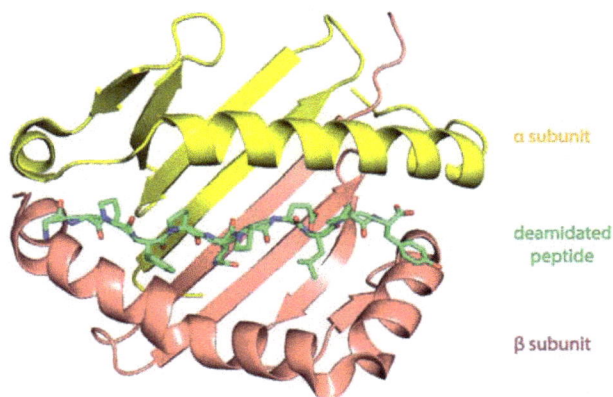

a subunit

deamidated peptide

β subunit

Figure 5. 3D reconstruction of DQ α^5-β^2-binding cleft with a deamidated α-gliadin peptide (green), using PyMOL (PBD ID 1S9V) [81].

Nowadays, it is clear that distinct gluten peptides are involved in celiac disease in a different manner. Peptides are divided into two groups: toxic and immunogenic. Toxic peptides are capable of inducing mucosal damage when administered in vivo on the intestine, whereas peptide is considered to be immunogenic if it is able to specifically stimulate HLA-DQ-restricted T cell lines isolated from peripheral blood of CD patients [82]. Peptides differ from each other in the degree of the immunogenicity. It is remarkable that some are immunodominant, meaning that they evoke strong T cell response in almost every CD patient, whereas the immunogenic do not. Immunogenicity is enhanced after tTG deamidation procedure. It is worth mentioning that tTG is more likely activated after inflammation, but it is still not clear whether the deamidation of peptides is by tTG initiates inflammation or vice versa [82].

All gluten proteins (gliadin and glutenin from wheat, hordein from barley, secalin from rye and avenin from oat) possess their own sets of toxic and immunogenic peptides (or epitopes) with distinct immunogenicities. However, gliadin peptides are known to be the most toxic and numerous, specifically derived from α- and γ-gliadin: the strongest and most common adaptive response to gluten is directed toward an α2-gliadin fragment of 33 amino acids in length [8]. Digestion of gliadin results in the emergence of two pieces: 25-mer (p31-55, it can be degraded to smaller peptides) and 33-mer (p57-89). Peptide p31-43 of α2-gliadin may directly induce interleukin-15 production from enterocytes and dendritic cells. Peptide p57-89 is deamidated by tTG and presented to T cells by HLA-DQ molecules. Glutenin peptides are also involved in T cell response [83]. Peptides may enter the cell by endocytosis, with their entrance into the cells requiring 37 °C temperature and Ca^{2+} in the media [84]. It has been shown that these peptides possess structural configuration characterized by a left-handed polyproline II helical conformation that is preferred by MHC class II ligands [85].

(1)   Properties of 33-mer peptide from α-gliadin

The α-gliadin 33-mer is one of the digestion-resistant gluten peptides that is highly reactive to isolated celiac T cells and is the main immunodominant toxic peptide in celiac patients. It is located in the *N*-terminal repetitive region of α-gliadin and contains six overlapping copies of three different DQ2-restricted epitopes (Figure 6) [86].

Using RNA-amplicon sequencing (NGS) technology it was shown that α-gliadins can be separated into six types and only one type contains all the immunogenic peptides and epitopes, whereas the other five types do not contain all the epitopes disabling 33-mer peptide formation [30]. Thus, distinct types of α-gliadins differ mainly in the number of repeat blocks consisting in interspersed motifs PFPPQQ and PYPQPQ.

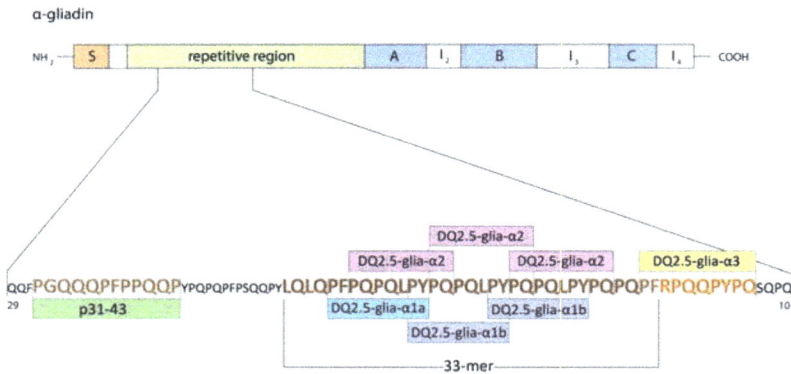

Figure 6. Fragment of α-gliadin protein sequence. Main immunogenic fragments: peptides p31-43, 33-mer and DQ2.5-glia-α3 are indicated.

Six epitopes of type 1 α-gliadin are DQ2.5-glia-α1a/b and DQ2.5-glia-α2 (Figure 6). There is also a partial overlap with 33-mer DQ2.5-glia-α3 epitope associated only with type 1 of gliadins. 33-mer is able to self-assemble in a concentration-dependent manner through structural transition [32]. It obtains polyproline II structure based on type II beta-turn with increase of peptide concentration.

33-mer reaches lamina propria and after deamidation plays a central role in the pathogenic cascade of celiac disease by activating the adaptive immune response. 33-mer enters the cell by intracellular pathway, excluding paracellular entrance. Gliadin-derived peptides can also be transcytosed from the apical of the intestinal epithelium to the basolateral side along with transferrin and IgA, avoiding entrance to the late endocytic compartment [87].

In vivo experiments revealed that 33-mer gliadin-derived peptide is undigested by enzymes of the intestinal brush border. Moreover, in a monkey model of gluten sensitivity, 33-mer peptide can be detected in the serum when the disease starts, indicating that this peptide can trespass the mucosa intact in vivo [88].

Then, 33-mer is deamidated by tTG present in the intestinal brush border and presented by dendritic cell to T cell (in mesenteric lymph nodes). T cells reach peripheral blood through the thoracic duct and product interferon-γ resulting in intestine epithelial cytotoxicity, while another peptide p31-43 has been reported to induce the innate immune response necessary to initiate the T-cell adaptive response through production of interleukin-15.

It has been shown that 33-mer of α-gliadin is very similar to protein Prn of *B. pertussis*, which causes pertussis. These results show that neither pertussis immunization nor disease induces production of antibodies reactive against the peptide, and thus it is unlikely that either pertussis immunization or disease contributes to CD pathogenesis on the basis of cross-reactive antibodies [89].

(2) Repertoire of gluten peptides active in CD

It has been established that deamidated forms of gluten peptides are more toxic than their amidated forms. tTG preferably deamidates sites QXP (X—any amino acid residue), which are abundant in immunodominant peptides. Interestingly, both DQ2 and DQ8 molecules lack the aspartic acid residue at β57 position present in other DQ molecules. DQ2 and DQ8 molecules possess positively charged pockets containing five anchor positions and a least three of them (P4, P6, and P7) prefer to bind negatively charged amino acids [90]. Crystallographic structure of DQ2 complexes with immunodominant epitope revealed that glutamic acid residue fits in the P4, P6 and P7 anchor positions and proline residue—in the P1, P3, P6 and P8 positions [91]. Analogous report regarding DQ8 complexes revealed only two glutamic acid-preferred positions (P1 and P9). This explains the lower number of gluten peptides active in DQ8 individuals.

Long-term T cell lines (TCL) or T cell clones (TCC) raised against gluten are used to identifying gluten immunogenic peptides. Anderson et al. established an approach that detects gluten-specific T cells in the peripheral blood (peripheral blood mononuclear cells, PBMC) after 3 days of consumption of gluten-containing food by an interferon-γ EliSpot assay [92]. A comprehensive, quantitative mapping of T cell epitopes was used to screen all the unique 20-mer sequences of gliadins, glutenins, hordeins, and secalins. Independently, this screening and EliSpot assay provided the set of immunodominant epitopes from wheat, barley, and rye (Table 3) [93,94]. Almost all DQ2 immunogenic peptides of α-gliadins map the N-terminal 57–89 region (33-mer). DQ2-restricted ω-gliadin peptides strictly related to α-gliadin 17-mer: it contains two overlapping copies of 9-mer epitopes. Immunogenic peptides of γ-gliadins are spread along all the sequences. Similarly, few DQ2-restricted sequences from secalin and hordein proteins were reported to stimulate intestinal CD4+ T cell lines or clones [75].

Table 3. Number of gluten immunogenic peptides currently identified within distinct gluten proteins.

Grain Species	Gluten Protein	Number of DQ2-Restricted Peptides Identified (Confirmed in Vitro on TCLs/TCCs or/and on PBMCs after in Vivo Challenge)	Number of DQ8-Restricted Peptides Identified (Confirmed in Vitro on TCLs/TCCs or/and on PBMCs after in Vivo Challenge)
Wheat	α-gliadins	3	3
	γ-gliadins	11	4
	ω-gliadins	3	4
	Glutenins	3	1
Barley	Hordeins	8	-
Rye	Secalins	11	-
Oat	Avenins	6	-

Only 3 DQ8-restricted epitopes were identified using T cell lines or T cell clones: two for α-gliadin, γ-gliadin and one for glutenin [95]. Additional peptides were discovered as a result of the work by Tye-Din et al. [93]. Furthermore, it was shown that HLA-DQ8-associated CD appears not to be exclusively dependent on deamidation by tTG [95].

Avenins differ from other groups of prolamins due to their low content of proline and glutamine residues. Nevertheless, a few gliadin-like and glutenin-like avenin-derived peptides were identified [96]. Avenin peptides were divided into three groups: low-stimulatory short peptides (six residues), stimulatory (27 and 10 residues) and peptides with upregulated stimulatory capacity (10 and 14 residues). Larger peptides (27 residues) are commensurable in size with 33-mer and induce response of dendritic cells in not only CD patients but also in control healthy patients. Whereas peptides with the appropriate size and disposition of amino acids residues (10 and 14 residues) are likely to go through a differential endocytic pathway.

Thus, immunogenic sequences were identified in all gluten proteins of *Triticeae* and oat. These studies revealed that amongst all the DQ2-restricted peptides of wheat, barley, rye and oat prolamins, there is a hierarchy of T cell recognition depending on the specific cereal ingested. Furthermore, an evident redundancy in DQ2-restricted peptide recognition occurs, i.e., activated by a dominant peptide T cells are capable of recognizing and responding to a large number of related gluten sequences and vice versa. However, there is no clear difference in the immunogenicity strength between DQ8-restricted peptides. Altogether, DQ8-type of HLA molecules are less strongly associated with celiac disease, compared to DQ2. Oat peptides possess the lowest immunogenic activity though avenin peptides are capable of inducing T cell response.

4.3. Wheat Allergy

Wheat flour triggers IgE-mediated food allergy and is one of the top eight food allergens. Wheat allergy commonly develops in childhood [97]. When an allergen specifically binds to IgE antibodies, it induces the activation of mast cells and basophils. In the case of wheat, it is believed that allergy occurs due to a breach in oral tolerance and as a consequence of Th2-biased immune dysregulation that induces sensitization and B-cell-specific allergen IgE production [98]. Gluten proteins causing allergy include some types of ω-gliadin as well as non-gluten protein of wheat such as profilin, serpin, α-purothionin, etc. Non-gluten flour proteins and some γ-, α/β-gliadins can cause an occupational respiratory allergy such as baker's asthma, which appears after the inhalation of flour by millers or bakers. ω5-gliadins trigger another type of allergy—food allergy—referred to as wheat-dependent exercise-induced anaphylaxis (WDEIA), which develops after the ingestion of wheat followed by intense physical exercise.

Recently, it was shown that γ-, α/β-, ω5-, ω1,2-gliadins contain IgE-binding epitopes as well as HMW and LMW subunits of glutenin [99] (Table 4). Nevertheless, major allergenic protein of wheat is ω5-gliadin possessing *N*-terminal sequence SRLL, which can be crucial for allergy pathogenesis, and repetitive region consists almost entirely of peptides FPQQQ and QQIPQQ [14].

Table 4. Currently identified IgE-binding epitopes in wheat gluten proteins. *—X—any amino acid.

Protein	IgE-Binding Epitope Motifs
α/β-gliadin	QQQFPGQQ, LQQQ
γ-gliadin	QPQQPFPQ
ω5-gliadin	QQXPXQQ *
ω1,2-gliadin	QQPXPXQ
HMW-GS	QQPGQ(GQQ)
LMW-GS	QQPIQQQP

γ-gliadin, α/β-gliadin and ω1,2-gliadin are causative allergens in both WDEIA patients and those with baker's asthma [100,101]. Epitopes QQPFP and PQQPF of gliadin are also involved in atopic dermatitis-related wheat allergy [102] as well as QQQPP motif in LMW-GS [103].

Nowadays, 3D structure of known IgE allergenic epitopes helps to elucidate its conformation and to produce recombinant allergens for further research.

4.4. Non-Celiac Gluten Sensitivity (NCGS)

The first reported NCGS cases were described as longstanding and previously unresolved history of abdominal pain, discomfort, bloating, altered bowel habit and fatigue with exclusion of celiac disease. NCGS is more frequently diagnosed in adults rather than in children [104]. In most cases, NCGS reveals itself a few hours after gluten digestion [104]. Similarly to CD patients, patients with NCGS suffer from nutritional deficiencies, coexisting autoimmunity, and a decreased bone mineral density compared with the general population. The prevalence of HLA-DQ2 and/or HLA-DQ8 genotypes is ~50% in NCGS comparable to the general population [105], but there is no anti-tTG2 antibodies identified. Gluten only triggered an innate immune response in NCGS and provoked an additional adaptive immune response with increased expression of IL-6, IL-21, IL-17 and IFN-γ [106]. However, gastrointestinal symptoms other than intestinal permeability and adaptive immune responses are not involved in the process. In NCGS, gliadins do not induce mucosal inflammation in vitro or the activation of basophils as seen in CD [107].

It has been suggested that in NCGS gluten-related peptides enter the systemic circulation and cause extraintestinal manifestations such as ataxia, neuropathy and encephalopathy [108]. Moreover, it has been proposed that gluten causes depression, anxiety, autism and schizophrenia in patients with NCGS [109], and also reported that psychosis might be a manifestation of NCGS [110].

Nowadays, gluten-related disorders have often been recognized as commonly mimicking irritable bowel syndrome (IBS) because of the similar symptoms such as abdominal pain, bloating, bowel habit abnormalities (either diarrhea or constipation) [111]. Indeed, both can coexist independently without necessarily sharing a common pathophysiological basis. Furthermore, the microbiome may also play a role in the pathogenesis of NCGS [112]. Gut microbiota composition and metabolomic profiles may influence the loss of gluten tolerance and subsequent onset of gluten intolerance in genetically-susceptible individuals [113]. Gut microbiota could become a target for further therapy [114].

Recently, a standardizing protocol was reported for the diagnostic confirmation of NCGS [3]. It implies assessment of the clinical response to GFD and consequent effect of the gluten challenge. It is important that patients are on a normal, gluten-containing diet for proper evaluation, which is not always possible. For these two assessment steps, a modified version of the Gastrointestinal Symptom Rating Scale (GSRS) is used. The GSRS protocol is based on reviews and the clinical experience and allows for evaluation of gastrointestinal and extra-intestinal symptoms. Patients name one to three symptoms and the Numerical Rating Scale (NRS) measures the severity score from 1 to 10. However, there are still difficulties in diagnosing and managing NCGS. Even though the precise mechanism and biochemical markers for the NCGS disease have still not identified, this protocol could be used to establish the prevalence of this condition.

5. Gluten Detoxification Strategies

5.1. Gluten Free Diet (GFD)

There is currently only one proven effective way of treating celiac disease and NCGS—a gluten free diet. It means the avoidance of gluten-containing food in gluten intolerance patients' ration. There is little information in the literature on minimal disease-eliciting doses of gluten, which would be safe for CD patients. Apparently, it should lie between 10 and 50–100 mg daily intake [115]. Starch-based gluten-free products contain trace amounts of gluten. However, a diet completely devoid of gluten is unrealistic. The diet is complicated due to cross-contamination and/or the presence of small amounts of the gluten in food and medicines.

GFD cannot be regarded as a healthy diet. Gluten-free products are usually made with starches or refined flours characterized by low fiber content. It is known that the consumption of adequate amounts of dietary fiber is related to important health benefits such as prevention of colon cancer, diabetes and cardiovascular disease [116]. Thus, GFD may lead to possible nutrient deficiencies in fiber resulting in consequent diseases. Several studies suggest using pseudo-cereal sources of fiber instead of gluten-free products in order to maintain the necessary fiber content level [117].

GFD also leads to deficiency in Vitamins C, B12, D and folic acid [118], which is associated not only with malabsorption caused by villi atrophy but also with low quality of GFD [117]. Consuming fruits and vegetables rich in vitamins and antioxidant substances up to five times a day is recommended. Some studies demonstrate that gluten-free cereal products contain lower amounts of folate compared to their gluten-containing counterparts, so there is a need for additional folate supplementation [119].

In CD patients, malabsorption and inflammation contribute to a low bone mineral density (BMD) [120]. CD patients have a 40% higher risk of having bone fractures compared with non-CD healthy people. Thus, the diet plays a critical role in the maintenance of proper bone mineralization. GFD appears to be unbalanced in terms of calcium, magnesium, zinc in male and iron in women, and additional supplementation required [121]. Zinc is an essential trace element involved in numerous reactions and biochemical functions. Zinc deficiency can affect protein synthesis and leads to growth arrest [122]. Magnesium is essential for several enzymatic reactions (for DNA and RNA polymerases, ionic pumps and calcium channels). Thus, it is recommended that gluten-free products are substituted with other cereals such as quinoa, sorghum and amaranth, which are safe and rich in folic acid, vitamins (riboflavin, Vitamin C and Vitamin E) and minerals [117].

At the same time, gluten-free diet contains high amounts of sugar and hydrogenated fats, which could result in the occurrence of hyperinsulinemia and an increased obesity risk [123].

Thus, GFD appears to be an unbalanced diet inadequate in terms of both macro- and micronutrients. In order to maintain the necessary level of all the nutrients an annual screening for nutrient status of a patient is required and there is a need for additional nutrient supplementation. Thus, GFD is not an optimal and healthy way to treat all the manifestations of gluten intolerance including CD, wheat allergy and NCGS. Even though a wheat free diet is optimal for wheat allergy treatment, patients can eat rye, barley and oat. A wheat free diet is also probably effective for NCGS treatment. Other directions of treatment of gluten intolerance need to be developed.

Many works focus on providing new medicinal approaches for effective gluten intolerance treatment. Two major directions exist: prevention and treatment of gluten related disorders. The prevention hypothesis implies that the time the gluten is introduced into the diet of infants at risk of CD may affect the disease incidence. The Prevent CD Family Study was held in 10 European countries. One thousand children and their mothers participated, and were followed up for a period of 1–3 years. It has been suggested that small quantities of gluten are administered gradually to induce oral immune tolerance to gluten. It is now accepted that gluten may be introduced into the infant's diet at any time between 4 and 12 months of age. In children at high risk of CD, an earlier introduction of gluten (4 vs. 6 months or 6 vs. 12 months) is associated with an earlier development of CD, but the cumulative incidence in later childhood is similar [124]. Recently, an analogous program in Italy was started to evaluate the at-risk infants age, at which CD-related autoimmune serological changes occur. Data obtained in this study indicate that delaying the gluten introduction into the infants' diet until the age of 12 months decreases the prevalence of CD [125]. Both studies need a much longer follow-up analysis to establish whether the timing of gluten exposure can really prevent CD or merely delay its onset.

5.2. Detoxification of Gluten Proteins with Enzymatic Therapy

This approach is based on the fact that gluten peptides are highly resistant to digestive pancreatic and brush border proteases. Fortunately, many organisms (e.g., bacteria, fungi, plants etc.) encode proteolytic enzymes possessing distinct features compared to endogenous proteases presented in human [126–128]. Thus, it has been proposed that exogenous enzymes can be employed for additional enzyme supplement therapy to promote the complete digestion of cereal proteins, and thus destroy T-cell gluten epitopes, in particular [129,130]. A number of peptidases possessing glutenase activities were isolated from germinating cereals (*Hordeum vulgare* L., *Triticum aestivum* L.), bacteria (*Flavobacterium meningosepticum*, *Sphingomonas capsulate*, *Myxococcus xanthus*), fungi (*Aspergillus niger*, *Aspergillus oryzae*), and stored-product pest yellow mealworm (*Tenebrio molitor*) [131–135]. One of them is ALV003 enzyme—modified recombinant EP-B2 enzyme from barley, and prolyl endopeptidase from bacteria *Sphingomonas capsulate*—was shown to be effective in vitro and in vivo, non-toxic and without allergic reactions [136,137]. Gluten-containing food can also be treated with bacterial-derived peptidases, in particular, proteases of certain lactobacilli present in sourdough are able to proteolyze proline-rich gluten peptides [138].

5.3. Modified Grains

There are several studies targeted at developing grains with reduced pathogenicity. On the basis of knowledge of peptide immunogenicity hierarchy, site-directed mutagenesis of wheat, which would not affect the baking properties, has also been proposed. However, hexaploidy of wheat seriously complicates this process. Nevertheless, successful transformation of bread wheat *Triticum aestivum* Butte 86 was reported [139]. In this paper, a subclass of ω-gliadins genes, encoding proteins that cause food IgE-mediated allergy, were silenced in order to decrease the level of ω5-gliadins in grain. Transgenic wheat has reduced allergenicity without influencing the dough quality. Similar work was performed to reduce the toxicity in CD patients of all gliadin proteins through the shutdown of these genes by RNA interference [140]. Genes of γ-, α- and ω-gliadins were down-regulated in these plant lines. This has led to the production of wheat lines with very low levels of toxicity for CD patients.

As discussed above, the gluten of barley and rye is also highly pathogenic for patients with gluten intolerance. Thus, a number of works describe modifications introduced into barley genome: for example, deletion of B and C hordeins resulted in 20-fold reduced immunotoxicity compared to wild type [141].

Nowadays, the wheat genome is modified in order to improve the dough quality. However, different modifications may introduce known or clinically cross-reactive allergens into genome. It was suggested that bioinformatic methods can be used to prevent such allergen introduction and assess the safety and allergenicity of modified crops, using a comprehensive database [142].

5.4. Corrections of Gluten Pathogenicity Pathways

tTG is very important in CD pathogenesis. For this reason, it has become a target for suppression by the design of potent and selective inhibitors. Inhibition of tTG2 by cystamine in vitro and in situ was confirmed by means of abolished reactivity of gliadin-specific T-cell response [143]. Recently, Keillor et al. reviewed the latest and most applicable inhibitors of tTG2 designed on the basis of the conformational effects and crystallographic structures of inhibited tTG2 [144].

Zonulin, one of the TJ regulatory proteins involved in the proper functioning of intestinal epithelial permeability, controls the passage through the mucosal barrier. The inhibition of zonulin overexpression can prevent it trespassing the gut barrier. The effective synthetic peptide inhibitor was developed and named as AT1001 or Larazotide acetate [145]. There is now a novel therapeutic agent targeting TJ regulation in patients with CD.

Peptides themselves are undoubtedly major CD participants. Peptide analogues of gliadin epitopes can be engineered with antagonistic effects of native peptides. Nexvax2® (Immusan T, Inc., Cambridge, MA, USA) is the peptide-based therapeutic vaccine based on desensitization therapy principles [146]. This product encompasses three peptides that respond to a substantial proportion of the T-cell reaction to gluten in HLA-DQ2-carring patients. Nexvax2 is currently undergoing clinical trials.

6. Conclusions

Nowadays, gluten intolerance is an important issue. The number of people diagnosed with gluten intolerance is increasing. Thus, there is a need for more effective and novel approaches to treat gluten-related disorders. Externally, it is caused by the consumption of gluten prolamin proteins present in wheat, barley and rye. In the present paper, we have summarized the knowledge on the classification, properties, structure, evolution and role of gluten proteins in the pathogenesis of gluten intolerance manifestations. Even though gluten proteins—gliadins, glutenins, hordeins, secalins and avenins—share similar features and evolutional origins, they possess different pathogenicities. A detailed understanding of the principal properties of gluten intolerance causative agents open ups the possibilities for the development of novel therapeutic approaches such as with improved low pathogenic wheat, barley and rye plant lines; renewed therapeutic enzymatic drugs and vaccines. This will obviate the need for GFD and improve the quality of life of people suffering from gluten intolerance.

Acknowledgments: We are very grateful to Jonathan McFarland for his editorial work throughout the preparation of this manuscript. This research was funded by the Russian Science Foundation (grant # 16-15-10410).

Author Contributions: All authors contributed to the preparation of this review article.

Conflicts of Interest: The authors declare no conflict of interest.

Abbreviations

CD	celiac disease
NCGS	non-celiac gluten sensitivity
HLA	human leukocyte antigen
MHC	major histocompatibility complex
tTG	tissue transglutaminase
IgA (IgG, IgE)	immunoglobulin A (G, E)
IEL	intraepithelial lymphocyte
TJ	tight junction
DC	dendritic cell
GA	gluten ataxia

HMW	high molecular weight
LMW	low molecular weight
HMW-GS	high molecular weight glutenin subunits
LMW-GS	low molecular weight glutenin subunits
HMW-SS	high molecular weight secalin subunits
SDS-PAGE	sodium dodecyl sulfate polyacrylamide gel electrophoresis
ER	endoplasmic reticulum
DNA	deoxyribonucleic acid
RNA	ribonucleic acid
FISH	fluorescence in situ hybridization
HPLC	high-performance liquid chromatography
PDB	protein data bank
NGS	next-generation sequencing
IFN-γ	interferon-γ
IL	interleukin
TCL	T cell line
TCC	T cell clone
PBMC	peripheral blood mononuclear cells
WDEIA	wheat-dependent exercise-induced anaphylaxis
GFD	gluten-free diet
IBS	irritable bowel syndrome
GSRS	gastrointestinal symptom rating scale
NRS	numerical rating scale
BMD	bone mineral density

References

1. Ferguson, A.; MacDonald, T.T.; McClure, J.P.; Holden, R.J. Cell-mediated immunity to gliadin within the small-intestinal mucosa in coeliac disease. *Lancet* **1975**, *1*, 895–897. [CrossRef]
2. Czaja-Bulsa, G. Non coeliac gluten sensitivity—A new disease with gluten intolerance. *Clin. Nutr.* **2015**, *34*, 189–194. [CrossRef] [PubMed]
3. Catassi, C.; Elli, L.; Bonaz, B.; Bouma, G.; Carroccio, A.; Castillejo, G.; Cellier, C.; Cristofori, F.; de Magistris, L.; Dolinsek, J.; et al. Diagnosis of Non-Celiac Gluten Sensitivity (NCGS): The Salerno Experts' Criteria. *Nutrients* **2015**, *7*, 4966–4977. [CrossRef] [PubMed]
4. Catassi, C.; Gatti, S.; Lionetti, E. World perspective and celiac disease epidemiology. *Dig. Dis.* **2015**, *33*, 141–146. [CrossRef] [PubMed]
5. Husby, S.; Koletzko, S.; Korponay-Szabo, I.R.; Mearin, M.L.; Phillips, A.; Shamir, R.; Troncone, R.; Giersiepen, K.; Branski, D.; Catassi, C.; et al. European Society for Pediatric Gastroenterology, Hepatology, and Nutrition guidelines for the diagnosis of coeliac disease. *J. Pediatr. Gastroenterol. Nutr.* **2012**, *54*, 136–160. [CrossRef] [PubMed]

6. Fasano, A.; Catassi, C. Clinical practice. Celiac disease. *N. Engl. J. Med.* **2012**, *367*, 2419–2426. [CrossRef] [PubMed]
7. Leffler, D.A.; Green, P.H.; Fasano, A. Extraintestinal manifestations of coeliac disease. *Nat. Rev. Gastroenterol. Hepatol.* **2015**, *12*, 561–571. [CrossRef] [PubMed]
8. Van Heel, D.A.; West, J. Recent advances in coeliac disease. *Gut* **2006**, *55*, 1037–1046. [CrossRef] [PubMed]
9. Wang, W.; Uzzau, S.; Goldblum, S.E.; Fasano, A. Human zonulin, a potential modulator of intestinal tight junctions. *J. Cell Sci.* **2000**, *113*, 4435–4440. [PubMed]
10. Schuppan, D. Current concepts of celiac disease pathogenesis. *Gastroenterology* **2000**, *119*, 234–242. [CrossRef] [PubMed]
11. Nilsen, E.M.; Jahnsen, F.L.; Lundin, K.E.; Johansen, F.E.; Fausa, O.; Sollid, L.M.; Jahnsen, J.; Scott, H.; Brandtzaeg, P. Gluten induces an intestinal cytokine response strongly dominated by interferon gamma in patients with celiac disease. *Gastroenterology* **1998**, *115*, 551–563. [CrossRef]
12. Dewar, D.; Pereira, S.P.; Ciclitira, P.J. The pathogenesis of coeliac disease. *Int. J. Biochem. Cell Biol.* **2004**, *36*, 17–24. [CrossRef]
13. Jacquenet, S.; Morisset, M.; Battais, F.; Denery-Papini, S.; Croizier, A.; Baudouin, E.; Bihain, B.; Moneret-Vautrin, D.A. Interest of ImmunoCAP system to recombinant omega-5 gliadin for the diagnosis of exercise-induced wheat allergy. *Int. Arch. Allergy Immunol.* **2009**, *149*, 74–80. [CrossRef] [PubMed]
14. Battais, F.; Mothes, T.; Moneret-Vautrin, D.A.; Pineau, F.; Kanny, G.; Popineau, Y.; Bodinier, M.; Denery-Papini, S. Identification of IgE-binding epitopes on gliadins for patients with food allergy to wheat. *Allergy* **2005**, *60*, 815–821. [CrossRef] [PubMed]
15. Rodrigo, L.; Hernandez-Lahoz, C.; Lauret, E.; Rodriguez-Pelaez, M.; Soucek, M.; Ciccocioppo, R.; Kruzliak, P. Gluten ataxia is better classified as non-celiac gluten sensitivity than as celiac disease: A comparative clinical study. *Immunol. Res.* **2016**, *64*, 558. [CrossRef] [PubMed]
16. Shewry, P.R.; Halford, N.G. Cereal seed storage proteins: Structures, properties and role in grain utilization. *J. Exp. Bot.* **2002**, *53*, 947–958. [CrossRef] [PubMed]
17. Kreis, M.; Forde, B.G.; Rahman, S.; Miflin, B.J.; Shewry, P.R. Molecular evolution of the seed storage proteins of barley, rye and wheat. *J. Mol. Biol.* **1985**, *183*, 499–502. [CrossRef]
18. Wieser, H. Chemistry of gluten proteins. *Food Microbiol.* **2007**, *24*, 115–119. [CrossRef] [PubMed]
19. Singh, H.; MacRitchie, F. Application of polymer science to properties of gluten. *J. Cereal Sci.* **2001**, *33*, 231–243. [CrossRef]
20. Muccilli, V.; Cunsolo, V.; Saletti, R.; Foti, S.; Masci, S.; Lafiandra, D. Characterization of B- and C-type low molecular weight glutenin subunits by electrospray ionization mass spectrometry and matrix-assisted laser desorption/ionization mass spectrometry. *Proteomics* **2005**, *5*, 719–728. [CrossRef] [PubMed]
21. Zilic, S.; Barac, M.; Pesic, M.; Dodig, D.; Ignjatovic-Micic, D. Characterization of proteins from grain of different bread and durum wheat genotypes. *Int. J. Mol. Sci.* **2011**, *12*, 5878–5894. [CrossRef] [PubMed]
22. Wrigley, C.W.; Shepherd, K.W. Electrofocusing of grain proteins from wheat genotypes. *Ann. N. Y. Acad. Sci.* **1973**, *209*, 154–162. [CrossRef] [PubMed]
23. Ferranti, P.; Mamone, G.; Picariello, G.; Addeo, F. Mass spectrometry analysis of gliadins in celiac disease. *J. Mass Spectrom.* **2007**, *42*, 1531–1548. [CrossRef] [PubMed]
24. Tatham, A.S.; Drake, A.F.; Shewry, P.R. A conformational study of a glutamine- and proline-rich cereal seed protein, C hordein. *Biochem. J.* **1985**, *226*, 557–562. [CrossRef] [PubMed]
25. Schofield, J.D.; Bottomley, R.C.; Timms, M.F.; Booth, M.R. The effect of heat on wheat gluten and the involvement of sulphydryl-disulphide interchange reactions. *J. Cereal Sci.* **1983**, *1*, 241–253. [CrossRef]
26. Rombouts, I.; Lagrain, B.; Brijs, K.; Delcour, J.A. β-Elimination reactions and formation of covalent cross-links in gliadin during heating at alkaline pH. *J. Cereal Sci.* **2010**, *52*, 362–367. [CrossRef]
27. Lagrain, B.; Rombouts, I.; Brijs, K.; Delcour, J.A. Kinetics of heat-induced polymerization of gliadin. *J. Agric. Food Chem.* **2011**, *59*, 2034–2039. [CrossRef] [PubMed]
28. Barak, S.; Mudgil, D.; Khatkar, B.S. Biochemical and functional properties of wheat gliadins: A review. *Crit. Rev. Food Sci. Nutr.* **2015**, *55*, 357–368. [CrossRef] [PubMed]
29. Hamer, R.J.; van Vliet, T. Understanding the structure and properties of gluten: An overview. In *Wheat Gluten*; Shewry, P.R., Tatham, A.S., Eds.; Royal Society of Chemistry: Cambridge, UK, 2000; pp. 125–131.

30. Ozuna, C.V.; Iehisa, J.C.; Gimenez, M.J.; Alvarez, J.B.; Sousa, C.; Barro, F. Diversification of the celiac disease alpha-gliadin complex in wheat: A 33-mer peptide with six overlapping epitopes, evolved following polyploidization. *Plant J.* **2015**, *82*, 794–805. [CrossRef] [PubMed]

31. Tatham, A.S.; Marsh, M.N.; Wieser, H.; Shewry, P.R. Conformational studies of peptides corresponding to the coeliac-activating regions of wheat alpha-gliadin. *Biochem. J.* **1990**, *270*, 313–318. [CrossRef] [PubMed]

32. Herrera, M.G.; Benedini, L.A.; Lonez, C.; Schilardi, P.L.; Hellweg, T.; Ruysschaert, J.M.; Dodero, V.I. Self-assembly of 33-mer gliadin peptide oligomers. *Soft Matter* **2015**, *11*, 8648–8660. [CrossRef] [PubMed]

33. Sato, N.; Matsumiya, A.; Higashino, Y.; Funaki, S.; Kitao, Y.; Oba, Y.; Inoue, R.; Arisaka, F.; Sugiyama, M.; Urade, R. Molecular assembly of wheat gliadins into nanostructures: A small-angle X-ray scattering study of gliadins in distilled water over a wide concentration range. *J. Agric. Food Chem.* **2015**, *63*, 8715–8721. [CrossRef] [PubMed]

34. Herrera, M.G.; Veuthey, T.V.; Dodero, V.I. Self-organization of gliadin in aqueous media under physiological digestive pHs. *Colloids Surf. B Biointerfaces* **2016**, *141*, 565–575. [CrossRef] [PubMed]

35. Banc, A.; Desbat, B.; Renard, D.; Popineau, Y.; Mangavel, C.; Navailles, L. Exploring the interactions of gliadins with model membranes: Effect of confined geometry and interfaces. *Biopolymers* **2009**, *91*, 610–622. [CrossRef] [PubMed]

36. Shewry, P.R.; Napier, J.A.; Tatham, A.S. Seed storage proteins: Structures and biosynthesis. *Plant Cell* **1995**, *7*, 945–956. [CrossRef] [PubMed]

37. Wellner, N.; Mills, E.N.; Brownsey, G.; Wilson, R.H.; Brown, N.; Freeman, J.; Halford, N.G.; Shewry, P.R.; Belton, P.S. Changes in protein secondary structure during gluten deformation studied by dynamic fourier transform infrared spectroscopy. *Biomacromolecules* **2005**, *6*, 255–261. [CrossRef] [PubMed]

38. Lawrence, G.J.; Shepherd, K.W. Chromosomal location of genes controlling seed proteins in species related to wheat. *Theor. Appl. Genet.* **1981**, *59*, 25–31. [PubMed]

39. Shewry, P.R.; Halford, N.G.; Tatham, A.S.; Popineau, Y.; Lafiandra, D.; Belton, P.S. The high molecular weight subunits of wheat glutenin and their role in determining wheat processing properties. *Adv. Food Nutr. Res.* **2003**, *45*, 219–302. [PubMed]

40. Payne, P.I.; Holt, L.M.; Jarvis, G.; Jackson, E.A. Two-dimensional fractionation of the endosperm proteins of bread wheat (*Triticum aestivum*): Biochemical and genetic studies. *Cereal Chem.* **1985**, *62*, 319–326.

41. Tosi, P.; D'Ovidio, R.; Napier, J.A.; Bekes, F.; Shewry, P.R. Expression of epitope-tagged LMW glutenin subunits in the starchy endosperm of transgenic wheat and their incorporation into glutenin polymers. *Theor. Appl. Genet.* **2004**, *108*, 468–476. [CrossRef] [PubMed]

42. Masci, S.; Egorov, T.A.; Ronchi, C.; Kuzmicky, D.D.; Kasarda, D.D.; Lafiandra, D. Evidence for the presence of only one cysteine residue in the D-type low molecular weight subunits of wheat glutenin. *J. Cereal Sci.* **1999**, *29*, 17–25. [CrossRef]

43. Gorg, A.; Postel, W.; Baumer, M.; Weiss, W. Two-dimensional polyacrylamide gel electrophoresis, with immobilized pH gradients in the first dimension, of barley seed proteins: Discrimination of cultivars with different malting grades. *Electrophoresis* **1992**, *13*, 192–203. [CrossRef] [PubMed]

44. Jensen, J.; Jorgensen, J.H.; Jensen, H.P.; Giese, H.; Doll, H. Linkage of the hordein loci Hor1 and Hor2 with the powdery mildew resistance loci Ml-k and Ml-a on Barley chromosome 5. *Theor. Appl. Genet.* **1980**, *58*, 27–31. [CrossRef] [PubMed]

45. Forde, B.G.; Kreis, M.; Williamson, M.S.; Fry, R.P.; Pywell, J.; Shewry, P.R.; Bunce, N.; Miflin, B.J. Short tandem repeats shared by B- and C-hordein cDNAs suggest a common evolutionary origin for two groups of cereal storage protein genes. *EMBO J.* **1985**, *4*, 9–15. [PubMed]

46. Anderson, O.D. The B-hordein prolamin family of barley. *Genome* **2013**, *56*, 179–185. [CrossRef] [PubMed]

47. Rechinger, K.B.; Simpson, D.J.; Svendsen, I.; Cameron-Mills, V. A role for gamma 3 hordein in the transport and targeting of prolamin polypeptides to the vacuole of developing barley endosperm. *Plant J.* **1993**, *4*, 841–853. [CrossRef] [PubMed]

48. Thompson, S.; Bishop, D.H.L.; Tatham, A.S.; Shewry, P.R. Exploring disulphide bond formation in a low molecular weight subunit of glutenin using a baculovirus expression system. *Gluten Proteins* **1994**, 345–355.

49. Faulks, A.J.; Shewry, P.R.; Miflin, B.J. The polymorphism and structural homology of storage polypeptides (hordein) coded by the Hor-2 locus in barley (*Hordeum vulgare* L.). *Biochem. Genet.* **1981**, *19*, 841–858. [CrossRef] [PubMed]

50. Tatham, A.S.; Shewry, P.R.; Belton, P.S. 13C-n.m.r. study of C hordein. *Biochem. J.* **1985**, *232*, 617–620. [PubMed]
51. I'Anson, K.J.; Morris, V.J.; Shewry, P.R.; Tatham, A.S. Small-angle X-ray-scattering studies of the C hordeins of barley (*Hordeum vulgare*). *Biochem. J.* **1992**, *287*, 183–185. [CrossRef] [PubMed]
52. Cameron-Mills, V.; von Wettstein, D. Protein body formation in the developing barley endosperm. *Carlsberg Res. Commun.* **1980**, *45*, 577–594. [CrossRef]
53. Halford, N.G.; Tatham, A.S.; Sui, E.; Daroda, L.; Dreyer, T.; Shewry, P.R. Identification of a novel beta-turn-rich repeat motif in the D hordeins of barley. *Biochim. Biophys. Acta* **1992**, *1122*, 118–122. [CrossRef]
54. Hull, G.; Sabelli, P.A.; Shewry, P.R. Restriction fragment analysis of the secalin loci of rye. *Biochem. Genet.* **1992**, *30*, 85–97. [CrossRef] [PubMed]
55. Salmanowicz, B.P.; Langner, M.; Kubicka-Matusiewicz, H. Variation of high-molecular-weight secalin subunit composition in Rye (*Secale cereale* L.) inbred lines. *J. Agric. Food Chem.* **2014**, *62*, 10535–10541. [CrossRef] [PubMed]
56. Miles, M.J.; Carr, H.J.; McMaster, T.; Belton, P.S.; Morris, V.J.; Field, J.M.; Shewry, P.R.; Tatham, A.S. Scanning tunnelling microscopy of a wheat gluten protein reveals details of a spiral supersecondary structure. *Proc. Natl. Acad. Sci. USA* **1991**, *88*, 68. [CrossRef] [PubMed]
57. Singh, N.K.; Shepherd, K.W.; McIntosh, R.A. Linkage mapping of genes for resistance to leaf, stem and stripe rusts and omega-secalins on the short arm of rye chromosome 1R. *Theor. Appl. Genet.* **1990**, *80*, 609–616. [CrossRef] [PubMed]
58. Clarke, B.C.; Mukai, Y.; Appels, R. The *Sec-1* locus on the short arm of chromosome 1R of rye (*Secale cereale*). *Chromosoma* **1996**, *105*, 269–275. [CrossRef] [PubMed]
59. Yamamoto, M.; Mukai, Y. High-resolution physical mapping of the secalin-1 locus of rye on extended DNA fibers. *Cytogenet. Genome Res.* **2005**, *109*, 79–82. [CrossRef] [PubMed]
60. Jiang, Q.T.; Wei, Y.M.; Andre, L.; Lu, Z.X.; Pu, Z.E.; Peng, Y.Y.; Zheng, Y.L. Characterization of ω-secalin genes from rye, triticale, and a wheat 1BL/1RS translocation line. *J. Appl. Genet.* **2010**, *51*, 403–411. [CrossRef] [PubMed]
61. Dennett, A.L.; Cooper, K.V.; Trethowan, R.M. The genotypic and phenotypic interaction of wheat and rye storage proteins in primary triticale. *Euphytica* **2013**, *194*, 235–242. [CrossRef]
62. Shewry, P.R. Plant storage proteins. *Biol. Rev. Camb. Philos. Soc.* **1995**, *70*, 375–426. [CrossRef] [PubMed]
63. Chesnut, R.S.; Shotwell, M.A.; Boyer, S.K.; Larkins, B.A. Analysis of avenin proteins and the expression of their mRNAs in developing oat seeds. *Plant Cell* **1989**, *1*, 913–924. [CrossRef] [PubMed]
64. Lapvetelainen, A.; Bietz, J.; Huebner, F. Reversed-phase high-performance liquid chromatography of oat proteins: Application of cultivar comparison and analysis of the effect of wet processing. *Cereal Chem.* **1995**, *72*, 259–264.
65. Egorov, T.A.; Musolyamov, A.K.; Andersen, J.S.; Roepstorff, P. The complete amino acid sequence and disulphide bond arrangement of oat alcohol-soluble avenin-3. *Eur. J. Biochem.* **1994**, *224*, 631–638. [CrossRef] [PubMed]
66. Real, A.; Comino, I.; de Lorenzo, L.; Merchan, F.; Gil-Humanes, J.; Gimenez, M.J.; Lopez-Casado, M.A.; Torres, M.I.; Cebolla, A.; Sousa, C.; et al. Molecular and immunological characterization of gluten proteins isolated from oat cultivars that differ in toxicity for celiac disease. *PLoS ONE* **2012**, *7*, e48365.
67. Lending, C.R.; Chesnut, R.S.; Shaw, K.L.; Larkins, B.A. Immunolocalization of avenin and globulin storage proteins in developing endosperm of *Avena sativa* L. *Planta* **1989**, *178*, 315–324. [CrossRef] [PubMed]
68. Qi, P.F.; Le, C.X.; Wang, Z.; Liu, Y.B.; Chen, Q.; Wei, Z.Z.; Xu, B.J.; Wei, Z.Y.; Dai, S.F.; Wei, Y.M.; et al. The gamma-gliadin-like gamma-prolamin genes in the tribe *Triticeae*. *J. Genet.* **2014**, *93*, 35–41. [CrossRef] [PubMed]
69. Vader, W.; Kooy, Y.; Van Veelen, P.; De Ru, A.; Harris, D.; Benckhuijsen, W.; Pena, S.; Mearin, L.; Drijfhout, J.W.; Koning, F. The gluten response in children with celiac disease is directed toward multiple gliadin and glutenin peptides. *Gastroenterology* **2002**, *122*, 1729–1737. [CrossRef] [PubMed]
70. Bushara, K.O. Neurologic presentation of celiac disease. *Gastroenterology* **2005**, *128*, S92–S97. [CrossRef] [PubMed]
71. Green, P.H.; Alaedini, A.; Sander, H.W.; Brannagan, T.H., 3rd; Latov, N.; Chin, R.L. Mechanisms underlying celiac disease and its neurologic manifestations. *Cell. Mol. Life Sci.* **2005**, *62*, 791–799.

72. Alaedini, A.; Okamoto, H.; Briani, C.; Wollenberg, K.; Shill, H.A.; Bushara, K.O.; Sander, H.W.; Green, P.H.; Hallett, M.; Latov, N. Immune cross-reactivity in celiac disease: Anti-gliadin antibodies bind to neuronal synapsin I. *J. Immunol.* **2007**, *178*, 6590–6595. [CrossRef] [PubMed]

73. Palosuo, K.; Alenius, H.; Varjonen, E.; Kalkkinen, N.; Reunala, T. Rye gamma-70 and gamma-35 secalins and barley gamma-3 hordein cross-react with omega-5 gliadin, a major allergen in wheat-dependent, exercise-induced anaphylaxis. *Clin. Exp. Allergy* **2001**, *31*, 466–473. [CrossRef] [PubMed]

74. Festenstein, G.W.; Hay, F.C.; Shewry, P.R. Immunochemical relationships of the prolamin storage proteins of barley, wheat, rye and oat. *Biochim. Biophys. Acta* **1987**, *912*, 371–383. [CrossRef]

75. Vader, L.W.; Stepniak, D.T.; Bunnik, E.M.; Kooy, Y.M.; de Haan, W.; Drijfhout, J.W.; Van Veelen, P.A.; Koning, F. Characterization of cereal toxicity for celiac disease patients based on protein homology in grains. *Gastroenterology* **2003**, *125*, 1105–1113. [CrossRef]

76. Hogberg, L.; Laurin, P.; Falth-Magnusson, K.; Grant, C.; Grodzinsky, E.; Jansson, G.; Ascher, H.; Browaldh, L.; Hammersjo, J.A.; Lindberg, E.; et al. Oats to children with newly diagnosed coeliac disease: A randomised double blind study. *Gut* **2004**, *53*, 649–654. [CrossRef] [PubMed]

77. Gatti, S.; Caporelli, N.; Galeazzi, T.; Francavilla, R.; Barbato, M.; Roggero, P.; Malamisura, B.; Iacono, G.; Budelli, A.; Gesuita, R.; et al. Oats in the diet of children with celiac disease: Preliminary results of a double-blind, randomized, placebo-controlled multicenter Italian study. *Nutrients* **2013**, *5*, 4653–4664. [CrossRef] [PubMed]

78. Wieser, H. Relation between gliadin structure and coeliac toxicity. *Acta Paediatr.* **1996**, *85*, 3–9. [CrossRef]

79. Hardy, M.Y.; Tye-Din, J.A.; Stewart, J.A.; Schmitz, F.; Dudek, N.L.; Hanchapola, I.; Purcell, A.W.; Anderson, R.P. Ingestion of oats and barley in patients with celiac disease mobilizes cross-reactive T cells activated by avenin peptides and immuno-dominant hordein peptides. *J. Autoimmun.* **2015**, *56*, 56–65. [CrossRef] [PubMed]

80. Hovhannisyan, Z.; Weiss, A.; Martin, A.; Wiesner, M.; Tollefsen, S.; Yoshida, K.; Ciszewski, C.; Curran, S.A.; Murray, J.A.; David, C.S.; et al. The role of HLA-DQ8 beta57 polymorphism in the anti-gluten T-cell response in coeliac disease. *Nature* **2008**, *456*, 534–538. [CrossRef] [PubMed]

81. Kim, B.T.; Mosekilde, L.; Duan, Y.; Zhang, X.Z.; Tornvig, L.; Thomsen, J.S.; Seeman, E. The structural and hormonal basis of sex differences in peak appendicular bone strength in rats. *J. Bone Miner. Res.* **2003**, *18*, 150–155. [CrossRef] [PubMed]

82. Ciccocioppo, R.; Di Sabatino, A.; Corazza, G.R. The immune recognition of gluten in coeliac disease. *Clin. Exp. Immunol.* **2005**, *140*, 408–416. [CrossRef] [PubMed]

83. Van de Wal, Y.; Kooy, Y.M.C.; van Veelen, P.; Vader, W.; August, S.A.; Drijfhout, J.W.; Pena, S.A.; Koning, F. Glutenin is involved in the glutendriven mucosal T cell response. *Eur. J. Immunol.* **1999**, *29*, 3133–3139. [CrossRef]

84. Barone, M.V.; Zimmer, K.P. Endocytosis and transcytosis of gliadin peptides. *Mol. Cell. Pediatr.* **2016**, *3*, 8. [CrossRef] [PubMed]

85. Herrera, M.G.; Zamarreno, F.; Costabel, M.; Ritacco, H.; Hutten, A.; Sewald, N.; Dodero, V.I. Circular dichroism and electron microscopy studies in vitro of 33-mer gliadin peptide revealed secondary structure transition and supramolecular organization. *Biopolymers* **2014**, *101*, 96–106. [CrossRef] [PubMed]

86. Shan, L.; Molberg, O.; Parrot, I.; Hausch, F.; Filiz, F.; Gray, G.M.; Sollid, L.M.; Khosla, C. Structural basis for gluten intolerance in celiac sprue. *Science* **2002**, *297*, 2275–2279. [CrossRef] [PubMed]

87. Lebreton, C.; Menard, S.; Abed, J.; Moura, I.C.; Coppo, R.; Dugave, C.; Monteiro, R.C.; Fricot, A.; Traore, M.G.; Griffin, M.; et al. Interactions among secretory immunoglobulin A, CD71, and transglutaminase-2 affect permeability of intestinal epithelial cells to gliadin peptides. *Gastroenterology* **2012**, *143*, 698–707. [CrossRef] [PubMed]

88. Mazumdar, K.; Alvarez, X.; Borda, J.T.; Dufour, J.; Martin, E.; Bethune, M.T.; Khosla, C.; Sestak, K. Visualization of transepithelial passage of the immunogenic 33-residue peptide from alpha-2 gliadin in gluten-sensitive macaques. *PLoS ONE* **2010**, *5*, e10228. [CrossRef] [PubMed]

89. He, Q.; Viljanen, M.K.; Hinkkanen, A.E.; Arvilommi, H.; Mertsola, J.; Viander, M. No evidence of cross-reactivity of human antibodies to a 33-mer peptide of the alpha-gliadin component of gluten with Bordetella pertussis pertactin. *Vaccine* **2005**, *23*, 3336–3340. [CrossRef] [PubMed]

90. Vartdal, F.; Johansen, B.H.; Friede, T.; Thorpe, C.J.; Stevanovic, S.; Eriksen, J.E.; Sletten, K.; Thorsby, E.; Rammensee, H.G.; Sollid, L.M. The peptide binding motif of the disease associated HLA-DQ (alpha 1* 0501, beta 1* 0201) molecule. *Eur. J. Immunol.* **1996**, *26*, 2764–2772. [CrossRef] [PubMed]

91. Arentz-Hansen, H.; McAdam, S.N.; Molberg, O.; Fleckenstein, B.; Lundin, K.E.; Jorgensen, T.J.; Jung, G.; Roepstorff, P.; Sollid, L.M. Celiac lesion T cells recognize epitopes that cluster in regions of gliadins rich in proline residues. *Gastroenterology* **2002**, *123*, 803–809. [CrossRef] [PubMed]

92. Anderson, R.P.; Degano, P.; Godkin, A.J.; Jewell, D.P.; Hill, A.V. In vivo antigen challenge in celiac disease identifies a single transglutaminase-modified peptide as the dominant A-gliadin T-cell epitope. *Nat. Med.* **2000**, *6*, 337–342. [CrossRef] [PubMed]

93. Tye-Din, J.A.; Stewart, J.A.; Dromey, J.A.; Beissbarth, T.; van Heel, D.A.; Tatham, A.; Henderson, K.; Mannering, S.I.; Gianfrani, C.; Jewell, D.P.; et al. Comprehensive, quantitative mapping of T cell epitopes in gluten in celiac disease. *Sci. Transl. Med.* **2010**, *2*, 41ra51. [CrossRef] [PubMed]

94. Beissbarth, T.; Tye-Din, J.A.; Smyth, G.K.; Speed, T.P.; Anderson, R.P. A systematic approach for comprehensive T-cell epitope discovery using peptide libraries. *Bioinformatics* **2005**, *21* (Suppl. 1), i29–i37. [CrossRef] [PubMed]

95. Camarca, A.; Del Mastro, A.; Gianfrani, C. Repertoire of gluten peptides active in celiac disease patients: Perspectives for translational therapeutic applications. *Endocr. Metab. Immune Disord. Drug Targets* **2012**, *12*, 207–219. [CrossRef] [PubMed]

96. Comino, I.; Bernardo, D.; Bancel, E.; de Lourdes Moreno, M.; Sanchez, B.; Barro, F.; Suligoj, T.; Ciclitira, P.J.; Cebolla, A.; Knight, S.C.; et al. Identification and molecular characterization of oat peptides implicated on coeliac immune response. *Food Nutr. Res.* **2016**, *60*, 30324. [CrossRef] [PubMed]

97. Patel, B.Y.; Volcheck, G.W. Food allergy: Common causes, diagnosis, and treatment. *Mayo Clin. Proc.* **2015**, *90*, 1411–1419. [CrossRef] [PubMed]

98. Chehade, M.; Mayer, L. Oral tolerance and its relation to food hypersensitivities. *J. Allergy Clin. Immunol.* **2005**, *115*, 3–12. [CrossRef] [PubMed]

99. Matsuo, H.; Yokooji, T.; Taogoshi, T. Common food allergens and their IgE-binding epitopes. *Allergol. Int.* **2015**, *64*, 332–343. [CrossRef] [PubMed]

100. Tatham, A.S.; Shewry, P.R. Allergens to wheat and related cereals. *Clin. Exp. Allergy* **2008**, *38*, 1712–1726. [PubMed]

101. Beyer, K.; Chung, D.; Schulz, G.; Mishoe, M.; Niggemann, B.; Wahn, U.; Sampson, H.A. The role of wheat omega-5 gliadin IgE antibodies as a diagnostic tool for wheat allergy in childhood. *J. Allergy Clin. Immunol.* **2008**, *122*, 419–421. [CrossRef] [PubMed]

102. Tanabe, S. IgE-binding abilities of pentapeptides, QQPFP and PQQPF, in wheat gliadin. *J. Nutr. Sci. Vitaminol. (Tokyo)* **2004**, *50*, 367–370. [CrossRef] [PubMed]

103. Tanabe, S.; Arai, S.; Yanagihara, Y.; Mita, H.; Takahashi, K.; Watanabe, M. A major wheat allergen has a Gln-Gln-Gln-Pro-Pro motif identified as an IgE-binding epitope. *Biochem. Biophys. Res. Commun.* **1996**, *219*, 290–293. [CrossRef] [PubMed]

104. Volta, U.; Bardella, M.T.; Calabro, A.; Troncone, R.; Corazza, G.R.; The Study Group for Non-Celiac Gluten Sensitivity. An Italian prospective multicenter survey on patients suspected of having non-celiac gluten sensitivity. *BMC Med.* **2014**, *12*, 85. [PubMed]

105. Aziz, I.; Lewis, N.R.; Hadjivassiliou, M.; Winfield, S.N.; Rugg, N.; Kelsall, A.; Newrick, L.; Sanders, D.S. A UK study assessing the population prevalence of self-reported gluten sensitivity and referral characteristics to secondary care. *Eur. J. Gastroenterol. Hepatol.* **2014**, *26*, 33–39. [CrossRef] [PubMed]

106. Sapone, A.; Lammers, K.M.; Casolaro, V.; Cammarota, M.; Giuliano, M.T.; De Rosa, M.; Stefanile, R.; Mazzarella, G.; Tolone, C.; Russo, M.I.; et al. Divergence of gut permeability and mucosal immune gene expression in two gluten-associated conditions: Celiac disease and gluten sensitivity. *BMC Med.* **2011**, *9*, 23. [CrossRef] [PubMed]

107. Bucci, C.; Zingone, F.; Russo, I.; Morra, I.; Tortora, R.; Pogna, N.; Scalia, G.; Iovino, P.; Ciacci, C. Gliadin does not induce mucosal inflammation or basophil activation in patients with nonceliac gluten sensitivity. *Clin. Gastroenterol. Hepatol.* **2013**, *11*, 1294–1299.e1. [CrossRef] [PubMed]

108. Aziz, I.; Hadjivassiliou, M.; Sanders, D.S. The spectrum of noncoeliac gluten sensitivity. *Nat. Rev. Gastroenterol. Hepatol.* **2015**, *12*, 516–526. [CrossRef] [PubMed]

109. Jackson, J.; Eaton, W.; Cascella, N.; Fasano, A.; Santora, D.; Sullivan, K.; Feldman, S.; Raley, H.; McMahon, R.P.; Carpenter, W.T., Jr.; et al. Gluten sensitivity and relationship to psychiatric symptoms in people with schizophrenia. *Schizophr. Res.* **2014**, *159*, 539–542. [CrossRef] [PubMed]

110. Lionetti, E.; Leonardi, S.; Franzonello, C.; Mancardi, M.; Ruggieri, M.; Catassi, C. Gluten Psychosis: Confirmation of a New Clinical Entity. *Nutrients* **2015**, *7*, 5532–5539. [CrossRef] [PubMed]

111. Sanders, D.S.; Aziz, I. Non-celiac wheat sensitivity: Separating the wheat from the chat! *Am. J. Gastroenterol.* **2012**, *107*, 1908–1912. [CrossRef] [PubMed]

112. Makharia, A.; Catassi, C.; Makharia, G.K. The overlap between irritable bowel syndrome and non-celiac gluten sensitivity: A clinical dilemma. *Nutrients* **2015**, *7*, 10417–10426. [CrossRef] [PubMed]

113. Leonard, M.M.; Camhi, S.; Huedo-Medina, T.B.; Fasano, A. Celiac disease genomic, environmental, microbiome, and metabolomic (CDGEMM) study design: Approach to the future of personalized prevention of celiac disease. *Nutrients* **2015**, *7*, 9325–9336. [CrossRef] [PubMed]

114. Leonard, M.M.; Fasano, A. The microbiome as a possible target to prevent celiac disease. *Expert Rev. Gastroenterol. Hepatol.* **2016**, *10*, 555–556. [CrossRef] [PubMed]

115. Hischenhuber, C.; Crevel, R.; Jarry, B.; Maki, M.; Moneret-Vautrin, D.A.; Romano, A.; Troncone, R.; Ward, R. Review article: Safe amounts of gluten for patients with wheat allergy or coeliac disease. *Aliment. Pharmacol. Ther.* **2006**, *23*, 559–575. [CrossRef] [PubMed]

116. Penagini, F.; Dilillo, D.; Meneghin, F.; Mameli, C.; Fabiano, V.; Zuccotti, G.V. Gluten-free diet in children: An approach to a nutritionally adequate and balanced diet. *Nutrients* **2013**, *5*, 4553–4565. [CrossRef] [PubMed]

117. Saturni, L.; Ferretti, G.; Bacchetti, T. The gluten-free diet: Safety and nutritional quality. *Nutrients* **2010**, *2*, 16–34. [CrossRef] [PubMed]

118. Hallert, C.; Grant, C.; Grehn, S.; Granno, C.; Hulten, S.; Midhagen, G.; Strom, M.; Svensson, H.; Valdimarsson, T. Evidence of poor vitamin status in coeliac patients on a gluten-free diet for 10 years. *Aliment. Pharmacol. Ther.* **2002**, *16*, 1333–1339. [CrossRef] [PubMed]

119. Hallert, C.; Svensson, M.; Tholstrup, J.; Hultberg, B. Clinical trial: B vitamins improve health in patients with coeliac disease living on a gluten-free diet. *Aliment. Pharmacol. Ther.* **2009**, *29*, 811–816. [CrossRef] [PubMed]

120. Pantaleoni, S.; Luchino, M.; Adriani, A.; Pellicano, R.; Stradella, D.; Ribaldone, D.G.; Sapone, N.; Isaia, G.C.; Di Stefano, M.; Astegiano, M. Bone mineral density at diagnosis of celiac disease and after 1 year of gluten-free diet. *Sci. World J.* **2014**, *2014*, 173082. [CrossRef] [PubMed]

121. Caruso, R.; Pallone, F.; Stasi, E.; Romeo, S.; Monteleone, G. Appropriate nutrient supplementation in celiac disease. *Ann. Med.* **2013**, *45*, 522–531. [CrossRef] [PubMed]

122. Vici, G.; Belli, L.; Biondi, M.; Polzonetti, V. Gluten free diet and nutrient deficiencies: A review. *Clin. Nutr.* **2016**, in press. [CrossRef] [PubMed]

123. Lamacchia, C.; Camarca, A.; Picascia, S.; Di Luccia, A.; Gianfrani, C. Cereal-based gluten-free food: How to reconcile nutritional and technological properties of wheat proteins with safety for celiac disease patients. *Nutrients* **2014**, *6*, 575–590. [CrossRef] [PubMed]

124. Szajewska, H.; Shamir, R.; Mearin, L.; Ribes-Koninckx, C.; Catassi, C.; Domellof, M.; Fewtrell, M.S.; Husby, S.; Papadopoulou, A.; Vandenplas, Y.; et al. Gluten introduction and the risk of coeliac disease: A position paper by the european society for pediatric gastroenterology, hepatology, and nutrition. *J. Pediatr. Gastroenterol. Nutr.* **2016**, *62*, 507–513. [CrossRef] [PubMed]

125. Fasano, A. Novel therapeutic/integrative approaches for celiac disease and dermatitis herpetiformis. *Clin. Dev. Immunol.* **2012**, *2012*, 959061. [CrossRef] [PubMed]

126. Zamyatnin, A.A., Jr. Plant proteases involved in regulated cell death. *Biochemistry* **2015**, *80*, 1701–1715. [CrossRef] [PubMed]

127. Yike, I. Fungal proteases and their pathophysiological effects. *Mycopathologia* **2011**, *171*, 299–323. [CrossRef] [PubMed]

128. Kantyka, T.; Shaw, L.N.; Potempa, J. Papain-like proteases of Staphylococcus aureus. *Adv. Exp. Med. Biol.* **2011**, *712*, 1–14. [PubMed]

129. Bethune, M.T.; Khosla, C. Oral enzyme therapy for celiac sprue. *Methods Enzymol.* **2012**, *502*, 241–271. [PubMed]

130. Wieser, H.; Koehler, P. Detoxification of gluten by means of enzymatic treatment. *J. AOAC Int.* **2012**, *95*, 356–363. [CrossRef] [PubMed]

131. Savvateeva, L.V.; Zamyatnin, A.A. Prospects of Developing Medicinal Therapeutic strategies and pharmaceutical design for effective gluten intolerance treatment. *Curr. Pharm. Des.* **2016**, *22*, 2439–2449. [CrossRef] [PubMed]

132. Savvateeva, L.V.; Gorokhovets, N.V.; Makarov, V.A.; Serebryakova, M.V.; Solovyev, A.G.; Morozov, S.Y.; Reddy, V.P.; Zernii, E.Y.; Zamyatnin, A.A., Jr.; Aliev, G. Glutenase and collagenase activities of wheat cysteine protease Triticain-alpha: Feasibility for enzymatic therapy assays. *Int. J. Biochem. Cell Biol.* **2015**, *62*, 115–124. [CrossRef] [PubMed]

133. Bethune, M.T.; Strop, P.; Tang, Y.; Sollid, L.M.; Khosla, C. Heterologous expression, purification, refolding, and structural-functional characterization of EP-B2, a self-activating barley cysteine endoprotease. *Chem. Biol.* **2006**, *13*, 637–647. [CrossRef] [PubMed]

134. Shan, L.; Marti, T.; Sollid, L.M.; Gray, G.M.; Khosla, C. Comparative biochemical analysis of three bacterial prolyl endopeptidases: Implications for coeliac sprue. *Biochem. J.* **2004**, *383*, 311–318. [CrossRef] [PubMed]

135. Goptar, I.A.; Semashko, T.A.; Danilenko, S.A.; Lysogorskaya, E.N.; Oksenoit, E.S.; Zhuzhikov, D.P.; Belozersky, M.A.; Dunaevsky, Y.E.; Oppert, B.; Filippova, I.Y.; et al. Cysteine digestive peptidases function as post-glutamine cleaving enzymes in tenebrionid stored-product pests. *Comp. Biochem. Physiol. B Biochem. Mol. Biol.* **2012**, *161*, 148–154. [CrossRef] [PubMed]

136. Lahdeaho, M.L.; Kaukinen, K.; Laurila, K.; Vuotikka, P.; Koivurova, O.P.; Karja-Lahdensuu, T.; Marcantonio, A.; Adelman, D.C.; Maki, M. Glutenase ALV003 attenuates gluten-induced mucosal injury in patients with celiac disease. *Gastroenterology* **2014**, *146*, 1649–1658. [CrossRef] [PubMed]

137. Tye-Din, J.A.; Anderson, R.P.; Ffrench, R.A.; Brown, G.J.; Hodsman, P.; Siegel, M.; Botwick, W.; Shreeniwas, R. The effects of ALV003 pre-digestion of gluten on immune response and symptoms in celiac disease in vivo. *Clin. Immunol.* **2010**, *134*, 289–295. [CrossRef] [PubMed]

138. Di Cagno, R.; De Angelis, M.; Auricchio, S.; Greco, L.; Clarke, C.; De Vincenzi, M.; Giovannini, C.; D'Archivio, M.; Landolfo, F.; Parrilli, G.; et al. Sourdough bread made from wheat and nontoxic flours and started with selected lactobacilli is tolerated in celiac sprue patients. *Appl. Environ. Microbiol.* **2004**, *70*, 1088–1096. [CrossRef] [PubMed]

139. Altenbach, S.B.; Allen, P.V. Transformation of the US bread wheat 'Butte 86' and silencing of omega-5 gliadin genes. *GM Crops* **2011**, *2*, 66–73. [CrossRef] [PubMed]

140. Gil-Humanes, J.; Piston, F.; Tollefsen, S.; Sollid, L.M.; Barro, F. Effective shutdown in the expression of celiac disease-related wheat gliadin T-cell epitopes by RNA interference. *Proc. Natl. Acad. Sci. USA* **2010**, *107*, 17023–17028. [CrossRef] [PubMed]

141. Tanner, G.J.; Howitt, C.A.; Forrester, R.I.; Campbell, P.M.; Tye-Din, J.A.; Anderson, R.P. Dissecting the T-cell response to hordeins in coeliac disease can develop barley with reduced immunotoxicity. *Aliment. Pharmacol. Ther.* **2010**, *32*, 1184–1191. [CrossRef] [PubMed]

142. Hileman, R.E.; Silvanovich, A.; Goodman, R.E.; Rice, E.A.; Holleschak, G.; Astwood, J.D.; Hefle, S.L. Bioinformatic methods for allergenicity assessment using a comprehensive allergen database. *Int. Arch. Allergy Immunol.* **2002**, *128*, 280–291. [CrossRef] [PubMed]

143. Molberg, O.; McAdam, S.; Lundin, K.E.; Kristiansen, C.; Arentz-Hansen, H.; Kett, K.; Sollid, L.M. T cells from celiac disease lesions recognize gliadin epitopes deamidated in situ by endogenous tissue transglutaminase. *Eur. J. Immunol.* **2001**, *31*, 1317–1323. [CrossRef]

144. Keillor, J.W.; Apperley, K.Y.; Akbar, A. Inhibitors of tissue transglutaminase. *Trends Pharmacol. Sci.* **2015**, *36*, 32–40. [CrossRef] [PubMed]

145. Paterson, B.M.; Lammers, K.M.; Arrieta, M.C.; Fasano, A.; Meddings, J.B. The safety, tolerance, pharmacokinetic and pharmacodynamic effects of single doses of AT-1001 in coeliac disease subjects: A proof of concept study. *Aliment. Pharmacol. Ther.* **2007**, *26*, 757–766. [CrossRef] [PubMed]

146. Larche, M.; Wraith, D.C. Peptide-based therapeutic vaccines for allergic and autoimmune diseases. *Nat. Med.* **2005**, *11*, S69–S76. [CrossRef] [PubMed]

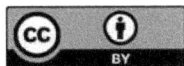

MDPI

Review

Effect of *Bifidobacterium breve* on the Intestinal Microbiota of Coeliac Children on a Gluten Free Diet: A Pilot Study

Andrea Quagliariello [1,†], Irene Aloisio [2,†], Nicole Bozzi Cionci [2], Donata Luiselli [1], Giuseppe D'Auria [3], Llúcia Martinez-Priego [3], David Pérez-Villarroya [3], Tomaž Langerholc [4], Maša Primec [4], Dušanka Mičetić-Turk [5] and Diana Di Gioia [2,*]

[1] Laboratory of Molecular Anthropology, Centre for Genome Biology Department of Biological, Geological and Environmental Sciences (BiGeA), University of Bologna, via Selmi 3, Bologna 40126, Italy; andrea.quagliariello@unibo.it (A.Q.); donata.luiselli@unibo.it (D.L.)
[2] Department of Agricultural Sciences, University of Bologna, viale Fanin 42, Bologna 40127, Italy; irene.aloisio@unibo.it (I.A.); nicole.bozzicionci@studio.unibo.it (N.B.C.)
[3] Sequencing and Bioinformatics Service, Fundación para el Fomento de la Investigación Sanitaria y Biomédica de la Comunidad Valenciana (FISABIO-Salud Pública), Valencia 46020, Spain; dauria_giu@gva.es (G.D.); martinez_lucpri@gva.es (L.M.-P.); enhancertrap@gmail.com (D.P.-V.)
[4] Department of Microbiology, Biochemistry, Molecular Biology and Biotechnology, Faculty of Agriculture and Life Sciences, University of Maribor, Pivola 10, Hoče 2311, Slovenia; tomaz.langerholc@um.si (T.L.); masa.primec@um.si (M.P.)
[5] Department of Pediatrics, Faculty of Medicine, University of Maribor, Taborska ulica 8, Maribor 2000, Slovenia; dusanka.micetic@um.si
* Correspondence: diana.digioia@unibo.it; Tel.: +39-051-2096269
† These authors contributed equally to this work.

Received: 10 August 2016; Accepted: 13 October 2016; Published: 22 October 2016

Abstract: Coeliac disease (CD) is associated with alterations of the intestinal microbiota. Although several *Bifidobacterium* strains showed anti-inflammatory activity and prevention of toxic gliadin peptides generation in vitro, few data are available on their efficacy when administered to CD subjects. This study evaluated the effect of administration for three months of a food supplement based on two *Bifidobacterium breve* strains (B632 and BR03) to restore the gut microbial balance in coeliac children on a gluten free diet (GFD). Microbial DNA was extracted from faeces of 40 coeliac children before and after probiotic or placebo administration and 16 healthy children (Control group). Sequencing of the amplified V3-V4 hypervariable region of 16S rRNA gene as well as qPCR of *Bidobacterium* spp., *Lactobacillus* spp., *Bacteroides fragilis* group *Clostridium sensu stricto* and enterobacteria were performed. The comparison between CD subjects and Control group revealed an alteration in the intestinal microbial composition of coeliacs mainly characterized by a reduction of the *Firmicutes/Bacteroidetes* ratio, of *Actinobacteria* and *Euryarchaeota*. Regarding the effects of the probiotic, an increase of *Actinobacteria* was found as well as a re-establishment of the physiological *Firmicutes/Bacteroidetes* ratio. Therefore, a three-month administration of *B. breve* strains helps in restoring the healthy percentage of main microbial components.

Keywords: coeliac disease; gluten free diet; probiotic; *Bifidobacterium breve*; intestinal microbiota; qPCR; next generation sequencing

1. Introduction

Coeliac disease (CD) is a chronic gastrointestinal tract disorder showing damages at the small intestine, which are hypothetically linked to an autoimmune response caused by gluten ingestion in genetically predisposed subjects. CD in Europe and North America is estimated to affect about 1% of the population, although its incidence in Western countries is increasing in the last decades [1,2]. CD is usually chronic but the lifelong adherence to a gluten-free diet (GFD) keeps the disease under control: the small intestine returns to its physiological condition and subsequent tests for CD specific autoantibodies are negative [3,4]. Even if the adherence to a GFD is the only effective solution against CD, patients risk suffering from an unbalanced nutritional intake and difficulties to adhere to the strict GFD are frequently reported.

The gut microbiota has a very close relation with the host contributing to the normal human physiology. It can provide a barrier for colonization of pathogens, synthesize vitamins and other beneficial compounds and stimulate the immune system. Environmental factors can lead to a disturbance of the microbiota composition, disrupting microbiota-host mutualism and shifting from a condition of homeostasis to a disease-associated profile [5]. In the last decade, CD has been associated to an altered composition of the intestinal microbiota even though studies reported in literature show that there is not a characteristic "coeliac intestinal microbiota" [6]. Some authors evidenced an intestinal dysbiosis in CD patients with active disease characterized by a remarkable reduction in Gram positive bacterial population in duodenal and faecal specimens facilitating the colonization of potentially harmful Gram negative bacteria within the mucosal surface of CD patients [7–9]. In particular, data obtained from duodenal biopsies revealed a reduction in the number of bifidobacteria [10] and changes in species distribution within the *Bifidobacterium* genus have been evidenced by Denaturing Gradient Gel Electrophoresis (DGGE) [11]. Moreover, symptom free CD patients adherent to a GFD at least for two years did not completely restore the microbiota composition and this condition can lead to a different metabolomics profile [9]. Bacteria belonging to the *Bifidobacterium* genus are well known for their health promoting properties and for their capability of stimulating cells to produce immune molecules and modulating the physiology of gut-associated lymphoid tissue (GALT) [12]. In particular, in vitro studies have been focused on the capability of bifidobacteria to increase the IL-10 secretion when co-incubated with mononuclear cells and faecal samples from CD patients [13]. Moreover, a *Bifidobacterium lactis* strain and a probiotic product containing *Lactobacillus* and *Bifidobacterium* strains resulted effective in reducing gliadin induced epithelial permeability through prevention of the toxic gliadin peptide generation during in vitro digestion [14–16].

Despite the encouraging data on the potential of probiotic strains, particularly bifidobacteria, in vivo studies in patients with CD remain still very scarce. Until now, only few studies have taken into account the direct administration of bifidobacteria in subjects affected by CD. Smecuol et al. [17] studied the effects of *Bifidobacterium infantis natren life start* strain in untreated CD patients or rather on a gluten containing diet. Authors found that *Bifidobacterium* administration may alleviate symptoms of untreated CD but it could not modify intestinal permeability. A second study [18] evaluated the administration of *Bifidobacterium longum* CECT 7347 in children on a GFD with newly diagnosed CD and it revealed a reduction of CD3+ T lymphocytes and TNF-α due to probiotic ingestion. To date, no studies on CD considered the administration of *Bifidobacterium breve* strains although this species has proven very successful in several paediatric trials regarding necrotizing enterocolitis, immunodeficiency and constipation [19–21].

This work is aimed at the assessment of the impact of the administration of two *Bifidobacterium breve* strains on the gut microbiota composition of coeliac patients compliant to a GFD and, at the same time, it evaluates the difference in the intestinal colonization of coeliac subjects on a GFD for several years with respect to healthy subjects.

2. Materials and Methods

2.1. Study Design and Samples Collection

The study was a double-blinded placebo controlled intervention including 40 patients affected by CD and 16 healthy children for the Control group recruited at a single centre, Department of

Paediatrics, University Clinical Center Maribor in a period from October 2013 to June 2014. Children with CD, aged between 1 and 19 years, were positive to serologic markers for CD and positive for small bowel biopsy, according to European Society for Paedriatric Gastroenterology Hepatology and Nutrition (ESPGHAN) criteria for CD [22]. More details about patients (Table S1) and inclusion/exclusion criteria of the recruiting process are available in Klemenak et al. [23]. The study was registered at https://www.clinicaltrials.gov (registration number: NCT02244047). Patients affected by CD have been randomly allocated into two groups: 20 in the Probiotic group and 20 in the Placebo group. The Probiotic group of patients received an experimental formulation containing *B. breve* for three months and the Placebo group received a placebo formulation for the same duration. Probiotic formulation was a mixture of 2 strains, *B. breve* BR03 (DSM 16604) and *B. breve* B632 (DSM 24706) (1:1), administered as lyophilized powder in a daily dosage of 10^9 Colony Forming Units (CFU) of each strain. Placebo was prepared with the same excipients without probiotic strains using an identical form of package. Each package of 2 g powder was mixed with fluids and ingested in the morning breakfast for three months.

Faecal samples of CD patients were collected twice, on enrolment (T0) and at the end of intervention with probiotic/placebo (T1). Members of Control group were sampled only once. Faecal samples were frozen immediately after collection at −80 °C, in numbered screw-capped plastic containers, until they were processed for DNA extraction. Researchers carrying out DNA extraction and molecular analyses (qPCR and sequencing) were blind to the group identity of patients (Control, Probiotic or Placebo group).

2.2. DNA Extraction from Faecal Samples

DNA was extracted from 200 mg of faeces (preserved at −80 °C after collection) were used using the QIAamp DNA Stool Mini Kit (Qiagen, West Sussex, UK) with a slight modification of the protocol: An additional incubation at 95 °C for 10 min of the stool sample with the lysis buffer was added to improve the bacterial cell rupture [24]. Extracted DNA was stored at −80 °C. The purity of extracted DNA was determined by measuring the ratio of the absorbance at 260 and 280 nm (Infinite®200 PRO NanoQuant, Tecan, Mannedorf, Switzerland) and the concentration was estimated by Qubit® 3.0 Fluorometer (Invitrogen, Life Technologies, Van Allen Way, Carlsbad, CA, USA).

2.3. Preparation of DNA Libraries for Illumina MiSeq Sequencing

The sample subjected to sequencing belonged to the following groups: 20 Probiotic group T0, 20 Probiotic group T1, 20 Placebo group T0, 20 Placebo group T1 and 16 Control group (Figure 1).

They were processed to amplify and sequence the V3-V4 region of the 16S rRNA gene. The amplicons, approximately 460 bp in length, were generated using the forward and reverse primers, respectively: 5′ TCGTCGGCAGCGTCAGATGTGTATAAGAGACAGCCTACGGGNGGCWGCAG 3′, 5′ CTCTCGTGGGCTCGGAGATGTGTATAAGAGACAGGACTACHVGGGTATCTAATCC 3′, already used in [25].

Each 25 μL PCR reaction contained 12.5 μL of HiFi HotStart ReadyMix (KAPA Biosystems, Woburn, MA, USA), 5 μL of each primer (0.2 μM) and microbial DNA (5 ng/μL). PCR amplification was performed using the following program: Heated lid at 110 °C, 95 °C for 3 min followed by 25 cycles at 95 °C for 30 s, 55 °C for 30 s, and 72 °C for 30 s, followed by a final elongation step at 72 °C for 5 min. PCR products were cleaned using the AMPure beads XP purification system (Beckman Coulter, UK) following Illumina 16S Ribosomal RNA Gene Amplicon instructions. Illumina sequencing adapters and dual-index barcodes were added to amplicons using the Nextera XT index kit (Illumina, San Diego, CA, USA). The following program was utilized for the second PCR amplification: 95 °C for 3 min followed by 8 cycles of 95 °C for 30 s, 55 °C for 30 s and 72 °C for 30 s and a final elongation at 72 °C for 5 min. A further clean up protocol using AMPure beads XP purification system (Beckman Coulter, UK) is performed. Amplicons were quantified using the Qubit® 2.0 Fluorometer (Invitrogen) and pooled equimolar to 4 nM. The pool was denatured with 0.2 M NaOH, further dilution with hybridization buffer to 20 pM and combined with denatured 30% PhiX. Samples were sequenced on the Illumina MiSeq platform at the Fundacion FISABIO (Valencia, Spain) facility using a 2 × 300 nucleotide paired reads protocol. Sequencing raw data were deposited at European Nucleotide Archive (ENA) and received the following ID: PRJEB14943.

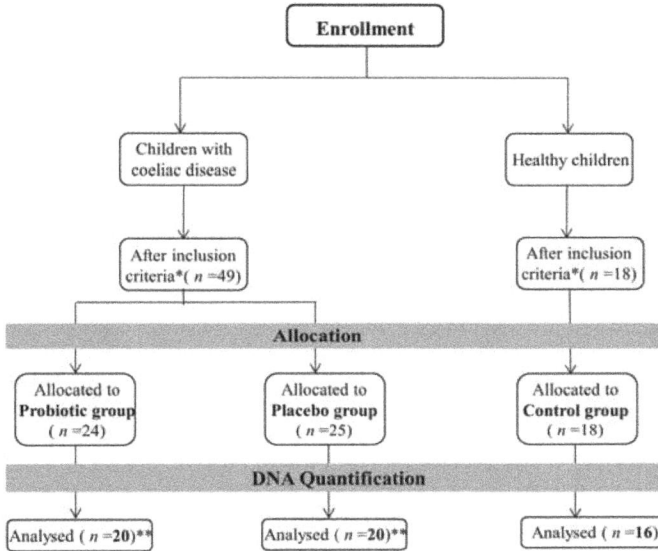

Figure 1. Summary of inclusion/exclusion criteria adopted for samples selection. Samples who showed the right DNA quantification level have been sequenced. * Inclusion criteria are summarized in Klemenak et al. [23]. ** Analysis was performed at the beginning of the study (T0) and after 3 months of treatment (T1).

2.4. Bioinformatics and Statistical Analyses of NGS Experiment

Several bioinformatics pipelines have been used to analyse the amount of data produced during this project. The first step of analysis was represented by quality controls of the generated raw data, which are essential to be confident of the quality of the experimental results. For this purpose, the FastQC 0.11.4 software (Babraham Bioinformatics) was used for a rapid visualization of sequences quality, then with the prinseq-lite.pl script sequences have been trimmed according to various quality criteria: first of all sequences with less than 50 bp were eliminated, then remaining reads were analyzed with a sliding-window approach of 20 bp, within this range each sequence with a mean quality lower than 20 was removed [26].

After that, the fastq-join tool from the ea-tools suite [27] was used to join forward and reverse sequences. The last quality control step was represented by the elimination of chimeric sequences using the Usearch tool (http://drive5.com/usearch/). Once high-quality double-stranded reads were obtained, they were aligned to the 16S reference sequences database at the RDP database project to identify the microbial community with the RDP classifier tool [28]. RDP classifier outputs have been then processed through several R software packages, such as *vegan*, *reshape2*, *RDPutils* and *phyloseq* in order to estimate various biodiversity indexes and to perform the principle statistics analyses on taxonomic profiles. Finally, data have been normalized and the function exactTest() of the *edgeR* package was used to evaluate the effective microbial differentiation among the studied groups [29].

2.5. Absolute Quantification of Selected Microbial Groups Using Quantitative PCR (qPCR)

Quantification of selected microbial groups i.e., *Bidobacterium* spp., *Lactobacillus* spp., *Bacteroides fragilis* group (comprising the species *B. fragilis*, *B. distasonis*, *B. ovatus*, *B. thetaiotaomicron*,

B. vulgatus), *Clostridium sensu stricto* or cluster I and total enterobacteria, was carried out with real-time PCR on DNA extracted from faecal samples. The assays were performed with a 20 μL PCR amplification mixture containing 10 μL of Fast SYBR® Green Master Mix (Applied Biosystems, Foster City, CA, USA), optimized concentrations of primers (Tables 1 and 2), H_2O molecular grade and 2 μL DNA extracted from faecal samples at a concentration of 2.5 ng/μL for all the assays. The primer concentrations were optimized through primer optimization matrices in a 48-well plate and evaluating the best Ct/Rn ratio. The different primers were also checked for their specificity using the database similarity search program nucleotide-nucleotide BLAST [30]. Moreover, to determine the specificity of amplification, analysis of product melting curve was performed after the last cycle of each amplification. The data obtained from the amplification were then transformed to obtain the number of bacterial Log CFU/g faeces according to the rRNA copy number available at the rRNA copy number database [31]. Standard curves were constructed using 16S rRNA PCR product of type strains of each target microorganism. PCR products were purified with a commercial kit DNA purification system (NucleoSpin® Extract II kit, MACHEREY-NAGEL GmbH & Co. KG, Duren, Germany) and the concentration measured at 260 nm. Serial dilutions were performed and 10^2, 10^3, 10^4, 10^5, 10^6, and 10^7 copies of the gene per reaction and were used for calibration.

Data of microbial counts were subjected to *T*-test in order to evidence significant differences between treated and Control group of subjects.

Table 1. Primer sequences and qPCR conditions used in the different assays.

Target Microorganisms	Primer Sequences (5'-3')	Amplicon Length (bp)	References	Annealing Temperature
Bifidobacterium spp. BifTOT-F BifTOT-R	TCGCGTCYGGTGTGAAAG CCACATCCAGCRTCCAC	243	[32]	55 °C
Lactobacillus spp. Lac-F Lac-R	GCAGCAGTAGGGAATCTTCCA GCATTYCACCGCTACACATG	349	[33]	60 °C
Bacteroides fragilis group Bfra-F Bfra-R	CGGAGGATCCGAGCGTTA CCGCAAACTTTCACAACTGACTTA	92	[34]	58 °C
Enterobacteria Eco 1457F Eco 1652R	CATTGACGTTACCCGCAGAAGAAGC CTCTACGAGACTCAAGCTGC	195	[35]	63 °C
Clostridium cluster I CI-F1 CI-F2	TACCHRAGGAGGAAGCCAC GTTCTTCCTAATCTCTACGCAT	232	[36]	52 °C

Table 2. qPCR amplification protocols and primer concentrations.

Target Microorganisms	Initial Denaturation	Denaturation	Annealing	Cycles	Fw nM	Rev nM
Bifidobacterium spp. BifTOT F/BifTOT-R	95 °C, 20 s	95 °C–30 s	60 °C–30 s	40	200	300
Lactobacillus spp. LAC-F/LAC-R	95 °C, 20 s	95 °C–30 s	63.5 °C–30 s	40	200	200
Bacteroides fragilis group Bfra-F/Bfra-R	95 °C, 20 s	95 °C–30 s	60 °C–30 s	40	300	300
Enterobacteria Eco-F/Eco-R	95 °C, 20 s	95 °C–30 s	60 °C–30 s	40	400	400
Clostridium cluster I CI-F1/CI-F2	95 °C, 20 s	95 °C–30 s	60 °C–30 s	40	200	200

Fw = Primer Forward, Rev = Primer Reverse.

3. Results

3.1 Metagenomic Analysis

The V3-V4 region of 16S rDNA gene was sequenced from 96 DNA samples using the Illumina MiSeq platform. A total dataset of 4,348,432 filtered high-quality joined reads (excluding the undetermined sequences) was thus generated, about 46,259 sequences per sample, with a mean quality between 30 and 35. Two samples were excluded from the whole dataset because they did not pass the established quality threshold.

Massive sequencing revealed the presence of six phyla (five belonging to Bacteria and one to Archaea) with a relative abundance higher than 1%: *Firmicutes, Bacteroidetes, Proteobacteria, Actinobacteria, Verrucomicrobia* and *Euryarchaeota*. The obtained phyla had a different distribution among the five groups of examined subjects as highlighted in the heat map (Figure 2), in particular in the *Firmicutes* and *Bacteroidetes* phyla.

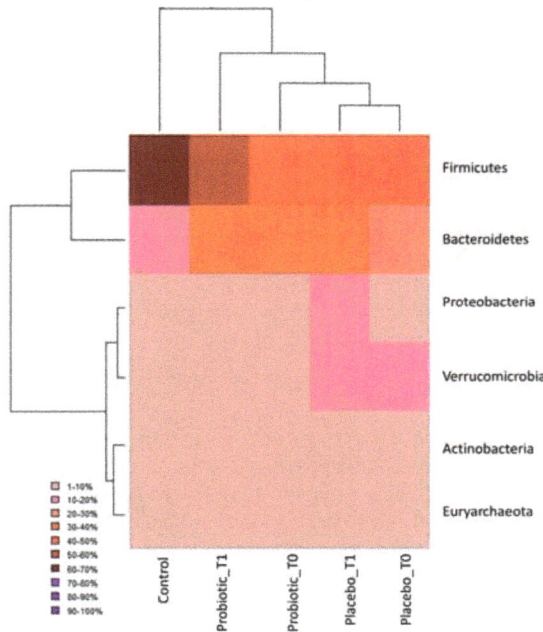

Figure 2. Hierarchically clustered heat map: Sample groups are reported in column, while phyla are reported in row.

In particular, the *Firmicutes* phylum showed the highest representativeness in the Control group (accounting for 60%–70% of the total microbial community), whereas it reached 50%–60% in Probiotic T1 and 40%–50% in the rest of CD patients (Probiotic T0, Placebo T0, and Placebo T1 groups).

On the other hand, the *Bacteroidetes* phylum was more abundant within CD subjects (20%–40%) than in the Control group subjects (10%–20%). The other phyla were more evenly distributed among groups, with the only difference for *Proteobacteria* and *Verrucomicrobia* that were more represented in the Placebo group (~10%–20%). Moreover, the hierarchical cluster analysis combined with the heat map pointed out that the Probiotic T1 group occupied an intermediate position between the Control group and the rest of CD individuals, being thus considered as an outlier with respect to the other disease clusters because of its closer relationship with control subjects.

From the comparison between the CD subjects and the Control group microbiota emerged a marked difference in the ratio of *Firmicutes/Bacteroidetes*. Figure 3 shows values of ratio *Firmicutes/Bacteroidetes* calculated for each group of subjects. CD subjects had a ratio values lower than the Control group thus meaning a high proportion of *Bacteroidetes* (Gram negative) with respect to *Firmicutes* (Gram positive). The administration of the probiotic for three months was found to increase the ratio value due to the higher level of *Firmicutes* phyla than *Bacteroidetes*.

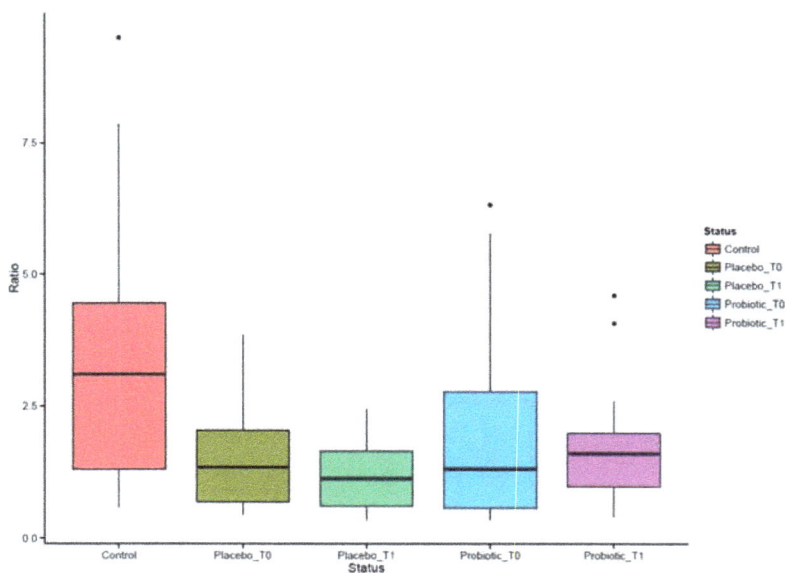

Figure 3. The *Firmicutes/Bacteroidetes* ratio.

Following the data normalization procedure and assignation of statistical significance described in Material and Method, several comparisons between pair of groups were performed in order to identify which phyla could distinguish the microbiota of Control group from that of CD patients not assuming the probiotic formulation, and from Probiotic T1 (Figure 4).

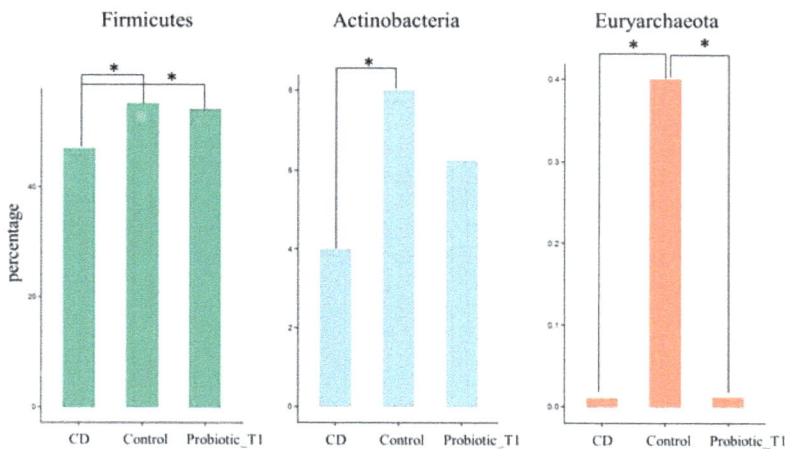

Figure 4. Relative abundance of the three phyla that show a statistical significance difference among CD, Control and Probiotic T1. CD group is composed of Probiotic T0, Placebo T0 and Placebo T1 samples. The * indicates $p < 0.01$. Supporting information on relative abundance and p-values is found in Tables S2 and S3.

Statistical analyses confirmed that *Firmicutes* were significantly lower in CD subjects not receiving the probiotic formulation compared to Controls and Probiotic group ($p < 0.01$). Similar results were found for *Actinobacteria* that were underrepresented in the CD group and increased after the administration of bifidobacteria, although not reaching the abundance found in the controls. A further discernment regarded the *Euryarchaeota* phylum belonging to *Archaea* that was almost exclusively present in the Control group. The same analysis was repeated comparing the microbial composition of the Control group with the Probiotic groups before and after the probiotic administration (respectively Probiotic T0 and Probiotic T1) (Figure 5). The comparison highlighted an increase in the relative abundance of *Firmicutes* ($p < 0.01$) and *Actinobacteria*, due to the effect of probiotic administration. On the other hand it was possible to observe a slight decrease of the abundance of *Proteobacteria* while the *Euryarchaeota* phylum kept unchanged after the treatment.

The same comparison was carried out at the family taxonomic level. Within the *Firmicutes* phylum, two families, which are poorly represented in the Probiotic T0 group, showed instead a higher level in both the Probiotic T1 and the Control groups: *Lactobacillaceae* and *Gracilibacteraceae*. In particular, both bacterial families showed a significant different abundance between Probiotic T0 and Probiotic T1 groups, whereas no differences were observed between Probiotic T1 and Control groups. In contrast, Probiotic T1 subjects demonstrated a high percentage of unclassified *Deltaproteobacteria* families. Moreover, this analysis enabled identifying the *Methanobacteriaceae* family as almost exclusively present within the Control group (Figure 6).

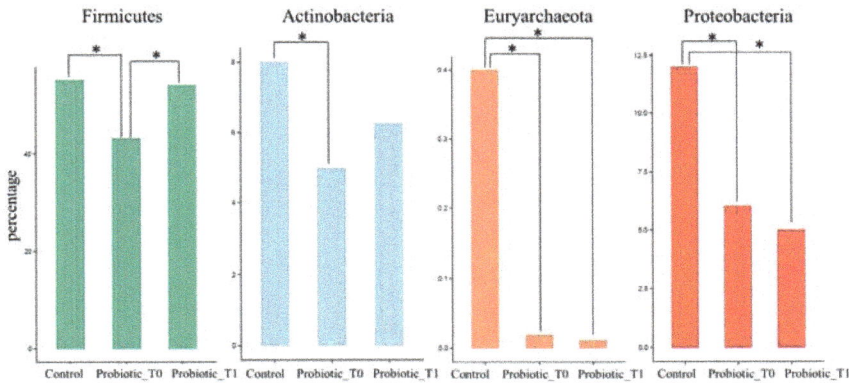

Figure 5. Significant differences in phyla relative abundance among Control, Probiotic T0 and Probiotic T1 groups. The * indicates $p < 0.01$. Supporting information on relative abundance and p-values is found in Tables S4 and S5.

The α-diversity indices (Observed, Chao1 and Shannon) were computed for all Operational Taxonomic Units (OTUs) founded in the five groups of samples as reported in Figure 7. No significant changes in OTUs composition among the studied groups were observed. Particularly, the observed raw biodiversity, as well as the Chao1 index, were slightly higher in the control samples than in all the other groups, but the differences were not significant. Even the Shannon index indicated similar trends among all groups, with a mean value of about 3. This similarity among groups was further confirmed by the application of Wilcoxon test on these indices, which indicated the totally absence of significant differences.

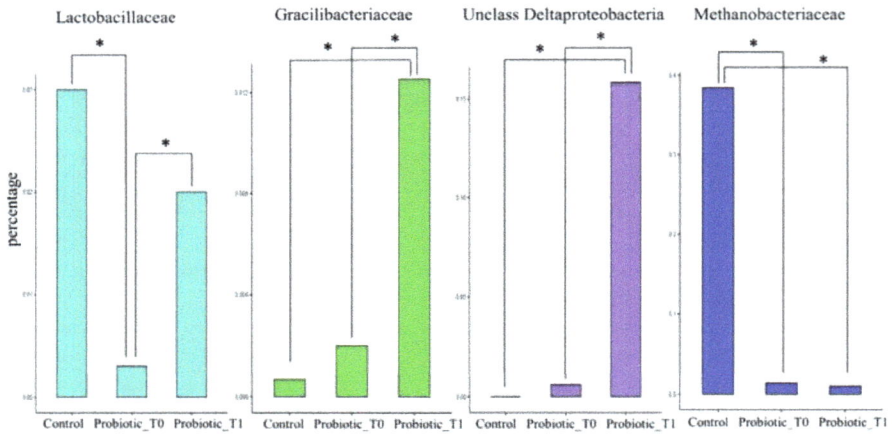

Figure 6. Statistical significant differences in families relative abundance among Control, Probiotic T0 and Probiotic T1 groups. The * indicates $p < 0.01$. Supporting information on relative abundance and p-values is found in Tables S6 and S7.

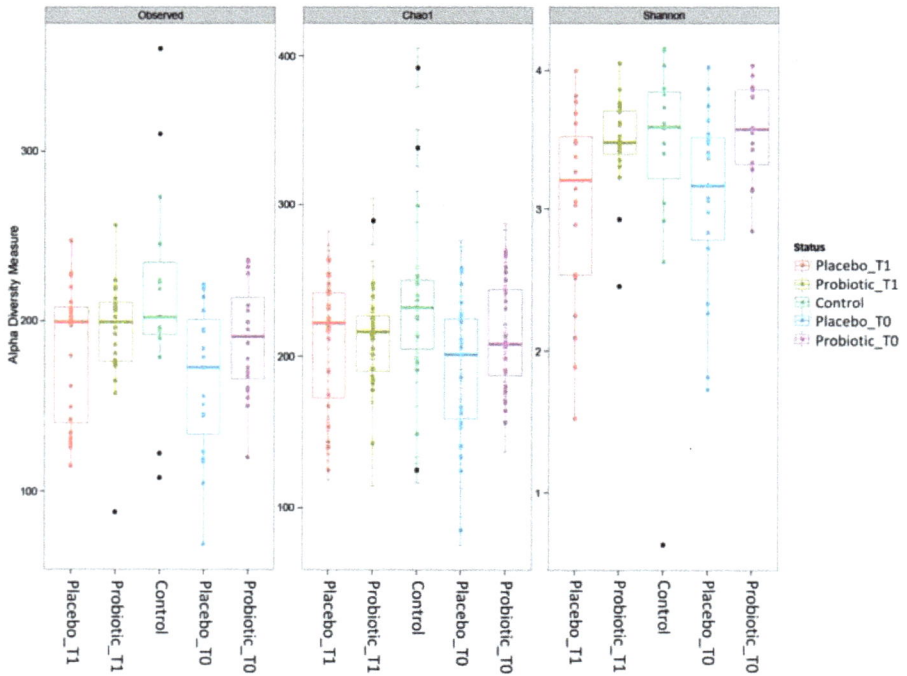

Figure 7. Alpha diversity indices among the studied groups.

3.2. Quantification of Selected Microbial Groups in Faecal Samples

qPCR analysis was carried out in order to obtain the absolute quantification of selected microbial groups as a supplementary information able to complete the microbial profile of the examined subjects. Faecal samples were collected and DNA extracted at two sampling times for CD subjects, on enrolment (Probiotic T0 + Placebo T0) and at the end of the three months intervention with probiotic or placebo (T1), and once for healthy individuals (control group). Quantification regarded specific microbial genera typical of the human gut, *Bifidobacterium* spp., *Clostridium sensu stricto*, *Bacteroides fragilis* group (comprising the most abundant species in human, i.e., *B. fragilis*, *B. distasonis*, *B. ovatus*, *B. thetaiotaomicron*, and *B. vulgatus*), and larger microbial group, *Lactobacillus* group, which include *Lactobacillus*, *Pediococcus*, *Leuconostoc* and *Weisella* species, and total enterobacteria comprehensives of a larger number of gram-negative intestinal bacteria. The average microbial counts obtained are shown in Table 3.

Quantification of *Bifidobacterium* spp. evidenced a slightly higher value in the subjects affected by CD at T0 with respect to the control group, although this difference was not significant. The comparison between subjects belonging to the probiotic group before and after the treatment showed that the administration of the probiotic formula containing *Bifidobacterium breve* led to a slight increase of bifidobacteria counts from 7.64 ± 1.01 to 8.06 ± 0.98 Log CFU/g of faeces. *Lactobacillus* spp. group analysis revealed that healthy subjects (Control group) had a higher presence of members of this group compared to CD patients, which on the contrary, showed a great heterogeneity in the distribution (Figure 8). ANOVA test revealed that the difference was statistically significant (emphp < 0.01). The opposite trend was found for members of *Bacteroides fragilis* group showing a higher median in CD subjects compared to healthy subjects, as shown in the box plot (Figure 9). The box plot relative to healthy subjects is shorter than the other one and it also shows a higher median value but a narrower distribution of the data. ANOVA test revealed that the difference is statistically significant ($p < 0.01$). CD patients showed more than 8.70 Log CFU/g of faeces of *Bacteroides fragilis* group bacteria. No significant differences were recorded concerning changes in the levels of *Bacteroides* due to treatment with probiotics.

With regard to enterobacteria, they were more abundant in the control group compared to CD patients: 8.29 ± 0.80 and 7.10 ± 1.24 CFU/g, respectively. This trend can also be outlined from the graphs reported in Figure 10, which clearly shows that the median value of control group is higher than CD groups, the latter showing a lower level of enterobacteria with a higher heterogeneity. Furthermore, after the three months of probiotic treatment it was possible to observe a decreased level of enterobacteria in Probiotic T1 (Figure 10 and Table 3). Regarding *Clostridium sensu stricto*, its quantification was lower than the other microbial groups (values from 5.83 to 6.19 Log CFU/g of faeces). No statistical differences resulted from the comparison between control and CD patients and between Probiotic and Placebo groups.

Table 3. Mean counts of different microbial groups analysed in stool samples expressed as Log CFU/g of faeces.

Target	Log No. CFU/g of Faeces				
	Probiotic Group		Placebo Group		Control Group
	T0	T1	T0	T1	T0
Bifidobacterium spp.	7.64 ± 1.01	8.06 ± 0.98	7.82 ± 0.80	7.74 ± 0.73	7.26 ± 0.92
Lactobacillus spp.	6.87 ± 1.08	6.92 ± 0.95	7.21 ± 0.80	7.04 ± 0.97	7.84 ± 0.58
B. fragilis group	8.73 ± 0.79	8.71 ± 0.77	8.74 ± 0.76	8.84 ± 1.03	7.46 ± 1.47
Enterobacteria	7.10 ± 1.24	6.75 ± 1.29	7.25 ± 1.81	7.63 ± 1.48	8.29 ± 0.80
Clostridium sensu stricto	5.97 ± 0.96	5.83 ± 0.87	6.17 ± 0.95	6.19 ± 0.81	5.86 ± 0.80

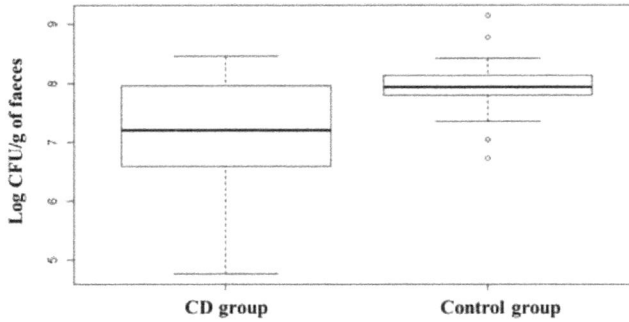

Figure 8. Box plots showing qPCR analysis of *Lactobacillus* group expressed in log CFU per gram of faecal sample relative to CD group and Control group. CD group is composed of Probiotic T0, Placebo T0 and Placebo T1 samples. Statistical difference between the two groups (p-values of < 0.01).

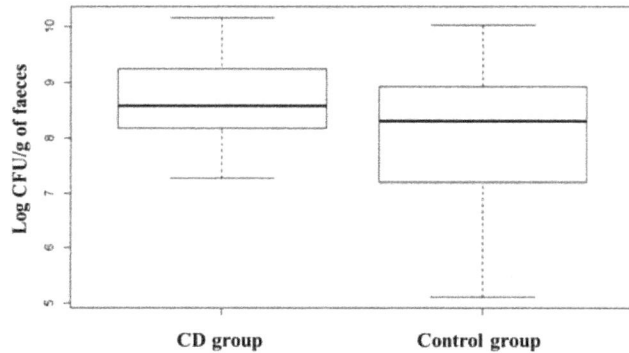

Figure 9. Box plots showing qPCR analysis of *Bacteroides fragilis* group expressed in log CFU per gram of faecal sample relative to CD group and Control group. CD group is composed of Probiotic T0, Placebo T0 and Placebo T1 samples. Statistical difference between the two groups (p-values of < 0.01).

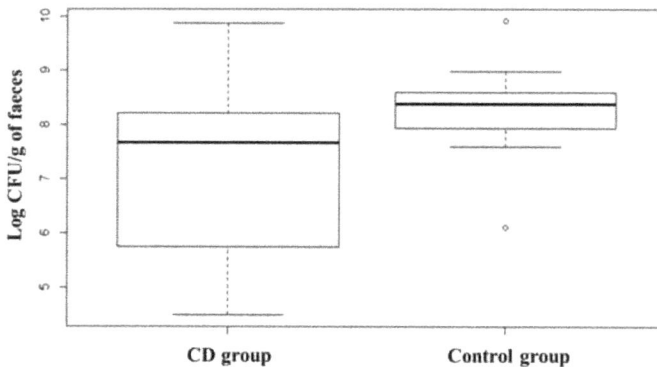

Figure 10. Box plots showing qPCR analysis of total enterobacteria expressed in log CFU per gram of faecal sample relative to CD group and Control group. CD group is composed of Probiotic T0, Placebo T0 and Placebo T1 samples. Statistical difference between the two groups (p-values of < 0.01).

4. Discussion

This work was focused on the characterization of the major changes occurring in the intestinal microbiota of CD patients on a GFD and on the evaluation of the effects that the administration of two *B. breve* strains (B632 and BR03) may have on these patients.

In the last few years a particular attention has been paid on the correlation between gut microbiota composition and CD. Several studies demonstrated an increase in gram-negative bacteria, mainly belonging to the *Bacteroidetes* phylum, at the expense of microorganisms of the *Actinobatceria* and *Firmicutes* phyla in subjects with active disease [7,8,10], in agreement with the results registered in other chronic inflammatory gastrointestinal diseases such as inflammatory bowel disease [37]. However, these differences did not allow identifying a coeliac microbiota signature directly linked to CD [6].

Although data regarding the health promoting properties of bifidobacteria and more in general of probiotic microorganisms are well documented, their role in the treatment of CD has been scarcely investigated. The two strains administered in this work, *B. breve* B632 and BR03, are known to possess anti-inflammatory activity stimulating intestinal cells in vitro to produce IL-6 and IL-10, respectively [38,39] and have been previously characterized for safety issues such as the absence of transmissible antibiotic resistance traits and toxicity towards gut epithelial cells. In addition, the two strains in combination showed a great capability of colonizing the gut of healthy children [40]. In relation to CD, a preliminary important outcome obtained from the administration of the described probiotic formulation to CD patients was the reduction of pro-inflammatory cytokine TNF-α in blood samples of CD subjects on a GFD after three months of treatment, as reported in Klemenak et al. [23].

The first interesting evidence that emerges from the present study is the absence of a severe intestinal dysbiosis in CD patients on a GFD diet, as shown by the comparison of the α-diversity similarity indices and the absence of statistically significant differences in OTU variability in the analysed cohort of CD patients with respect to the Control group. On the contrary, literature data related to active disease patients non-adherent to a GFD showed the presence of extensive changes in the microbial composition [8]. Therefore, the strict adherence to the GFD partially recovers the intestinal equilibrium status.

However, the results obtained in this study showed a significant quantitative difference in some microbial groups by qPCR and by metagenomic analysis in CD patients with respect to the Control group. The elaboration of the microbial relative abundance data obtained by Illumina MiSeq sequencing were able to clearly separate CD subjects from the Control group ones. The lower number of *Bacteroidetes* phylum in CD patients with respect to the Control group was supported by *B. fragilis* group quantification by qPCR and it is consistent with the results of another study on CD patients on GFD [7]. The obtained results are also in agreement with the observation that CD subjects present an imbalance in the *Firmicutes/Bacteroidetes* ratio, usually lower in CD patients, and this ratio is not completely restored in patients under a GFD [41]. Moreover, the probiotic administration induced an evident increase of *Firmicutes* abundance while maintaining a similar percentage of *Bacteroidetes*, thus resulting in a higher value of the *Firmicutes/Bacteroidetes* ratio. In addition, the Control group microbiota seems to be characterized by a higher percentage of *Actinobacteria* and *Euryarchaeota*. The association between CD disease status and a lower presence of *Actinobacteria* has already been described [42]. Particularly interesting, although not yet described in the literature, is the result regarding the *Euryarchaeota* phylum, which is highly represented in the Control group, but almost absent in the coeliac subjects. The same applies for the *Methanobacteriaceae* family. This evidence could conceivably be linked to differences in the dietary habits of the two groups of subjects. Recent research works focused on *Euryarchaeota* highlighted their ability to promote polysaccharide degradation and absorption of fatty acids, thus they seem to play a role in energy extraction from degradation of organic compounds [43]. Grain is the most common source of polysaccharides in modern human populations, thus the important reduction of archaea microorganisms within coeliac group on GFD is linked to their different nutritional status, in particular to the compliance of the GFD and the consequent lower polysaccharide intake.

Focusing on the effects of the administration of the *B. breve* strains on microbial composition, an increase of members of the *Actinobacteria* phylum (NGS) and bifidobacteria (qPCR) have been detected in the CD subjects after three months of probiotic supplementation, although the increase was not statistically significant. One of the possible reasons could be the short duration of the treatment, furthermore it is already known that, after the weaning period, the microbiota is resilient to changes [44]. The treatment with the *B. breve* strains has therefore not caused major changes at the level of the genus or phylum to which the probiotic belongs, as it might have been expected, but the intake of the probiotic has nevertheless acted as a "trigger" element for the increase of *Firmicutes* and the restoration of the physiological *Firmicutes/Bacteroidetes* ratio. By reaching the microbial family level of analysis, it was possible to get more details on the effect of probiotic administration, allowing to reach the conclusion that two *Firmicutes* families (*Lactobacillaceae* and *Gracilibacteraceae*) changed their relative abundances upon probiotic treatment (Probiotic T1 group), particularly *Lactobacillaceae* that reached almost the values that characterized the Control group. Other studies have also observed a lower presence of *Lactobacillaceae* in CD patients, indicating a close relationship between this pathological condition and the bacterial family [9]. This means that the probiotic has restored the normal amount of *Lactobacillaceae* members belonging to these families within the treated individuals. It remains to be explained why the administration of such a *Bifidobacterium* strain have affected *Lactobacillaceae* species. This could be related to a high ability of *Bifidobacterium* to deep influence gut microflora composition, by enhancing the blooming of some species and antagonizing others probably by the effect of the production of metabolites such as acetic acid [45]. In particular, there are evidences that *Bifidobacterium* support *Lactobacillaceae* development [46]. Moreover, it is highly probable that the decrease of TNF-α observed within treated individuals is closely linked to the increase of lactobacilli, with their anti-inflammatory function promoted by the administration of *Bifidobacterium* [47,48].

5. Conclusions

In conclusion, the present study demonstrated that three months administration of *B. breve* strains could make the intestinal microbiota of coeliac patients more similar to that of healthy individuals, restoring the abundance of some microbial communities that characterize the typical physiological condition.

Supplementary Materials: The following are available online at http://www.mdpi.com/2072-6643/8/10/660/s1, Table S1: Description of the study groups at the beginning of intervention, Table S2: *p*-values among groups. Table S3: Mean values of relative abundance with standard deviation, Table S4: *p*-values among groups, Table S5: Mean values of relative abundance with standard deviation, Table S6: *p*-values among groups, Table S7: Mean values of relative abundance with standard deviation.

Acknowledgments: We are grateful to Probiotical S.p.A. (Novara, Italy) for providing probiotic formulation free of charge and to parents of children enrolled in the study for the cooperation in the research. This work was done in the framework of the VII FP TRAFOON (Traditional food network to improve the transfer of knowledge for innovation), grant agreement No. 613912, which covered the cost to publish in open access. The study was partially funded by the University of Bologna, Program RFO 2014 (J32I15000830005), code number RFO14DIGIO.

Author Contributions: D.D.G. and T.L. conceived and designed the study; M.P. and D.M.-T. were responsible for patients recruitment; I.A. and N.B.C. performed the qPCR experiments and analyzed the data; G.D. and L.P.-M. contributed with reagents/materials/analysis tools for the NGS experiment; A.Q. performed the NGS experiment and analyzed the data; D.V.-P. contributed to statistical analysis; I.A., A.Q. and D.D.G. wrote the paper; and D.D.G. and D.L. critically revised and approved the final manuscript.

Conflicts of Interest: The authors declare no conflict of interest.

References

1. Reilly, N.R.; Fasano, A. Presentation of Celiac Disease. *Gastrointest. Endosc. Clin. N. Am.* **2012**, *22*, 613–621. [CrossRef] [PubMed]
2. Ludvigsson, J.F.; Rubio-Tapia, A.; van Dyke, C.T.; Melton, L.J.; Zinsmeister, A.R.; Lahr, B.D.; Murray, J.A. Increasing incidence of celiac disease in a North American population. *Am. J. Gastroenterol.* **2013**, *108*, 818–824. [CrossRef] [PubMed]

3. Rubio-Tapia, A.; Hill, I.D.; Kelly, C.P.; Calderwood, A.H.; Murray, J.A. ACG clinical guidelines: Diagnosis and management of celiac disease. *Am. J. Gastroenterol.* **2013**, *108*, 656–676. [CrossRef] [PubMed]
4. Pagliari, D.; Urgesi, R.; Frosali, S.; Riccioni, M.E.; Newton, E.E.; Landolfi, R.; Pandolfi, F.; Cianci, R. The Interaction among Microbiota, Immunity, and Genetic and Dietary Factors Is the *Condicio Sine Qua Non* Celiac Disease Can Develop. *J. Immunol. Res.* **2015**, *2015*, 1–10.
5. Candela, M.; Biagi, E.; Maccaferri, S.; Turroni, S.; Brigidi, P. Intestinal microbiota is a plastic factor responding to environmental changes. *Trends Microbiol.* **2012**, *20*, 385–391. [CrossRef] [PubMed]
6. Verdu, E.F.; Galipeau, H.J.; Jabri, B. Novel players in coeliac disease pathogenesis: Role of the gut microbiota. *Nat. Rev. Gastroenterol. Hepatol.* **2015**, *12*, 497–506. [CrossRef] [PubMed]
7. Collado, M.C.; Donat, E.; Ribes-Koninckx, C.; Calabuig, M.; Sanz, Y. Specific duodenal and faecal bacterial groups associated with paediatric coeliac disease. *J. Clin. Pathol.* **2009**, *62*, 264–269. [CrossRef] [PubMed]
8. De Palma, G.; Nadal, I.; Medina, M.; Donat, E.; Ribes-koninckx, C.; Calabuig, M.; Sanz, Y. Intestinal dysbiosis and reduced immunoglobulin-coated bacteria associated with coeliac disease in children. *BMC Microbiol.* **2010**, *10*, 63. [CrossRef] [PubMed]
9. Di Cagno, R.; de Angelis, M.; de Pasquale, I.; Ndagijimana, M.; Vernocchi, P.; Ricciuti, P.; Gagliardi, F.; Laghi, L.; Crecchio, C.; Guerzoni, M.; et al. Duodenal and faecal microbiota of celiac children: Molecular, phenotype and metabolome characterization. *BMC Microbiol.* **2011**, *11*, 219. [CrossRef] [PubMed]
10. Nadal, I.; Donant, E.; Ribes-Koninckx, C.; Calabuig, M.; Sanz, Y. Imbalance in the composition of the duodenal microbiota of children with coeliac disease. *J. Med. Microbiol.* **2007**, *56*, 1669–1674. [CrossRef] [PubMed]
11. Carmen, C.M.; Hernández, M. Identification and differentiation of Lactobacillus, Streptococcus and *Bifidobacterium species* in fermented milk products with bifidobacteria. *Microbiol. Res.* **2007**, *162*, 86–92. [CrossRef] [PubMed]
12. Preidis, G.A.; Versalovic, J. Targeting the Human Microbiome With Antibiotics, Probiotics, and Prebiotics: Gastroenterology Enters the Metagenomics Era. *Gastroenterology* **2009**, *136*, 2015–2031. [CrossRef] [PubMed]
13. Medina, M.; de Palma, G.; Ribes-Koninckx, C.; Calabuig, M.; Sanz, Y. *Bifidobacterium* strains suppress in vitro the pro-inflammatory milieu triggered by the large intestinal microbiota of coeliac patients. *J. Inflamm. (Lond.)* **2008**, *5*, 19. [CrossRef] [PubMed]
14. Lindfors, K.; Blomqvist, T.; Juuti-Uusitalo, K.; Stenman, S.; Venalainen, J.; Maki, M.; Kaukinen, K. Live probiotic *Bifidobacterium lactis* bacteria inhibit the toxic effects induced by wheat gliadin in epithelial cell culture. *Clin. Exp. Immunol.* **2008**, *152*, 552–558. [CrossRef] [PubMed]
15. Laparra, J.M.; Sanz, Y. Interactions of gut microbiota with functional food components and nutraceuticals. *Pharmacol. Res.* **2010**, *61*, 219–225. [CrossRef] [PubMed]
16. De Angelis, M.; Rizzello, C.G.; Fasano, A.; Clemente, M.G.; Simone, C.; de Silano, M.; Vincenzi, M.; de Losito, I.; Gobbetti, M. VSL#3 probiotic preparation has the capacity to hydrolyze gliadin polypeptides responsible for Celiac Sprue. *Biochim. Biophys. Acta Mol. Basis Dis.* **2006**, *1762*, 80–93.
17. Smecuol, E.; Hwang, H.J.; Sugai, E.; Corso, L.; Cherñavsky, A.C.; Bellavite, F.P.; González, A.; Vodánovich, F.; Moreno, M.L.; Vázquez, H.; et al. Exploratory, Randomized, Double-blind, Placebo-controlled Study on the Effects of *Bifidobacterium* infantis Natren Life Start Strain Super Strain in Active Celiac Disease. *J. Clin. Gastroenterol.* **2013**, *47*, 139–147. [CrossRef] [PubMed]
18. Olivares, M.; Castillejo, G.; Varea, V.; Sanz, Y. Double-blind, randomised, placebo-controlled intervention trial to evaluate the effects of *Bifidobacterium longum* CECT 7347 in children with newly diagnosed coeliac disease. *Br. J. Nutr.* **2014**, *112*, 30–40. [CrossRef] [PubMed]
19. Braga, T.D.; Alves, G.; Israel, P.; Lira, C.; de Lima, M.D.C. Efficacy of *Bifidobacterium breve* and Lactobacillus casei oral supplementation on necrotizing enterocolitis in very-low-birth-weight preterm infants: A double-blind, randomized, controlled trial 1–3. *J. Clin.* **2011**, *93*, 81–86. [CrossRef] [PubMed]
20. Tabbers, M.M.; de Milliano, I.; Roseboom, M.G.; Benninga, M.A. Is *Bifidobacterium breve* effective in the treatment of childhood constipation? Results from a pilot study. *Nutr. J.* **2011**, *10*, 19. [CrossRef] [PubMed]
21. Wada, M.; Nagata, S.; Saito, M.; Shimizu, T.; Yamashiro, Y.; Matsuki, T.; Asahara, T.; Nomoto, K. Effects of the enteral administration of *Bifidobacterium breve* on patients undergoing chemotherapy for pediatric malignancies. *Support. Care Cancer* **2010**, *18*, 751–759. [CrossRef] [PubMed]

22. Husby, S.; Koletzko, S.; Korponay-Szabó, I.R.; Mearin, M.L.; Phillips, A.; Shamir, R.; Troncone, R.; Giersiepen, K.; Branski, D.; Catassi, C.; et al. European Society for Pediatric Gastroenterology, Hepatology, and Nutrition guidelines for the diagnosis of coeliac disease. *JPGN* **2012**, *54*, 136–160. [CrossRef] [PubMed]

23. Klemenak, M.; Dolinšek, J.; Langerholc, T.; Di Gioia, D.; Mičetić-Turk, D. Administration of *Bifidobacterium breve* Decreases the Production of TNF-α in Children with Celiac Disease. *Dig. Dis. Sci.* **2015**, *60*, 3386–3392. [CrossRef] [PubMed]

24. Aloisio, I.; Mazzola, G.; Corvaglia, L.T.; Tonti, G.; Faldella, G.; Biavati, B.; di Gioia, D. Influence of intrapartum antibiotic prophylaxis against group B Streptococcus on the early newborn gut composition and evaluation of the anti-Streptococcus activity of *Bifidobacterium* strains. *Appl. Microbiol. Biotechnol.* **2014**, *98*, 6051–6060. [CrossRef] [PubMed]

25. Klindworth, A.; Pruesse, E.; Schweer, T.; Peplies, J.; Quast, C.; Horn, M.; Glockner, F.O. Evaluation of general 16S ribosomal RNA gene PCR primers for classical and next-generation sequencing-based diversity studies. *Nucleic Acids Res.* **2013**, *41*, 1–11. [CrossRef] [PubMed]

26. Schmieder, R.; Edwards, R. Quality control and preprocessing of metagenomic datasets. *Bioinformatics* **2011**, *27*, 863–864. [CrossRef] [PubMed]

27. Aronest, E. Command-Line Tools for Processing Biological Sequencing Data, Ea-Utils. Available online: https://github.com/earonesty/ea-utils (accessed on 25 June 2015).

28. Lan, Y.; Wang, Q.; Cole, J.R.; Rosen, G.L. Using the RDP classifier to predict taxonomic novelty and reduce the search space for finding novel organisms. *PLoS ONE* **2012**, *7*, 1–15. [CrossRef] [PubMed]

29. McMurdie, P.J.; Holmes, S. Waste Not, Want Not: Why Rarefying Microbiome Data Is Inadmissible. *PLoS Comput. Biol.* **2014**, *10*, e1003531. [CrossRef] [PubMed]

30. Altschul, S.F.; Gish, W.; Miller, W.; Myers, E.W.; Lipman, D.J. Basic local alignment search tool. *J. Mol. Biol.* **1990**, *215*, 403–410. [CrossRef]

31. Lee, Z.M.P.; Bussema, C.; Schmidt, T.M. rrn DB: Documenting the number of rRNA and tRNA genes in bacteria and archaea. *Nucleic Acids Res.* **2009**, *37*, 489–493. [CrossRef] [PubMed]

32. Rinttila, T.; Kassinen, A.; Malinen, E.; Krogius, L.; Palva, A. Development of an extensive set of 16S rDNA-targeted primers for quantification of pathogenic and indigenous bacteria in faecal samples by real-time PCR. *J. Appl. Microbiol.* **2004**, *97*, 1166–1177. [CrossRef] [PubMed]

33. Castillo, M.; Martín-Orúe, S.M.; Manzanilla, E.G.; Badiola, I.; Martín, M.; Gasa, J. Quantification of total bacteria, enterobacteria and lactobacilli populations in pig digesta by real-time PCR. *Vet. Microbiol.* **2006**, *114*, 165–170. [CrossRef] [PubMed]

34. Penders, J.; Thijs, C.; Vink, C.; Stelma, F.F.; Snijders, B.; Kummeling, I.; van den Brandt, P.A.; Stobberingh, E.E. Factors influencing the composition of the intestinal microbiota in early infancy. *Pediatrics* **2006**, *118*, 511–521. [CrossRef] [PubMed]

35. Bartosch, S.; Fite, A.; Macfarlane, G.T.; McMurdo, M.E.T. Characterization of Bacterial Communities in Feces from Healthy Elderly Volunteers and Hospitalized Elderly Patients by Using Real-Time PCR and Effects of Antibiotic Treatment on the Fecal Microbiota. *Appl. Environ. Microbiol.* **2004**, *70*, 3575–3581. [CrossRef] [PubMed]

36. Song, Y.; Liu, C.; McTeague, M.; Summanen, P.; Finegold, S. *Clostridium bartlettii* sp. nov., isolated from human faeces. *Anaerobe* **2004**, *10*, 179–184. [CrossRef] [PubMed]

37. Collins, S.M.; Surette, M.; Bercik, P. The interplay between the intestinal microbiota and the brain. *Nat. Rev. Microbiol.* **2012**, *10*, 735–742. [CrossRef] [PubMed]

38. Aloisio, I.; Santini, C.; Biavati, B.; Dinelli, G.; Cenčič, A.; Chingwaru, W.; Mogna, L.; di Gioia, D. Characterization of *Bifidobacterium* spp. strains for the treatment of enteric disorders in newborns. *Appl. Microbiol. Biotechnol.* **2012**, *96*, 1561–1576. [CrossRef] [PubMed]

39. Drago, L.; de Vecchi, E.; Gabrieli, A.; de Grandi, R.; Toscano, M. Immunomodulatory effects of Lactobacillus salivarius LS01 and *Bifidobacterium breve* BR03, alone and in combination, on peripheral blood mononuclear cells of allergic asthmatics. *Allergy Asthma Immunol. Res.* **2015**, *7*, 409–413. [CrossRef] [PubMed]

40. Mogna, L.; del Piano, M.; Mogna, G. Capability of the two microorganisms *Bifidobacterium breve* B632 and *Bifidobacterium breve* BR03 to colonize the intestinal microbiota of children. *J. Clin. Gastroenterol.* **2014**, *48*, S37–S39. [CrossRef] [PubMed]

41. Sanz, Y. Effects of a gluten-free diet on gut microbiota and immune function in healthy adult humans. *Gut Microbes* **2010**, *1*, 135–137. [CrossRef] [PubMed]

42. De Palma, G.; Capilla, A.; Nova, E.; Castillejo, G.; Varea, V.; Pozo, T.; Garrote, J.A.; Polanco, I.; López, A.; Ribes-Koninckx, C.; et al. Influence of milk-feeding type and genetic risk of developing coeliac disease on intestinal microbiota of infants: The PROFICEL study. *PLoS ONE* **2012**, *7*, e30791. [CrossRef] [PubMed]
43. Samuel, B.S.; Gordon, J.I. A humanized gnotobiotic mouse model of host-archaeal-bacterial mutualism. *Proc. Natl. Acad. Sci. USA* **2006**, *103*, 10011–10016. [CrossRef] [PubMed]
44. Rodriguez, J.M.; Murphy, K.; Stanton, C.; Ross, R.P.; Kober, O.I.; Juge, N.; Avershina, E.; Rudi, K.; Narbad, A.; Jenmalm, M.C.; et al. The composition of the gut microbiota throughout life, with an emphasis on early life. *Microb. Ecol. Health Dis.* **2015**, *26*, 26050. [CrossRef] [PubMed]
45. Li, Y.; Shimizu, T.; Hosaka, A.; Kaneko, N.; Ohtsuka, Y.; Yamashiro, Y. Effects of *Bifidobacterium breve* supplementation on intestinal flora of low birth weight infants. *Pediatr. Int.* **2004**, *46*, 509–515. [CrossRef] [PubMed]
46. Ohtsuka, Y.; Ikegami, T.; Izumi, H.; Namura, M.; Ikeda, T.; Ikuse, T.; Baba, Y.; Kudo, T.; Suzuki, R.; Shimizu, T. Effects of *Bifidobacterium breve* on inflammatory gene expression in neonatal and weaning rat intestine. *Pediatr. Res.* **2012**, *71*, 46–53. [CrossRef] [PubMed]
47. Servin, A.L. Antagonistic activities of lactobacilli and bifidobacteria against microbial pathogens. *FEMS Microbiol. Rev.* **2004**, *28*, 405–440. [CrossRef] [PubMed]
48. Tien, M.; Girardin, S.E.; Regnault, B.; le Bourhis, L.; Dillies, M.; Coppée, J.; Bourdet-sicard, R.; Sansonetti, P.J. Anti-inflammatory effect of lactobacillus casei on shigella-infected human intestinal epithelial cells. *J. Immunol.* **2016**, *176*, 1228–1237. [CrossRef]

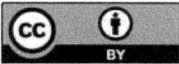

nutrients

MDPI

Article

Dietary Gluten-Induced Gut Dysbiosis Is Accompanied by Selective Upregulation of microRNAs with Intestinal Tight Junction and Bacteria-Binding Motifs in Rhesus Macaque Model of Celiac Disease

Mahesh Mohan [1], Cheryl-Emiliane T. Chow [2], Caitlin N. Ryan [2], Luisa S. Chan [2], Jason Dufour [3], Pyone P. Aye [1,3], James Blanchard [3], Charles P. Moehs [4] and Karol Sestak [5,6,*]

[1]   Division of Comparative Pathology, Tulane National Primate Research Center, Covington, LA 70433, USA; mmohan@tulane.edu (M.M.); paye@tulane.edu (P.P.A.)
[2]   Second Genome Inc., San Francisco, CA 94080, USA; cheryl@secondgenome.com (C.-E.T.C.); caitlin@secondgenome.com (C.N.R.); luisa@secondgenome.com (L.S.C.)
[3]   Division of Veterinary Resources, Tulane National Primate Research Center, Covington, LA 70433, USA; jdufour@tulane.edu (J.D.); jblanch1@tulane.edu (J.B.)
[4]   Arcadia Biosciences Inc., Seattle, WA 98119, USA; max.moehs@arcadiabio.com
[5]   Division of Microbiology, Tulane National Primate Research Center, Covington, LA 70433, USA
[6]   PreCliniTria LLC, Mandeville, LA 70471, USA
*   Correspondence: ksestak@tulane.edu; Tel.: +1-985-871-6409

Received: 29 August 2016; Accepted: 18 October 2016; Published: 28 October 2016

Abstract: The composition of the gut microbiome reflects the overall health status of the host. In this study, stool samples representing the gut microbiomes from 6 gluten-sensitive (GS) captive juvenile rhesus macaques were compared with those from 6 healthy, age- and diet-matched peers. A total of 48 samples representing both groups were studied using V4 16S rRNA gene DNA analysis. Samples from GS macaques were further characterized based on type of diet administered: conventional monkey chow, i.e., wheat gluten-containing diet (GD), gluten-free diet (GFD), barley gluten-derived diet (BOMI) and reduced gluten barley-derived diet (RGB). It was hypothesized that the GD diet would lower the gut microbial diversity in GS macaques. This is the first report illustrating the reduction of gut microbial alpha-diversity ($p < 0.05$) following the consumption of dietary gluten in GS macaques. Selected bacterial families (e.g., *Streptococcaceae* and *Lactobacillaceae*) were enriched in GS macaques while *Coriobacteriaceae* was enriched in healthy animals. Within several weeks after the replacement of the GD by the GFD diet, the composition (beta-diversity) of gut microbiome in GS macaques started to change ($p = 0.011$) towards that of a normal macaque. Significance for alpha-diversity however, was not reached by the day 70 when the feeding experiment ended. Several inflammation-associated microRNAs (miR-203, -204, -23a, -23b and -29b) were upregulated ($p < 0.05$) in jejunum of 4 biopsied GS macaques fed GD with predicted binding sites on 16S ribosomal RNA of *Lactobacillus reuteri* (accession number: NR_025911), *Prevotella stercorea* (NR_041364) and *Streptococcus luteciae* (AJ297218) that were overrepresented in feces. Additionally, claudin-1, a validated tight junction protein target of miR-29b was significantly downregulated in jejunal epithelium of GS macaques. Taken together, we predict that with the introduction of effective treatments in future studies the diversity of gut microbiomes in GS macaques will approach those of healthy individuals. Further studies are needed to elucidate the regulatory pathways of inflammatory miRNAs in intestinal mucosa of GS macaques and to correlate their expression with gut dysbiosis.

Keywords: celiac; gluten; gut; microbiome; microbiota; dysbiosis; rhesus; macaque; metagenomics; 16S rRNA; miRNA; chronic inflammation

1. Introduction

The human gastrointestinal (GI) tract contains approximately 10^{14} microorganisms [1] that colonize a surface of >30 m^2 [2]. The gut microbiome co-exists with its host as a super-organism, in a mutualistic manner [3–5], affecting the host's metabolism, immunity and overall fitness [6,7]. Diet, age, gender, genetics, usage of antibiotics, and multiple other factors influence the composition of the gut microbiome [8–17].

Non-human primates, owing to their close biological similarity with humans, are a valuable resource in biomedical research [18]. An earlier study by McKenna and colleagues identified important similarities but at the same time unique differences between human and rhesus gut microbiomes [19]. For example, *Treponema* sp. spirochetes were found to be abundant in macaques [19]. Recent studies with rural African human populations revealed an overabundance of intestinal *Treponoma* and *Prevotella* sp. compared to populations consuming a Western type of diet [16,20,21]. McKenna and colleagues documented an alteration in the composition of the gut microbiome, i.e., intestinal dysbiosis in rhesus monkeys, due to chronic colitis [19]. In another study, utilizing infant macaques that were either breast- or bottle-fed, differences in immune responsiveness and accumulation of metabolites were noted and linked to changes in gut microbiome composition [22]. In Japanese macaques (*Macaca fuscata*), consumption of a high-fat maternal diet resulted in displacement of potentially harmful gut microflora such as *Campylobacter* sp. [15]. Finally, inulin treatment successfully resolved idiopathic chronic diarrhea and restored gut microflora in dysbiotic macaques [23,24].

A loss of gut microbial diversity as one of the hallmarks of dysbiosis is commonly found in patients with Inflammatory Bowel Disease (IBD). While many obligate anaerobic commensal microorganisms are lost during IBD, an increase of aerotolerant *Enterobacteriaceae* and expansion of the *Prevotellaceae* takes place [25–30]. Intestinal dysbiosis has also been observed in patients with celiac disease (CD) [31–35]. Investigations that focused on pediatric patients during and after the Swedish CD outbreak, suggested that rod-shaped intestinal bacteria might have predisposed children to CD [36–38]. It has been reported that bacteria most involved in gluten metabolism belong to phylum *Firmicutes*, mainly from the *Lactobacillus* genus, followed by *Streptococcus*, *Staphylococcus* and *Clostridium* genera [39]. It was shown that GFD treatment significantly alters proportions of these bacterial populations [31]. It was suggested that increased presence of some of the bacteria involved in gluten metabolism might be associated with enteritis [39]. An unrelated report showed that *Proteobacteria* and not *Firmicutes* is the most abundant phylum in celiacs, with members of the *Neisseria* genus being the most represented [40]. Regardless of the exact reflection of intestinal dysbiosis that appears may vary in different categories of CD patients, it was observed that dietary gluten-induced dysbiosis is not easily restored by GFD treatment [35]. Although in GS rhesus macaques the progression of enteropathy is linked with the gradually decreasing presence of mucosal barrier-maintaining interleukins (IL)-17, IL-22 [41] and various other functions, alterations in gut microbiota are yet to be studied in this model. Since a recent study demonstrated that fecal miRNAs secreted by intestinal epithelial cells could enter luminal bacterial cells and regulate their growth via post-transcriptional gene regulation [42], we profiled miRNA expression in jejunum of GS macaques. Thirteen differentially expressed (DE) miRNAs were identified, with eight containing specific binding motifs to dysbiotic bacterial species and intestinal tight junction (TJ) proteins. In summary, our main objective was to determine if dysbiosis takes place in GS macaques fed a gluten-containing diet and if it can be restored upon administration of GFD. Results indicate that the diversity of the gut microbiome of GS macaques is significantly lower than that of healthy, age-matched peers and dysbiosis is linked with upregulation of pro-inflammatory miRNAs. Future studies shall focus on restoration of gut microbiome diversity and composition—by a long-term dietary and/or other therapeutic interventions.

2. Experimental Section

2.1. Ethics Approval

This study was performed using samples collected from normal healthy and GS non-human primates. Ethics approval for veterinary procedures was obtained from the Tulane University Animal Care and Use Committee, Animal Welfare Assurance A-4499-01. Tulane National Primate Research Center (TNPRC) is accredited by the Association for Assessment and Accreditation of Laboratory Animal Care (AAALAC). Steps were taken to ameliorate animal suffering in accordance with the recommendations of the Guide to the Care and Use of Laboratory Animals (NIH) 78-23 (Revised, 2011).

2.2. Rhesus Macaques, Diets and Samples Collected

Forty-eight stool samples were obtained via fecal loops from 12 juvenile (1–3-years-old, 6 healthy controls and 6 GS) captive rhesus macaques (*Macaca mulatta*) of Indian origin. As described, the GS and control macaques were stationed in a dedicated bio-security level 2 facility, physically separated from the rest of the colony as well as from the same study animals on different, dietary gluten-modified diets, to prevent contamination of each chow with undesirable gluten sources [43]. The 12 animals were selected irrespective of sex. All animals were seronegative and free of viral, bacterial or parasitic pathogens including the simian retrovirus type D, simian T lymphotropic virus type 1, simian immunodeficiency virus and herpes B virus [41,44]. Tuberculin skin tests were negative for each individual. The 6 GS macaques had previously been reported with celiac-like GS, i.e., an equivalent of human CD [45]. Approximately 0.5 g of stool were obtained from at least 3 representative macaques at each time point when fed gluten-modified diets: conventional monkey chow, i.e., wheat gluten-containing diet (GD), gluten-free diet (GFD), conventional barley gluten-derived diet (BOMI) and reduced gluten barley-derived diet (RGB) (Supplementary Materials Table S1). Samples from GS macaques were obtained at multiple time points while samples from healthy control macaques were obtained only once. Immediately upon collection, stools were suspended in 1.0 mL of phosphate saline buffer and then stored at −80 °C until processed for DNA extraction.

2.3. DNA Extraction, Library Preparation and Profiling

Frozen stool samples were thawed at room temperature prior to DNA extraction. Approximately 0.25 g (wet weight) of stool was measured for each sample and DNA was extracted using the MoBio PowerMag Microbiome kit (Mo Bio Laboratories Inc., Carlsbad, CA, USA) according to the manufacturer's guidelines and optimized for high-throughput processing. All samples were quantified using the Qubit Quant-iT dsDNA High Sensitivity Kit (Invitrogen, Life Technologies, Grand Island, NB, USA). To enrich samples for bacterial 16S V4 rDNA region, DNA was amplified utilizing fusion primers designed against the surrounding conserved regions tailed with sequences to incorporate Illumina (San Diego, CA, USA) adapters and indexing barcodes [46]. Each sample was PCR amplified with two differently bar coded V4 fusion primers. Samples that met the post-PCR quantification minimum were advanced for pooling and sequencing. For each sample, amplified products were concentrated using a solid-phase reversible immobilization method for the purification of PCR products and quantified by qPCR. An amplicon pool containing 16S V4 enriched, amplified, barcoded samples, was sequenced for 2 × 250 cycles on an Illumina MiSeq (San Diego, CA, USA). Samples were processed in a Good Laboratory Practices (GLP) compliant service laboratory running Quality Management Systems for sample and data tracking.

2.4. Operational Taxonomic Unit (OTU) Selection

Sequenced paired-end reads were merged using USEARCH and the resulting sequences were compared as described [47,48]. Briefly, all sequences matching a unique strain with an identity $\geq$99% were assigned a strain OTU. To ensure specificity of the strain hits, a difference of $\geq$0.25% between the identity of the best hit and the second hit was required (e.g., 99.75 vs. 99.5). For each strain OTU, one of the matching reads was selected as a representative and all sequences were mapped by USEARCH (usearch_global) against the strain OTU representative sequence to calculate strain abundance. The remaining non-strain sequences were quality filtered and de-replicated with USEARCH. Resulting unique sequences were then clustered at 97% by UPARSE de novo OTU clustering and a representative consensus sequence per de novo OTU was determined. The UPARSE clustering algorithm includes a chimera filtering step. Representative OTU sequences were classified via mothur's Bayesian classifier with a threshold of 80% confidence; the classifier was trained against the Greengenes reference database (v13.5, greengenes.lbl.gov) [49] of 16S rRNA sequences clustered at 99% similarity. Spurious OTUs were removed.

2.5. Alpha- (within Sample) and Beta- (between Samples) Diversity

"Observed" diversity reflects the number of unique OTUs within each sample while Shannon diversity reflects the richness of a sample along with the relative abundance of present OTUs. Both Observed and Shannon diversities were used to assess alpha-diversity. The Bray-Curtis dissimilarity index was evaluated to determine beta-diversity.

2.6. Ordination and Clustering

Dendrograms were constructed to graphically summarize the inter-sample relationships based on Bray-Curtis dissimilarity using hierarchical clustering by Ward's method.

2.7. Whole Microbiome and Taxon Significance Testing

Permutational Analysis of Variance (PERMANOVA) was utilized for whole microbiome beta-diversity differences among discrete categorical or continuous variables [50]. Univariate differential abundance of OTUs was tested using a negative binomial noise model for the overdispersion and Poisson process intrinsic to this data, as implemented in the DESeq2 package [51], and described for microbiome applications [52].

2.8. miRNA Profiling, Real Time qRT-PCR and Confocal Microscopy

Proximal jejunum biopsy tissues from 4 GS and 6 healthy control macaques fed GD for at least one year (long-term GD) were collected and processed as described [45]. Half of the collected biopsies were preserved in 5 mL of RNA-later solution (Qiagen Inc., Valencia, CA, USA) while second half was embedded in paraffin and 7 µm sections were used for immunofluorescent staining, i.e., confocal microscopy.

Total RNA from intact jejunal tissue samples was isolated using the miRNeasy total RNA isolation kit (Qiagen Inc.) following the manufacturer's protocol. The 100 ng of total RNA was first reverse transcribed using the miRNA reverse transcription reaction kit and loaded onto the TaqMan® OpenArray® Human MicroRNA Panel, QuantStudio™ 12K Flex system (Thermo-Fisher, Waltham, MA, USA) and processed as described previously [53].

TJ protein (Claudin-1, Claudin-3 and Occludin gene expression in jejunum samples was quantified by Power SYBR Green RNA to C_T One-Step RT-PCR assay (Thermo-Fisher). Each qRT-PCR reaction (20 µL) contained the following: 2X Power SYBR Green Master Mix (12.5 µL), 200 nM forward and reverse primer (Supplementary Materials Table S2) and 200 ng of total RNA. Comparative real-time PCR was performed and relative change in gene expression was calculated using the ΔΔCT method. Data was normalized to a combination of three endogenous controls (Beta-Actin, 18S rRNA and GAPDH).

Immunofluorescence studies for the detection of Claudin-1 (1 in 50) (Abcam, Cambridge, UK) was done as described earlier [53]. Cytokeratin (Biocare, Concord, CA, USA) (1 in 500) and Topro-3 (1 in 2000) was employed as a marker for intestinal epithelial cells and nuclei, respectively. Positive signals were detected using appropriate Alexa fluor conjugated secondary antibodies (Thermo-Fisher, Waltham, MA, USA).

2.9. Data Analysis

QuantStudio™ run files from GS (n = 4) and control macaques (n = 5) were analyzed simultaneously using ExpressionSuite software v1.0.3 (Thermo-Fisher) as described previously [54]. Since Expression Suite software is not equipped to perform non-parametric analysis, the output file containing five columns (well, sample, detector, task and C_T values) were saved as a tab-delimited text file, imported and analyzed by non-parametric Wilcoxon's rank sum test for independent samples using RealTime STATMINER™ package (Integromics on Spotfire DecisionSite) designed to compare samples using the $\Delta\Delta C_T$ method for relative quantification of gene expression. miRNA expression data was normalized to a combination of two endogenous controls (RNU44 and RNU48). In all experiments, the C_T upper limit was set to 28 meaning that all miRNA detectors with a C_T value greater than or equal to 28 were excluded. TaqMan OpenArray® microRNA data files were deposited with the National Center for Biotechnology Information database (GEO, Accession number: GSE89170, http://www.ncbi.nlm.nih.gov/geo/query/acc.cgi?acc=GSE89170).

For TJ protein mRNA qRT-PCR studies, one GS macaque with the highest ΔC_T value served as the calibrator/reference and assigned a value of 1. All DE mRNAs in GS and other macaques in the normal healthy control group are shown as an n-fold difference relative to this macaque. mRNA qRT-PCR data was analyzed by non-parametric Wilcoxon's rank sum test for independent samples using RealTime STATMINER™ package. A p value of less than 0.05 was considered significant.

3. Results

3.1. Gut Microbiomes Differ Significantly between Healthy and GS Macaques

In order to compare gut microbiomes between healthy and GS macaques that were fed conventional, gluten-containing monkey chow (GD) for at least one year, we measured alpha-diversity, relative abundance of top bacterial families and performed clustering analyses.

Alpha-diversity (Shannon diversity index) was significantly higher in healthy compared to GS macaques (p = 0.02), despite that the observed number of OTUs did not differ (p = 0.07) (Figure 1, Supplementary Materials Table S3). Proportionally, two of the top 8 families (*Streptococcaceae* and *Lactobacillaceae*) were enriched in GS macaques, while one family (*Coriobacteriaceae*) was enriched in healthy macaques (Figure 2, Supplementary Materials Table S4). When gut microbial diversity metrics were compared between the GS and healthy animals with consideration of sex, there were similar differences as there were without such consideration.

Hierarchical clustering (Supplementary Materials Figure S1) and weighted ordination analyses showed good separation of represented bacterial families between samples collected from healthy control and GS macaques. The 157 OTUs differed significantly in relative abundance between healthy and GS macaques (Figure 3). Approximately 89 out of the 157 significant OTUs belonged to the phylum *Firmicutes*. Genera enriched in GS animals included *Anaerostipes*, *Coprococcus*, *Dorea*, *Feacalibacterium*, *Fibrobacter*, *Lachnospira*, *Lactobacillus*, *Oscillospira*, *Peptococcus*, *Prevotella*, *Ruminococcus*, *Sarcina*, *Streptococcus*, and YRC22. Genera enriched in healthy rhesus macaques included *Anaerofustis*, *Corynebacterium*, *Dehalobacterium*, *Methanobrevibacter*, *Methanosphaera*, *Prevotella*, *Ruminococcus*, *Treponema*, and *Weissella*.

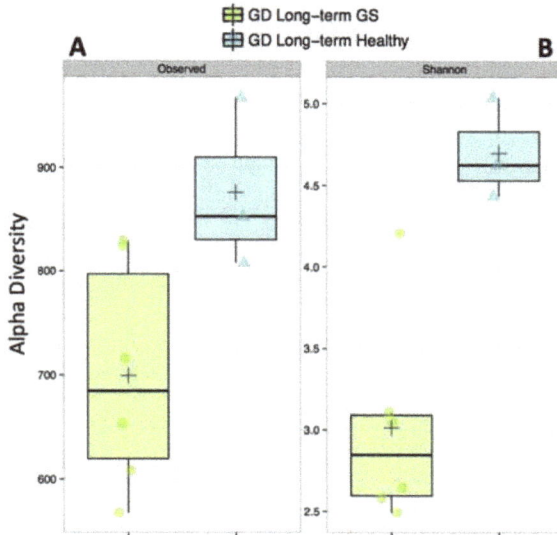

Figure 1. Alpha-diversity of the gut microbiome is decreased in gluten-sensitive (GS) macaques. Observed (**A**) corresponds to total number of Operational Taxonomic Units (OTUs) present in sample; Shannon, (**B**) corresponds to Shannon Diversity Index that accounts for both the abundance and evenness of OTUs. **Green** color represents GS juvenile macaques on GD (long-term) diet while **blue** indicates age- and gluten-containing diet (GD) diet-matched healthy controls.

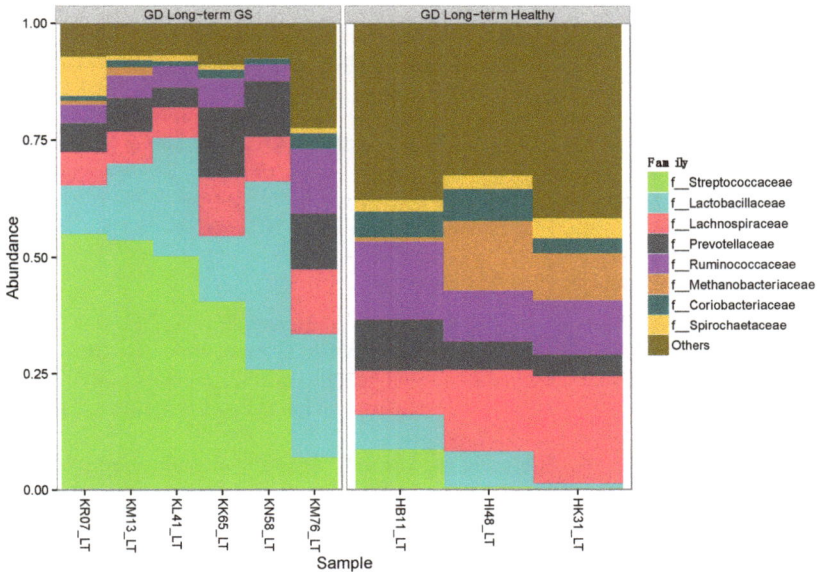

Figure 2. Proportional abundance of microbial taxa in GS and control macaques. Plot shows the most abundant taxa at the family level. **Left** panel represents GS juvenile macaques on GD diet while **right** panel indicates age- and diet-matched healthy control macaques.

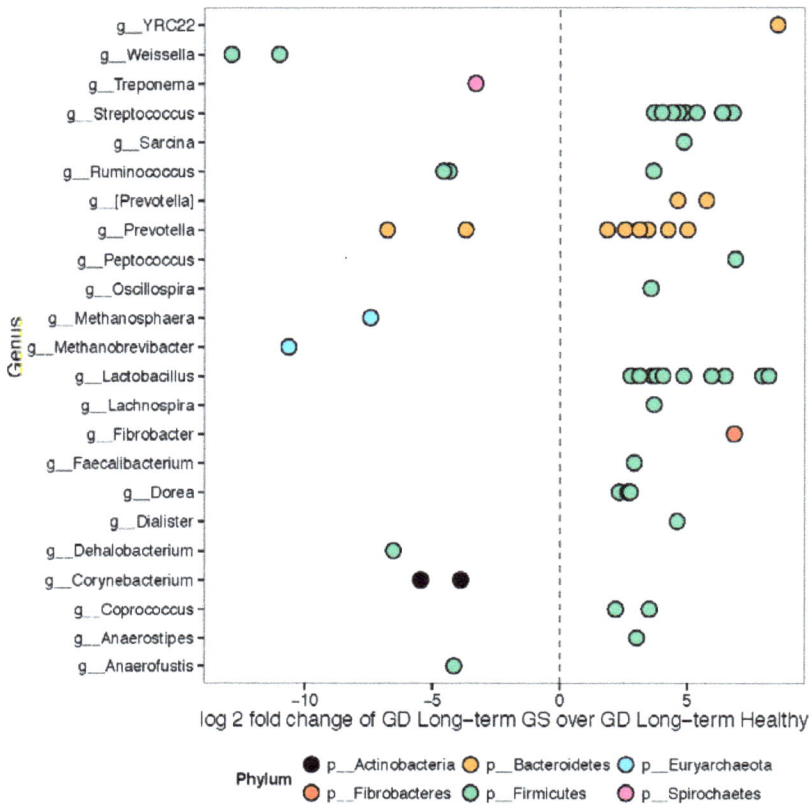

Figure 3. Differentially abundant features: GS macaques vs. healthy controls on GD. Each point represents an OTU belonging to each Genus. Only significant OTUs assigned at genus-level are shown. Features were considered significant if their FDR-corrected *p*-value was less than or equal to 0.05. There were 157 significantly different OTUs detected out of 1263 tested. Fifty-six OTUs had genus-level annotations.

3.2. Gut Microbiomes of GS Macaques Are Influenced by GFD

After placing the GS macaques on GFD, alpha-diversity and relative OTU abundances were evaluated at days 14, 28, 42 and 70 to assess the extent of potential improvement, i.e., restoration of gut microbiome composition to that observed in normal healthy controls (Figure 4 and Supplementary Materials Figure S2). No significant differences were observed in alpha-diversity metrics by day 70 of GFD (Supplementary Materials Figure S2A,B).

Nevertheless, 145 of 1212 OTUs were significantly different in their abundance when the individual GFD time-points were tested (Figure 4). Many of the significant OTUs (23) belonged to families *Ruminococcaceae* and *Lachnospiraceae* (8) within the phylum *Firmicutes* (Figure 4, Supplementary Materials Table S5). In addition, there were no significant differences in alpha-diversity between BOMI and RGB diets (Supplementary Materials Figure S2C,D). Irrespective of the diet fed to GS macaques, the phylum *Firmicutes* comprised majority of the microbial species (mean = 64.7%). The phylum *Proteobacteria* was in a few instances dominant (mean = 7.8%) over *Firmicutes*. The relative abundances of the top 8 most abundant phyla did not differ significantly when comparing the GFD, BOMI and RGB diets. However, *Firmicutes*, followed by *Bacteroidetes* and *Proteobacteria* were dominant (Figure 5).

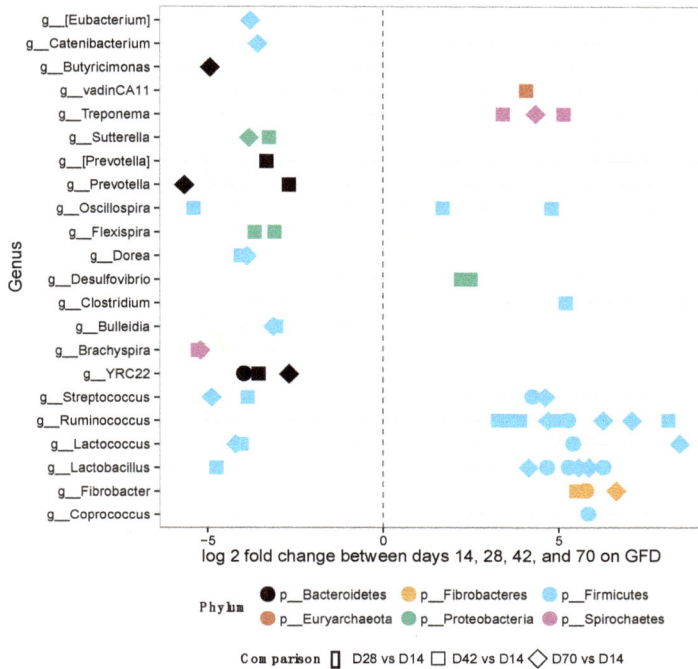

Figure 4. Differentially abundant features in GS macaques while on GFD. One hundred forty-five significantly different OTUs belonging to each genus out of 1212 tested were identified in GS macaques while on GFD. Overall increase of beneficial bacterial groups is seen in GS macaques while on GFD. Most of the significant features were from the phylum *Firmicutes*, particularly the family *Ruminococcaceae*.

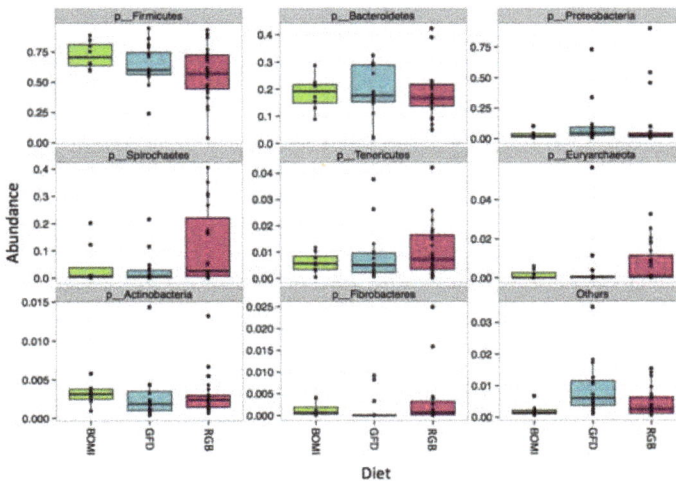

Figure 5. Composition at the phylum level. Irrespective of diet, the phylum *Firmicutes* comprised the majority of the gut microbiome in GS macaques.

While on GFD, significant changes in abundance of individual OTUs were detected in GS macaques (Figure 4): 145 differentially abundant OTUs of 1212 tested were identified. Overall, increase of beneficial bacterial groups was also seen in GS macaques while on GFD. Most of the significant OTUs were from the phylum *Firmicutes*, particularly the family *Ruminococcaceae*. The greatest number of significantly differential OTUs occurred between day 14 and 42 of GFD. Only 17 OTUs differed between day 14 and 28. Eleven OTUs were classified to a strain-level as *Brachyspira pilosicoli*, *Clostridium bartletti*, *Clostridium perfringens*, *Coprococcus eutactus*, *Desulfovibrio piger*, *Eubacterium biforme*, *Eubacterium siraeum*, *Flexispira/Helicobacter fennelliae*, *Oscillospira/Ruminococcaceae* bacterium D16, *Ruminococcus champanellensis*, and *Treponema berlinense*.

3.3. Inflammation-Associated miRNAs Are Upregulated in Jejunum of GS Macaques and Have Predicted Binding Sites on Bacterial 16S Ribosomal RNA

We profiled miRNA expression in jejunum of four GS macaques and identified thirteen DE ($p < 0.05$) miRNAs (Figure 6). Out of these, 8 were upregulated and 5 downregulated (Figure 6).

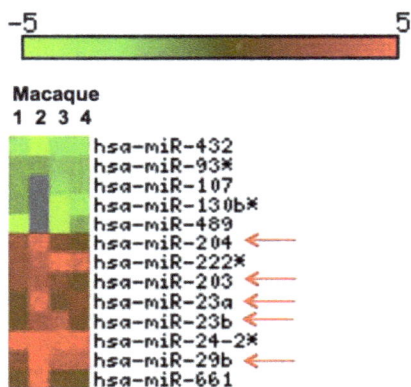

Figure 6. Heat Map of differentially expressed (DE) miRNAs in GS macaques. Values corresponding to jejunum of four GS macaques normalized against average of 5 normal healthy controls are shown. Eight out of 13 DE miRNAs were significantly upregulated (**red**) and the remaining five were downregulated (**green**) ($p < 0.05$). **Red** arrows indicate miRNAs previously reported and linked to inflammatory disorders [55–61].

We next scanned the bacterial 16S rRNA sequence of four bacterial species, namely, *Lactobacillus reuteri* (accession number (No.) NR_025911), *Prevotella copri* (accession No. AB244773), *P. stercorea* (accession No. NR_041364), *Streptococcus luteciae* (accession No. AJ297218) that were found to be overrepresented in feces of GS macaques (Figure 3) for potential binding sites for these DE miRNAs using the RNAhybrid algorithm [62]. As observed and reported previously by Liu et al. [42], using the RNAhybrid algorithm, we identified binding sites for miR-204, miR-29b and miR-107 on the 16S rRNA sequence of *P. copri* and *P. stercorea* that showed perfect Watson and Crick base pairing in the miRNA seed region (nucleotide positions 2 to 7 on 5′ end) with very low minimum free energy (MFE) (Figure 7). Additionally, miR-29b and miR-204 were also found to have binding sites on the 16S rRNA sequence of *L. reuteri* and *S. leuticeae*, respectively.

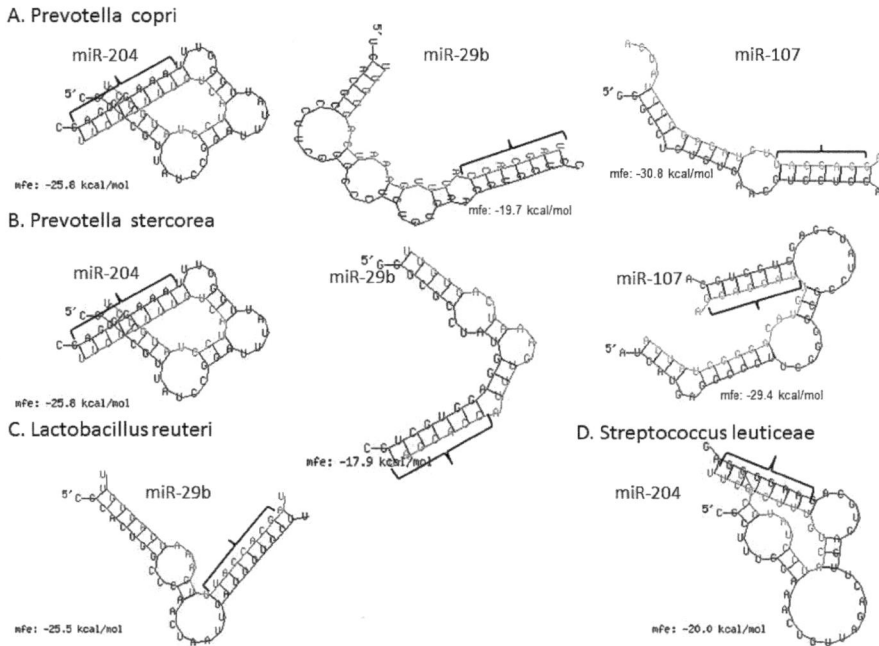

Figure 7. miRNA (**green**) vs. 16S ribosomal RNA (violet) (rRNA) pairing using RNAhybrid algorithm. Note the perfect Watson and Crick base pairing in miRNA 5′ seed nucleotides (nts) 2–7 (bracket) and extra homology in 3′ region of miR-204, miR-29b and miR-107 with 16S rRNA of *P. copri* (**A**); and *P. stercorea* (**B**); In addition, notice the significantly good homology between miR-204 and miR-29b seed nts and 16s rRNA of *L. reuteri* (**C**); and *S. leuticeae* (**D**), respectively.

3.4. Claudin-1, an Epithelial Tight Junction Protein and A Validated Target of miR-29b Is Significantly Downregulated in Jejunum of GS Macaques

MiRNAs and RNA binding proteins are known to regulate TJ protein expression [63,64]. Recent studies in IBD and IBS have demonstrated miR-122 and miR-29b to directly target and downregulate the expression of occludin [65] and claudin-1 [55] expression, respectively. Using the TargetScan 7.1 [66] and RNAhybrid [62] algorithm, we identified a *perfect* Watson-Crick *match* to the *seed nucleotides* 2–7 of three upregulated miRNAs, namely, miR-203, miR-204 and miR-29b on the 3′ UTR of claudin-1 mRNA (Supplementary Materials Figure S3) that are highly conserved across multiple mammalian species that includes chimpanzees and rhesus macaques [66]. These in silico findings strengthen the possibility of direct post-transcriptional silencing of claudin-1 by three different miRNAs. Since miR-29b has already been validated to directly target claudin-1 expression [55], we next investigated claudin-1 protein expression in the jejunum of GS macaques.

Consistent with miR-203, miR-204 and miR-29b upregulation, downregulation of claudin-1, a TJ protein that regulates intestinal epithelial permeability was observed (Figure 8). The miRNA expression of three TJ proteins, namely, claudin-1, -3 and occludin was significantly diminished in GS relative to normal healthy control macaques (Figure 8A). The decreased RNA expression was corroborated by the confocal microscopy of claudin-1 protein expression (Figure 8B,C) directly in the jejunal villous enterocytes of GS macaque compared to the healthy control. These findings suggest that dysregulated miRNA expression in response to chronic inflammation could enhance epithelial permeability by downregulating TJ protein which in turn would facilitate systemic translocation of dysbiotic bacteria in GS macaques.

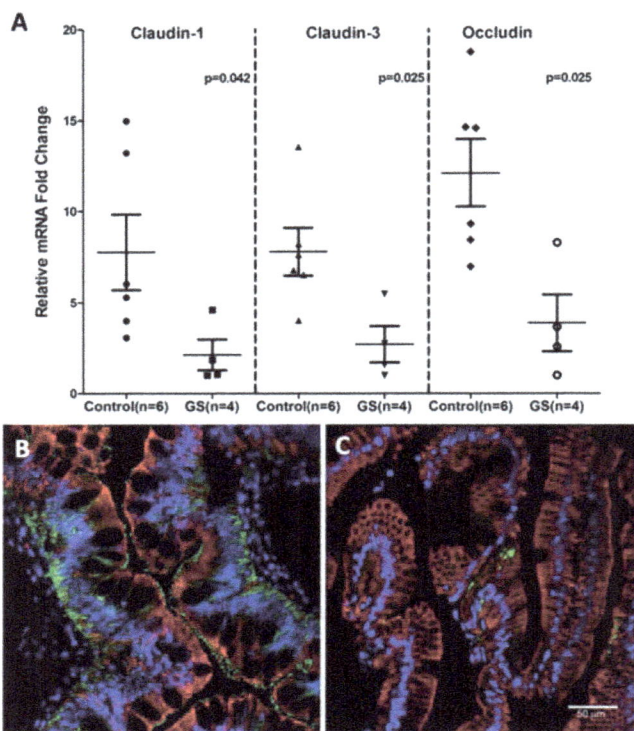

Figure 8. Tight junction protein expression in jejunum of GS macaques. mRNA expression of Claudin-1,-3 and Occludin is significantly decreased ($p < 0.05$) in jejunum of GS ($n = 4$) relative to normal healthy control macaques ($n = 6$) (**A**); Data was normalized to a combination of three endogenous controls (Beta-Actin, 18S rRNA, GAPDH) and analyzed using non-parametric Wilcoxon's rank sum test for independent samples. The error bars represent standard error of mean fold change within each group. While Claudin-1 (**green**) protein is well expressed in jejunum epithelial cells (**red**) from normal healthy macaque (**B**); its signal is very low or absent in jejunum from GS animal (**C**). Both B and C panels are triple labels with claudin-1 in **green**, cytokeratin in **red** and nuclear labeling with Topro3 in **blue**.

In summary, a non-significant increase in alpha-diversity was observed in GS macaques while on GFD (Supplementary Materials Figure S2A,B), raising the proposition that with further progression of time and continued feeding of GFD, gut microbiomes of GS macaques might revert towards normal, healthy controls. Remarkably, the PERMANOVA results for GFD and RGB time points confirmed that gut microbiome composition (beta-diversity) was changing in GS macaques with progression of time: It was determined that beta-diversity values differed significantly between the time points when GS macaques were switched from gluten-containing to gluten-free ($p = 0.011$) or gluten-reduced ($p < 0.05$) diets. In contrast, alpha-diversity metrics attributed to samples associated with GFD, BOMI and RGB diets did not change significantly during the short-term (1–2.5 months) periods of experimental feeding although their average values were increasing (Supplementary Materials Figure S2C,D). miRNA data demonstrated significant dysregulation in the intestines of GS macaques (Figures 6 and 7) and as previously demonstrated [42], allude to the possibility that dysregulated miRNAs could potentially regulate the intestinal microbiome in GS macaques via post transcriptional gene regulation [42].

4. Discussion

Non-human primates are being used in translational research involving infectious, immune-mediated, metabolic and other disorders where the scientific objectives cannot be fully accomplished by the use of other animal models [43,67–69]. The gut microbiomes of two biologically distinct (GS and healthy) groups of captive rhesus macaques were for the first time compared. A recent work by Yasuda and colleagues demonstrated that rhesus stool microbiome is a suitable proxy for both large and small intestine microbiomes [70]. In the present study, representative stool samples were characterized by amplifying V4 region of the 16S rRNA gene [19,32,34,35,37]. It was hypothesized that disease progression in GS macaques is associated with a loss of gut microbial diversity which can potentially lead to increased epithelial permeability thereby exacerbating intestinal inflammation [25–29]. Our findings clearly demonstrate that microbiomes in GS and healthy macaques differ significantly while on long-term (≥one year) conventional, gluten-containing diet, i.e., GD. Since the gut microbiomes of GS macaques have not been studied before, findings reported here are novel and provide directions for potential future studies. The GS macaques can be used in preclinical studies to evaluate if novel dietary or other therapeutic interventions can reverse gut dysbiosis. In studies with unrelated, chronic bacterial colitis-affected macaques, an overgrowth of *Pasteurellaceae* and *Enterobacteriaceae*, as well as decreased microbial diversity was observed. Taken together, our findings also corroborate that gluten sensitivity can contribute to chronic bacterial enterocolitis e.g., one of the major health concerns of polyfactorial origin in captive macaques [24,44,71,72].

As noted by McKenna and colleagues [19], a distinctive feature of the macaque gut microbiome is the abundance of intestinal Spirochetes from the *Treponema* lineage. In agreement with those observations, in the present study, intestinal Spirochetes were abundant in healthy controls, while GS macaques had lower loads of these bacteria. This finding suggests that a thriving population of intestinal Spirochetes is indeed an indicator of robust health in macaques. It is also consistent with the findings of Zeller and Takeuchi [73], who pointed out the presence of intestinal Spirochetes in healthy macaques. Our group previously reported that intestinal Spirochetes, despite their high prevalence, were not among intestinal bacteria linked with chronic enterocolitis [44].

One of the key similarities between human and rhesus gut microbiomes is that *Firmicutes* and *Bacteroidetes* are the two prominent phyla. It was established that the ratio between these two can be in humans affected by "western" and "low-calorie/high-fiber" types of diets [74,75]. Consistent with these findings, *Firmicutes* followed by *Bacteroidetes*, were amongst the most abundant phyla represented in our study macaques. Nonetheless, several differences in composition were observed between GS and healthy control macaques. While GS macaques exhibited dysbiosis, several groups of intestinal bacteria were differentially abundant when compared with healthy controls. The over-abundant groups included two major families belonging to the phylum *Firmicutes*, i.e., *Streptococcaceae* and *Lactobacillaceae*. Previously, it was reported by Caminero et al., that both *Lactobacillaceae* and *Streptococcaceae* play an important role in metabolism of gluten [39]. While it is obvious that the presence of *Streptococcaceae* represents potential to contain pathogenic strains, the biological significance underlying the increased presence of *Lactobacillaceae* in GS macaques is less certain. Clearly, *Lactobacillus* spp. have the capacity to degrade gluten resulting in decreased immunotoxicity of its major immunogens such as the 33-mer of alpha-gliadin [76]. At the same time, however, the full pathogenic potential of dysbiotic bacterial taxa including *Lactobacillaceae*, *Streptococcaceae* and others in GS individuals still needs to be elucidated. Interestingly, and in concordance with our study, Ardeshir and colleagues (2014) independently reported that chronic intestinal enterocolitis is in rhesus macaques associated with an over-abundance of intestinal *Lactobacillaceae* [24], suggesting that not all of the *Lactobacilli* spp. act as a health-promoting probiotics. According to their study, *Lactobacillaceae* overgrowth can be reduced in macaques by inulin treatment [24]. Less abundant taxa in GS macaques were mostly represented by *Coriobacteriaceae* that belong to phylum *Actinobacteria*. *Actinobacteria* were recognized as the producers of host-beneficial metabolites with antibacterial, antifungal, immunomodulatory and other functions [66,77]. Reduced abundance of *Bacteroidetes* has been previously reported in human celiac infants [33]. Similar studies that utilized different technologies, and focused on different types of (biopsy) samples, have not always produced consistent results [32,34,35,37]. In our study, a few of the bacterial taxa belonging to *Bacteroidetes* were less abundant in GS macaques while others, namely *Prevotella* sp., were overabundant compared to healthy controls. One group of patients where GS occurs with higher frequency and in parallel with neurodevelopmental disorders, are the patients with Autism Spectrum Disorder [78,79]. It has been reported that Autism and Parkinson's disease patients lack beneficial gut microflora [80,81]. In this context, we previously reported that up-regulation of the Autism Spectrum Disorder-associated gene CADPS2, and other neurodevelopmental disorder-related genes (BACE2 and DSCR5) were detected in GS macaques [82]. Despite that these associations and links are still largely under-explored, they offer clues for potential future studies.

While microbial dysbiosis is a hallmark of chronic inflammatory diseases of the gastrointestinal tract, the potential mechanisms underlying these alterations remain unknown. A recent study demonstrated that fecal miRNAs secreted by intestinal epithelial cells could enter luminal bacterial cells and regulate their growth via post-transcriptional gene regulation [42]; suggesting a critical mechanism by which the host could not only shape but also potentially dysregulate its intestinal microbiome. Additionally, miRNAs have also been demonstrated to regulate the intestinal epithelial barrier in inflammatory bowel disease (IBD) and irritable bowel syndrome (IBS) via post-transcriptional regulation of TJ proteins [54,83]. Notable miRNAs associated with inflammation in our study included miR-203 and miR-29b that have previously been reported to be upregulated in IBD and IBS [54–56]. More importantly, the inverse relationship between miR-203, -204 and -29b expression and their predicted/validated claudin-1 target protein expression, suggests an important post-transcriptional mechanism regulating the intestinal epithelial barrier that could promote translocation of dysbiotic intestinal bacteria leading to adverse systemic inflammation/immune dysregulation in GS macaques and celiac disease patients. Similarly, dysregulation of miR-204 and miR-23a/b has been reported in various other inflammatory conditions [58–61].

Although we identified several DE miRNAs previously associated with various chronic inflammatory diseases to have binding sites on the 16S rRNA sequence of *Lactobacillus*, *Prevotella* and *Streptococcus* species in GS macaques with gut dysbiosis, further studies are needed to corroborate presence of these miRNAs in feces of GS individuals and to correlate their expression levels with changes in the bacterial flora. Data from such analyses will pave the way for in vitro mechanistic/growth kinetic studies [42] to elucidate the novel concept of whether dietary gluten-induced dysbiosis involves selective modulation of the GI microbiota via luminal shedding of intestinal epithelial miRNAs.

5. Conclusions

This is the first report illustrating the reduction of gut microbial diversity following the consumption of dietary gluten in GS macaques. Although administration of GFD to GS macaques was expected to restore composition of dysbiotic gut microbiomes to normal, diversity metrics did not corroborate such expectation. These findings are consistent with studies of celiac patients whose gut microbiome composition was not restored even after "long-term" treatment with GFD [84]. Notwithstanding, we believe that further extension of GFD feeding regimen and/or inclusion of additional treatments such as anti-inflammatory compounds would result in more complete restoration of intestinal microbiota in GS subjects. Thus, the present study has set the stage for future experiments, in which the effects of novel treatment strategies will be assessed. These approaches will include oral probiotics, microbiome restitution, gluten-modified diets, recombinant glutenases and anti-inflammatory drugs. The gut microbiome and miRNA metrics are expected to provide useful evaluative tools in these studies.

Supplementary Materials: The following are available online at http://www.mdpi.com/2072-6643/8/11/684/s1, Figure S1: Hierarchical clustering by GS status. Microbiomes were clustered by the Ward Method and Bray-Curtis Distance. The two clusters (control healthy = blue and GS = green) of macaques, all fed GD diet, are differentiated by GS status, except for KM76. KM76 macaque had a lower proportion of Strepococcaceae (6.8%), similar to healthy controls, Figure S2: Alpha-diversity estimates (Observed and Shannon) in GS macaques while on GFD (A,B); as well as comparisons between BOMI, GFD and RGB diets (C,D), Figure S3: miRNA (green) vs. claudin-1 mRNA 3′ UTR (red) pairing using RNAhybrid algorithm. Note the perfect Watson and Crick base pairing in miRNA 5′ seed nucleotides (nts) 2–7 (bracket) and extra homology in 3′ region of miR-203, miR-204 and miR-29b with claudin-1 mRNA 3′ UTR, Table S1: Rhesus macaque stool sample descriptions, Table S2: Primer sequences used for real time SYBR Green One-step qRT-PCR. Table S3. Kruskal-Wallis rank sum test—alpha-diversity metrics, Table S4: Kruskal-Wallis rank sum test—8 most abundant families, Table S5: Selected time points of GFD: D14–D70.

Acknowledgments: The authors would like to thank Hazel Thwin, Diane Pattison and Xavier Alvarez (Tulane University) for their technical support, and Daniel Morton (Second Genome) for his help with study design. Research reported in this publication was supported by the National Institute of Diabetes and Digestive and Kidney Diseases and National Institute on Drug Abuse of the National Institutes of Health under Award Numbers R42DK097976, R01DK083929, R01DA042524 as well as the NIH base grant of the Tulane National Primate Research Center OD011104-54. The content is solely the responsibility of the authors and does not necessarily represent the official views of the National Institutes of Health. The study was completed as part of the collaboration between Arcadia Biosciences, Second Genome Inc., PreCliniTria LLC., and Tulane University.

Author Contributions: Mahesh Mohan was responsible for miRNA-related work (miRNA profiling, tight junction protein analysis and miRNA-bacterial 16S rRNA homology analysis), participated in study design and manuscript preparation. Cheryl-Emiliane T. Chow and Caitlin N. Ryan performed sequence and statistical analyses, interpreted the data and assisted with manuscript preparation. Luisa S. Chan managed sample processing, assisted with study design, data interpretation and manuscript preparation. Jason Dufour provided veterinary care and participated in coordination of dietary regimens. Pyone P. Aye and James Blanchard helped with preparation and coordination of animal studies. Charles P. Moehs was responsible for preparation of the experimental diets as well as for the study's overall coordination and manuscript preparation. Karol Sestak formulated the study, coordinated the work, participated in data interpretation and wrote the manuscript.

Conflicts of Interest: The authors declare no conflict of interests.

References

1. Atarashi, K.; Honda, K. Microbiota in autoimmunity and tolerance. *Curr. Opin. Immunol.* **2011**, *23*, 761–768. [CrossRef] [PubMed]

2. Helander, H.F.; Fandriks, L. Surface area of the digestive tract-revisited. *Scand. J. Gastroenterol.* **2014**, *49*, 681–689. [CrossRef] [PubMed]

3. Lederberg, J. Infectious history. *Science* **2000**, *288*, 287–293. [CrossRef] [PubMed]

4. Turnbaugh, P.J.; Ley, R.E.; Hamady, M.; Fraser-Liggett, C.; Knight, R.; Gordon, J.I. The human microbiome project: Exploring the microbial part of ourselves in a changing world. *Nature* **2007**, *449*, 804–810. [CrossRef] [PubMed]

5. Li, M.; Wang, B.; Zhang, M.; Rantalainen, M.; Wang, S.; Zhou, H.; Zhang, Y.; Shen, J.; Pang, X.; Zhang, M.; et al. Symbiotic gut microbes modulate human metabolic phenotypes. *Proc. Natl. Acad. Sci. USA* **2008**, *105*, 2117–2122. [CrossRef] [PubMed]

6. Dethlefsen, L.; McFall-Ngai, M.; Relman, D.A. An ecological and evolutionary perspective on human-microbe mutualism and disease. *Nature* **2007**, *449*, 811–818. [CrossRef] [PubMed]

7. Nicholson, J.K.; Holmes, E.; Kinross, J.; Burcelin, R.; Gibson, G.; Jia, W.; Pettersson, S. Host-gut microbiota metabolic interactions. *Science* **2012**, *336*, 1262–1267. [CrossRef] [PubMed]

8. Ley, R.E.; Hamady, M.; Lozupone, C.; Turnbaugh, P.; Ramey, R.R.; Bircher, J.S.; Schlegel, M.L.; Tucker, T.A.; Schrenzel, M.D.; Knight, R.; et al. Evolution of mammals and their gut microbes. *Science* **2008**, *320*, 1647–1651. [CrossRef] [PubMed]

9. Zoetendal, E.; Rajilić-Stojanović, M.; De Vos, W. High-throughput diversity and functionality analysis of the gastrointestinal tract microbiota. *Gut* **2008**, *57*, 1605–1615. [CrossRef] [PubMed]

10. Arumugam, M.; Raes, J.; Pelletier, E.; Le Paslier, D.; Yamada, T.; Mende, D.R.; Fernandes, G.R.; Tap, J.; Bruls, T.; Batto, J.M.; et al. Enterotypes of the human gut microbiome. *Nature* **2011**, *473*, 174–180. [CrossRef] [PubMed]

11. Wu, G.D.; Chen, J.; Hoffmann, C.; Bittinger, K.; Chen, Y.Y.; Keilbaugh, S.A.; Bewtra, M.; Knights, D.; Walters, W.A.; Knight, R.; et al. Linking long-term dietary patterns with gut microbial enterotypes. *Science* **2011**, *334*, 105–108. [CrossRef] [PubMed]

12. Yatsunenko, T.; Rey, F.E.; Manary, M.J.; Trehan, I.; Dominguez-Bello, M.G.; Contreras, M.; Magris, M.; Hidalgo, G.; Baldassano, R.N.; Anokhin, A.P.; et al. Human gut microbiome viewed across age and geography. *Nature* **2012**, *486*, 222–227. [CrossRef] [PubMed]

13. Tyakht, A.V.; Kostryukova, E.S.; Popenko, A.S.; Belenikin, M.S.; Pavlenko, A.V.; Larin, A.K.; Karpova, I.Y.; Selezneva, O.V.; Semashko, T.A.; Ospanova, E.A.; et al. Human gut microbiota community structures in urban and rural populations in Russia. *Nat. Commun.* **2013**. [CrossRef] [PubMed]

14. Bergström, A.; Skov, T.H.; Bahl, M.I.; Roager, H.M.; Christensen, L.B.; Ejlerskov, K.T.; Mølgaard, C.; Michaelsen, K.F.; Licht, T.R. Establishment of intestinal microbiota during early life: A longitudinal, explorative study of a large cohort of Danish infants. *Appl. Environ. Microbiol.* **2014**, *80*, 2889–2900. [CrossRef] [PubMed]

15. Ma, J.; Prince, A.L.; Bader, D.; Hu, M.; Ganu, R.; Baquero, K.; Blundell, P.; Harris, R.A.; Frias, A.E.; Grove, K.L.; et al. High-fat maternal diet during pregnancy persistently alters the offspring microbiome in a primate model. *Nat. Commun.* **2014**, *5*. [CrossRef] [PubMed]

16. Schnorr, S.L.; Candela, M.; Rampelli, S.; Centanni, M.; Consolandi, C.; Basaglia, G.; Turroni, S.; Biagi, E.; Peano, C.; Severgnini, M.; et al. Gut microbiome of the Hadza hunter-gatherers. *Nat. Commun.* **2014**, *5*, 3654. [CrossRef] [PubMed]

17. David, L.A.; Materna, A.C.; Friedman, J.; Campos-Baptista, M.I.; Blackburn, M.C.; Perrotta, A.; Erdman, S.E.; Alm, E.J. Host lifestyle affects human microbiota on daily timescales. *Genome Biol.* **2014**, *15*, R8. [CrossRef] [PubMed]

18. Martin, M.E.; Bhatnagar, S.; George, M.D.; Paster, B.J.; Canfield, D.R.; Eisen, J.A.; Solnick, J.V. The impact of *Helicobacter pylori* infection on the gastric microbiota of the rhesus macaque. *PLoS ONE* **2013**, *8*, e76375. [CrossRef] [PubMed]

19. McKenna, P.; Hoffmann, C.; Minkah, N.; Aye, P.P.; Lackner, A.; Liu, Z.; Lozupone, C.A.; Hamady, M.; Knight, R.; Bushman, F.D. The macaque gut microbiome in health, lentiviral infection, and chronic enterocolitis. *PLoS Pathog.* **2008**, *4*, e20. [CrossRef] [PubMed]

20. De Filippo, C.; Cavalieri, D.; Di Paola, M.; Ramazzotti, M.; Poullet, J.B.; Massart, S.; Collini, S.; Pieraccini, G.; Lionetti, P. Impact of diet in shaping gut microbiota revealed by a comparative study in children from Europe and rural Africa. *Proc. Natl. Acad. Sci. USA* **2010**, *107*, 14691–14696. [CrossRef] [PubMed]

21. Ou, J.; Carbonero, F.; Zoetendal, E.G.; DeLany, J.P.; Wang, M.; Newton, K.; Gaskins, H.R.; O'Keefe, S.J. Diet, microbiota, and microbial metabolites in colon cancer risk in rural Africans and African Americans. *Am. J. Clin. Nutr.* **2013**, *98*, 111–120. [CrossRef] [PubMed]

22. Ardeshir, A.; Narayan, N.R.; Méndez-Lagares, G.; Lu, D.; Rauch, M.; Huang, Y.; Van Rompay, K.K.; Lynch, S.V.; Hartigan-O'Connor, D.J. Breast-fed and bottle-fed infant rhesus macaques develop distinct gut microbiotas and immune systems. *Sci. Transl. Med.* **2014**, *6*, 252ra120. [CrossRef] [PubMed]

23. Broadhurst, M.J.; Ardeshir, A.; Kanwar, B.; Mirpuri, J.; Gundra, U.M.; Leung, J.M.; Wiens, K.E.; Vujkovic-Cvijin, I.; Kim, C.C.; Yarovinsky, F.; et al. Therapeutic helminth infection of macaques with idiopathic chronic diarrhea alters the inflammatory signature and mucosal microbiota of the colon. *PLoS Pathog.* **2012**, *8*, e1003000. [CrossRef] [PubMed]

24. Ardeshir, A.; Sankaran, S.; Oslund, K.; Hartigan-O'Connor, D.; Lerche, N.; Hyde, D.; Dandekar, S. Inulin treatment leads to changes in intestinal microbiota and resolution of idiopathic chronic diarrhea in rhesus macaques. *Ann. Am. Thorac. Soc.* **2014**, *11*, S75–S75. [CrossRef]

25. Lupp, C.; Robertson, M.L.; Wickham, M.E.; Sekirov, I.; Champion, O.L.; Gaynor, E.C.; Finlay, B.B. Host-mediated inflammation disrupts the intestinal microbiota and promotes the overgrowth of Enterobacteriaceae. *Cell Host Microbe* **2007**, *2*, 119–129. [CrossRef] [PubMed]

26. Sokol, H.; Seksik, P. The intestinal microbiota in inflammatory bowel diseases: Time to connect with the host. *Curr. Opin. Gastroenterol.* **2010**, *26*, 327–331. [CrossRef] [PubMed]

27. Morgan, X.C.; Tickle, T.L.; Sokol, H.; Gevers, D.; Devaney, K.L.; Ward, D.V.; Reyes, J.A.; Shah, S.A.; LeLeiko, N.; Snapper, S.B.; et al. Dysfunction of the intestinal microbiome in inflammatory bowel disease and treatment. *Genome Biol.* **2012**, *13*, R79. [CrossRef] [PubMed]

28. Tong, M.; Li, X.; Parfrey, L.W.; Roth, B.; Ippoliti, A.; Wei, B.; Borneman, J.; McGovern, D.P.; Frank, D.N.; Li, E.; et al. A modular organization of the human intestinal mucosal microbiota and its association with Inflammatory Bowel Disease. *PLoS ONE* **2013**, *8*, e80702. [CrossRef] [PubMed]

29. Walujkar, S.A.; Dhotre, D.P.; Marathe, N.P.; Lawate, P.S.; Bharadwaj, R.S.; Shouche, Y.S. Characterization of bacterial community shift in human Ulcerative Colitis patients revealed by Illumina based 16S rRNA gene amplicon sequencing. *Gut Path.* **2014**, *6*, 22. [CrossRef] [PubMed]

30. Lucke, K.; Miehlke, S.; Jacobs, E.; Schuppler, M. Prevalence of *Bacteroides* and *Prevotella* spp. in ulcerative colitis. *J. Med. Microbiol.* **2006**, *55*, 617–624. [CrossRef] [PubMed]

31. De Palma, G.; Nadal, I.; Collado, M.C.; Sanz, Y. Effects of a gluten-free diet on gut microbiota and immune function in healthy adult human subjects. *Br. J. Nutr.* **2009**, *102*, 1154–1160. [CrossRef] [PubMed]

32. De Palma, G.; Capilla, A.; Nova, E.; Castillejo, G.; Varea, V.; Pozo, T.; Garrote, J.A.; Polanco, I.; López, A.; Ribes-Koninckx, C.; et al. Influence of milk-feeding type and genetic risk of developing coeliac disease on intestinal microbiota of infants: The PROFICEL study. *PLoS ONE* **2012**, *7*, e30791. [CrossRef] [PubMed]

33. Sellitto, M.; Bai, G.; Serena, G.; Fricke, W.F.; Sturgeon, C.; Gajer, P.; White, J.R.; Koenig, S.S.; Sakamoto, J.; Boothe, D.; et al. Proof of concept of microbiome-metabolome analysis and delayed gluten exposure on celiac disease autoimmunity in genetically at-risk infants. *PLoS ONE* **2012**, *7*, e33387. [CrossRef] [PubMed]

34. Cheng, J.; Kalliomäki, M.; Heilig, H.G.; Palva, A.; Lähteenoja, H.; de Vos, W.M.; Salojärvi, J.; Satokari, R. Duodenal microbiota composition and mucosal homeostasis in pediatric celiac disease. *BMC Gastroenterol.* **2013**, *13*, 113. [CrossRef] [PubMed]

35. Sánchez, E.; Donat, E.; Ribes-Koninckx, C.; Fernández-Murga, M.L.; Sanz, Y. Duodenal-mucosal bacteria associated with celiac disease in children. *Appl. Environ. Microbiol.* **2013**, *79*, 5472–5479. [CrossRef] [PubMed]

36. Ivarsson, A.; Persson, L.Å.; Nyström, L.; Ascher, H.; Cavell, B.; Danielsson, L.; Dannaeus, A.; Lindberg, T.; Lindquist, B.; Stenhammar, L.; et al. Epidemic of coeliac disease in Swedish children. *Acta Paediatr.* **2000**, *89*, 165–171. [CrossRef] [PubMed]

37. Ou, G.; Hedberg, M.; Hörstedt, P.; Baranov, V.; Forsberg, G.; Drobni, M.; Sandström, O.; Wai, S.N.; Johansson, I.; Hammarström, M.L.; et al. Proximal small intestinal microbiota and identification of rod-shaped bacteria associated with childhood celiac disease. *Am. J. Gastroenterol.* **2009**, *104*, 3058–3067. [CrossRef] [PubMed]

38. Sjöberg, V.; Sandström, O.; Hedberg, M.; Hammarström, S.; Hernell, O.; Hammarström, M.L. Intestinal T-cell responses in celiac disease—Impact of celiac disease associated bacteria. *PLoS ONE* **2013**, *8*, e53414. [CrossRef] [PubMed]

39. Caminero, A.; Herrán, A.R.; Nistal, E.; Pérez-Andrés, J.; Vaquero, L.; Vivas, S.; de Morales, J.M.; Albillos, S.M.; Casqueiro, J. Diversity of the cultivable human gut microbiome involved in gluten metabolism: Isolation of microorganisms with potential interest for coeliac disease. *FEMS Microbiol. Ecol.* **2014**, *88*, 309–319. [CrossRef] [PubMed]

40. D'Argenio, V.; Casaburi, G.; Precone, V.; Pagliuca, C.; Colicchio, R.; Sarnataro, D.; Discepolo, V.; Kim, S.M.; Russo, I.; Blanco, G.D.; et al. Metagenomics reveals dysbiosis and a potentially pathogenic N. *flavescens* strain in duodenum of adult celiac patients. *Am. J. Gastroenterol.* **2016**, *111*, 879–890. [CrossRef] [PubMed]

41. Xu, H.; Feely, S.L.; Wang, X.; Liu, D.X.; Borda, J.T.; Dufour, J.; Li, W.; Aye, P.P.; Doxiadis, G.G.; Khosla, C.; et al. Gluten-sensitive enteropathy coincides with decreased capability of intestinal T cells to secrete IL-17 and IL-22 in a macaque model for celiac disease. *Clin. Immunol.* **2013**, *147*, 40–49. [CrossRef] [PubMed]

42. Liu, S.; da Cunha, A.P.; Rezende, R.M.; Cialic, R.; Wei, Z.; Bry, L.; Comstock, L.E.; Gandhi, R.; Weiner, H.L. The Host Shapes the Gut Microbiota via Fecal MicroRNA. *Cell Host Microbe* **2016**, *19*, 32–43. [CrossRef] [PubMed]

43. Sestak, K.; Thwin, H.; Dufour, J.; Aye, P.P.; Liu, D.X.; Moehs, C.P. The effects of reduced gluten barley diet on humoral and cell-mediated systemic immune responses of gluten-sensitive rhesus macaques. *Nutrients* **2015**, *7*, 1657–1671. [CrossRef] [PubMed]

44. Sestak, K.; Merritt, C.K.; Borda, J.; Saylor, E.; Schwamberger, S.R.; Cogswell, F.; Didier, E.S.; Didier, P.J.; Plauche, G.; Bohm, R.P.; et al. Infectious agent and immune response characteristics of chronic enterocolitis in captive rhesus macaques. *Infect. Immun.* **2003**, *71*, 4079–4086. [CrossRef] [PubMed]

45. Sestak, K.; Thwin, H.; Dufour, J.; Liu, D.X.; Alvarez, X.; Laine, D.; Clarke, A.; Doyle, A.; Aye, P.P.; Blanchard, J.; et al. Supplementation of reduced gluten barley diet with oral prolyl endopeptidase effectively abrogates enteropathy-associated changes in gluten-sensitive macaques. *Nutrients* **2016**, *8*, 1–13. [CrossRef] [PubMed]

46. Caporaso, J.G.; Lauber, C.L.; Walters, W.A.; Berg-Lyons, D.; Lozupone, C.A.; Turnbaugh, P.J.; Fierer, N.; Knight, R. Global patterns of 16S rRNA diversity at a depth of millions of sequences per sample. *Proc. Natl. Acad. Sci. USA* **2011**, *108* (Suppl. 1), 4516–4522. [CrossRef] [PubMed]

47. McDonald, D.; Price, M.N.; Goodrich, J.; Nawrocki, E.P.; DeSantis, T.Z.; Probst, A.; Andersen, G.L.; Knight, R.; Hugenholtz, P. An improved Greengenes taxonomy with explicit ranks for ecological and evolutionary analyses of bacteria and archaea. *ISME J.* **2012**, *6*, 610–618. [CrossRef] [PubMed]

48. Edgar, R.C. UPARSE: Highly accurate OTU sequences from microbial amplicon reads. *Nat. Methods* **2013**, *10*, 996–998. [CrossRef] [PubMed]

49. DeSantis, T.Z.; Hugenholtz, N.; Larsen, N.; Rojas, M.; Brodie, E.L.; Keller, K.; Huber, T.; Dalevi, D.; Hu, P.; Andersen, G.L. Greengenes, a chimera-checked 16S rRNA gene database and workbench compatible with ARB. *Appl. Environ. Microbiol.* **2006**, *72*, 5069–5072. [CrossRef] [PubMed]

50. Anderson, M.J. A new method for non-parametric multivariate analysis of variance. *Aust. Ecol.* **2001**, *26*, 32–46.

51. Love, M.; Huber, W.; Anders, S. Moderated estimation of fold change and dispersion for RNA-seq data with DESeq2. *Genome Biol.* **2014**, *15*. [CrossRef] [PubMed]

52. McMurdie, P.J.; Holmes, S. Waste Not, Want Not: Why Rarefying Microbiome Data Is Inadmissible. *PLoS Comput. Biol.* **2014**, *10*, e1003531. [CrossRef] [PubMed]

53. Mohan, M.; Kumar, V.; Lackner, A.A.; Alvarez, X. Dysregulated miR-34a-SIRT1-acetyl p65 axis is a potential mediator of immune activation in the colon during chronic simian immunodeficiency virus infection of rhesus macaques. *J. Immunol.* **2015**, *194*, 291–306. [CrossRef] [PubMed]

54. Chandra, L.C.; Kumar, V.; Torben, W.; Stouwe, C.V.; Winsauer, P.; Amedee, A.; Molina, P.E.; Mohan, M. Chronic administration of Δ9-tetrahydrocannabinol induces intestinal anti-inflammatory microRNA expression during acute SIV infection of rhesus macaques. *J. Virol.* **2015**, *89*, 1168–1181. [CrossRef] [PubMed]

55. Zhou, Q.; Costinean, S.; Croce, C.M.; Brasier, A.R.; Merwat, S.; Larson, S.A.; Basra, S.; Verne, G.N. MicroRNA 29 targets nuclear factor-κB-repressing factor and Claudin 1 to increase intestinal permeability. *Gastroenterology* **2015**, *148*, 158–169. [CrossRef] [PubMed]

56. Ke, X.F.; Fang, J.; Wu, X.N.; Yu, C.H. MicroRNA-203 accelerates apoptosis in LPS-stimulated alveolar epithelial cells by targeting PIK3CA. *Biochem. Biophys. Res. Commun.* **2014**, *450*, 1297–1303. [CrossRef] [PubMed]

57. Peck, B.C.; Weiser, M.; Lee, S.E.; Gipson, G.R.; Iyer, V.B.; Sartor, R.B.; Herfarth, H.H.; Long, M.D.; Hansen, J.J.; Isaacs, K.L.; et al. MicroRNAs Classify Different Disease Behavior Phenotypes of Crohn's Disease and May Have Prognostic Utility. *Inflamm. Bowel Dis.* **2015**, *21*, 2178–2187. [CrossRef] [PubMed]

58. Li, G.; Luna, C.; Qiu, J.; Epstein, D.L.; Gonzalez, P. Role of miR-204 in the regulation of apoptosis, endoplasmic reticulum stress response, and inflammation in human trabecular meshwork cells. *Investig. Ophthalmol. Vis. Sci.* **2011**, *52*, 2999–3007. [CrossRef] [PubMed]

59. Zhang, B.; Liu, S.Q.; Li, C.; Lykken, E.; Jiang, S.; Wong, E.; Gong, Z.; Tao, Z.; Zhu, B.; Wan, Y.; et al. MicroRNA-23a Curbs Necrosis during Early T Cell Activation by Enforcing Intracellular Reactive Oxygen Species Equilibrium. *Immunity* **2016**, *44*, 568–581. [CrossRef] [PubMed]

60. Zhu, S.; Pan, W.; Song, X.; Liu, Y.; Shao, X.; Tang, Y.; Liang, D.; He, D.; Wang, H.; Liu, W.; et al. The microRNA miR-23b suppresses IL-17-associated autoimmune inflammation by targeting TAB2, TAB3 and IKK-α. *Nat. Med.* **2012**, *18*, 1077–1086. [CrossRef] [PubMed]

61. Chapman, C.G.; Pekow, J. The emerging role of miRNAs in inflammatory bowel disease: A review. *Ther. Adv. Gastroenterol.* **2015**, *8*, 4–22. [CrossRef] [PubMed]

62. Krüger, J.; Rehmsmeier, M. RNAhybrid: microRNA target prediction easy, fast and flexible. *Nucl. Acids Res.* **2006**, *34*, 451–454. [CrossRef] [PubMed]

63. Cichon, C.; Sabharwal, H.; Rüter, C.; Schmidt, M.A. MicroRNAs regulate tight junction proteins and modulate epithelial/endothelial barrier functions. *Tissue Barriers* **2014**, *2*, e944446. [CrossRef] [PubMed]

64. Yang, H.; Rao, J.N.; Wang, J.Y. Posttranscriptional Regulation of Intestinal Epithelial Tight Junction Barrier by RNA-binding Proteins and microRNAs. *Tissue Barriers* **2014**, *2*, e28320. [CrossRef] [PubMed]

65. Bressan, W. Biological control of maize seed pathogenic fungi by use of actinomycetes. *BioControl* **2003**, *48*, 233–240. [CrossRef]

66. Agarwal, V.; Bell, G.W.; Nam, J.W.; Bartel, D.P. Predicting effective microRNA target sites in mammalian mRNAs. *eLife* **2015**, *4*. [CrossRef] [PubMed]

67. Pound, L.D.; Kievit, P.; Grove, K.L. The nonhuman primate as a model for type 2 diabetes. *Curr. Opin. Endocrinol. Diabetes Obes.* **2014**, *21*, 89–94. [CrossRef] [PubMed]

68. Sui, Y.; Gordon, S.; Franchini, G.; Berzofsky, J.A. Nonhuman primate models for HIV/AIDS vaccine development. *Curr. Protoc. Immunol.* **2013**, *102*, 12–14.

69. Beaudoin-Gobert, M.; Sgambato-Faure, V. Serotonergic pharmacology in animal models: From behavioral disorders to dyskinesia. *Neuropharmacology* **2014**, *81*, 15–30. [CrossRef] [PubMed]

70. Yasuda, K.; Oh, K.; Ren, B.; Tickle, T.L.; Franzosa, E.A.; Wachtman, L.M.; Miller, A.D.; Westmoreland, S.V.; Mansfield, K.G.; Vallender, E.J.; et al. Biogeography of the intestinal mucosal and luminal microbiome in the rhesus macaque. *Cell Host Microbe* **2015**, *17*, 385–391. [CrossRef] [PubMed]

71. Dassanayake, R.P.; Zhou, Y.; Hinkley, S.; Stryker, C.J.; Plauche, G.; Borda, J.T.; Sestak, K.; Duhamel, G.E. Characterization of cytolethal distending toxin of Campylobacter species isolated from captive macaque monkeys. *J. Clin. Microbiol.* **2005**, *43*, 641–649. [CrossRef] [PubMed]

72. Ardeshir, A.; Oslund, K.L.; Ventimiglia, F.; Yee, J.; Lerche, N.W.; Hyde, D.M. Idiopathic microscopic colitis of rhesus macaques: Quantitative assessment of colonic mucosa. *Anat. Rec.* **2013**, *296*, 1169–1179. [CrossRef] [PubMed]

73. Zeller, J.; Takeuchi, A. Infection of the colon of the rhesus monkey by spiral-shaped organisms. *Vet. Pathol. Suppl.* **1982**, *7*, 26–32. [CrossRef] [PubMed]

74. Ley, R.E.; Turnbaugh, P.J.; Klein, S.; Gordon, J.I. Human gut microbes associated with obesity. *Nature* **2006**, *444*, 1022–1023. [CrossRef] [PubMed]

75. Honda, K.; Littman, D.R. The microbiome in infectious disease and inflammation. *Ann. Rev. Immunol.* **2012**, *30*, 759–795. [CrossRef] [PubMed]

76. Caminero, A.; Galipeau, H.J.; McCarville, J.L.; Johnston, C.W.; Bernier, S.P.; Russell, A.K.; Jury, J.; Herran, A.R.; Casqueiro, J.; Tye-Din, J.A.; et al. Duodenal bacteria from patients with celiac disease and healthy subjects distinctly affect gluten breakdown and immunogenicity. *Gastroenterology* **2016**, *151*, 670–683. [CrossRef] [PubMed]

77. Mahajan, G.B.; Balachandran, L. Antibacterial agents from actinomycetes—A Review. *Front. Biosci.* **2012**, *4*, 240–253. [CrossRef]

78. Barcia, G.; Posar, A.; Santucci, M.; Parmeggiani, A. Autism and coeliac disease. *J. Autism Dev. Disord.* **2008**, *38*, 407–408. [CrossRef] [PubMed]

79. Gilbert, J.A.; Krajmalnik-Brown, R.; Porazinska, D.L.; Weiss, S.J.; Knight, R. Toward effective probiotics for Autism and other neurodevelopmental disorders. *Cell* **2013**, *155*, 1446–1448. [CrossRef] [PubMed]

80. Scheperjans, F.; Aho, V.; Pereira, P.A.; Koskinen, K.; Paulin, L.; Pekkonen, E.; Haapaniemi, E.; Kaakkola, S.; Eerola-Rautio, J.; Pohja, M.; et al. Gut microbiota are related to Parkinson's disease and clinical phenotype. *Mov. Disord.* **2014**, *30*, 350–358. [CrossRef] [PubMed]

81. Kang, D.W.; Park, J.G.; Ilhan, Z.E.; Wallstrom, G.; LaBaer, J.; Adams, J.B.; Krajmalnik-Brown, R. Reduced incidence of *Prevotella* and other fermenters in intestinal microflora of autistic children. *PLoS ONE* **2013**, *8*, e68322. [CrossRef] [PubMed]

82. Sestak, K.; Conroy, L.; Aye, P.P.; Mehra, S.; Doxiadis, G.G.; Kaushal, D. Improved xenobiotic metabolism and reduced susceptibility to cancer in gluten-sensitive macaques upon introduction of a gluten-free diet. *PLoS ONE* **2011**, *6*, e18648. [CrossRef] [PubMed]

83. Ye, D.; Guo, S.; Al-Sadi, R.; Ma, T.Y. MicroRNA regulation of intestinal epithelial tight junction permeability. *Gastroenterology* **2011**, *141*, 1323–1333. [CrossRef] [PubMed]

84. Wacklin, P.; Laurikka, P.; Lindfors, K.; Collin, P.; Salmi, T.; Lähdeaho, M.L.; Saavalainen, P.; Mäki, M.; Mättö, J.; Kurppa, K.; et al. Altered duodenal microbiota composition in celiac disease patients suffering from persistent symptoms on a long-term gluten-free diet. *Am. J. Gastroenterol.* **2014**, *109*, 1933–1941. [CrossRef] [PubMed]

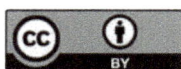

Article

Prevalence and Characterization of Self-Reported Gluten Sensitivity in The Netherlands

Tom van Gils [1,*], Petula Nijeboer [1], Catharina E. IJssennagger [1], David S. Sanders [2], Chris J. J. Mulder [1] and Gerd Bouma [1]

[1]   Celiac Center Amsterdam, Department Gastroenterology and Hepatology, VU University Medical Center, P.O. Box 7057, 1007 MB Amsterdam, The Netherlands; p.nijeboer@vumc.nl (P.N.); c.ijssennagger@vumc.nl (C.E.I.); cjmulder@vumc.nl (C.J.J.M.); g.bouma@vumc.nl (G.B.)
[2]   Academic Unit of Gastroenterology, Royal Hallamshire Hospital, Sheffield S10 2JF, UK; David.Sanders@sth.nhs.uk
*   Correspondence: t.vangils@vumc.nl; Tel.: +31-20-444-0613; Fax: +31-20-444-0554

Received: 20 September 2016; Accepted: 3 November 2016; Published: 8 November 2016

Abstract: Background: A growing number of individuals reports symptoms related to the ingestion of gluten-containing food in the absence of celiac disease. Yet the actual prevalence is not well established. Methods: Between April 2015 and March 2016, unselected adults visiting marketplaces, dental practices and a university in The Netherlands were asked to complete a modified validated questionnaire for self-reported gluten sensitivity (srGS). Results: Among the 785 adults enquired, two had celiac disease. Forty-nine (6.2%) reported symptoms related to the ingestion of gluten-containing food. These individuals were younger, predominantly female and lived more frequently in urban regions compared with the other respondents. Symptoms reported included bloating (74%), abdominal discomfort (49%) and flatulence (47%). A total of 23 (47%) srGS individuals reported having had tried a gluten-free or gluten-restricted diet. Abdominal discomfort related to fermentable oligosaccharide, disaccharide, monosaccharide and polyol (FODMAP)-containing food was more often reported in srGS individuals compared with the other respondents (73.5% vs. 21.7%, $p < 0.001$). Conclusion: Self-reported GS is common in The Netherlands, especially in younger individuals, females and urban regions, although the prevalence was lower than in a comparable recent UK study. It cannot be excluded that FODMAPs are in part responsible for these symptoms.

Keywords: gluten; non-celiac gluten sensitivity; non-celiac wheat sensitivity; celiac disease; irritable bowel syndrome; FODMAPs

1. Introduction

The concept of a causal relationship between the ingestion of gluten and the occurrence of symptoms in the absence of celiac disease (CD) and wheat allergy was first described in the late 1970s by Cooper and Ellis [1,2]. This clinical entity has been termed non-celiac gluten or wheat sensitivity (NCGS or NCWS) [3,4]. Over the past several years, NCWS has gained significant interest and the number of individuals embracing a gluten-free diet is rapidly growing [5]. The discussion of whether or not gluten can cause symptoms in the absence of CD is confused by a popular phenomenon of people who avoid gluten-containing food in the light of a healthier lifestyle which is related to the fast growth of the gluten-free market [6]. This theory that grains by means of their composition are unhealthy, should be distinguished from the question as to whether gluten can cause symptoms in the absence of CD and wheat allergy.

As defined by the 2015 Salerno Expert's Criteria [4], NCWS includes both intestinal and extra-intestinal symptoms which are related to the ingestion of gluten-containing food after exclusion of CD and wheat allergy. Most common symptoms include bloating, abdominal pain, diarrhea, tiredness and headache [4]. These symptoms display a significant overlap with the irritable bowel syndrome (IBS), which is one of the most common disorders in daily practice [7,8]. Although NCWS patients report that their symptoms are induced by gluten, it has been hypothesized that their symptoms may in fact be induced by other compounds in grains, among which a group of carbohydrates, referred to as fermentable oligo-, di-, monosaccharides and polyols (FODMAPs) have gained substantial interest [9].

Despite the overwhelming current interest in NCWS, the actual prevalence is difficult to establish in the absence of a gold standard. The number of studies that have addressed this question are sparse and the outcome varied widely between 0.6% and 13% [3,10–16].

Here, we studied the population prevalence of self-reported gluten sensitivity (srGS) in a large cohort of adults in the Dutch population.

2. Materials and Methods

2.1. Participants

Between April 2015 and March 2016, individuals visiting markets, dental practices and a university in The Netherlands were asked to participate in a survey from the Gastroenterology and Hepatology department of the VU University Medical Center, Amsterdam (The Netherlands). There was no referral to the subject of the study during recruiting respondents. Participants completed a modified version of a previously validated questionnaire as described elsewhere [12]. Participation was anonymous and informed consent was given by completing the survey. Exclusion criteria included individuals under 18 years of age. At all sites a trained person was available to support the respondents when necessary.

2.2. Questionnaire

The questionnaire was divided in four sections. The first comprised basic demographic information, including age, sex and education level. Living area was divided in urban and rural region based on the location where the respondents completed the questionnaire. Urban region was defined as the *Randstad*, a megalopolis in The Netherlands consisting of the four largest Dutch cities (Amsterdam, Rotterdam, The Hague and Utrecht). Rural area was defined as the area outside the *Randstad* and all these sites included small to middle-large villages with less than 20,000 inhabitants (Figure 1). A high education level was defined as having completed at least a higher professional education level or university education level.

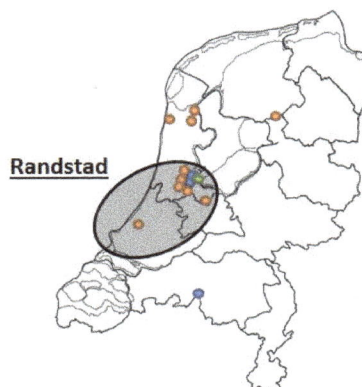

Figure 1. Sites where participants were recruited in The Netherlands. Orange: dental practice. Blue: market. Green: university. Circled: *Randstad* (considered as urban region).

The second section screened for symptoms consistent with irritable bowel syndrome (IBS) in accordance with the Rome III criteria: recurrent abdominal pain or discomfort during the last six months. These should be present on three or more days a month together with two or three of the following situations: improvement with defecation, onset associated with a change in frequency of stool and/or onset associated with a change in shape of stool [7]. Participants were also asked about their medical history.

The third section of the survey enquired about srGS and recognized related symptoms to gluten, as demonstrated by previous studies and those of expert opinions. In this section we also asked about the use of a GFD and other grain products in srGS as well as healthcare visits due to gluten-related symptoms. Respondents who did not reported gluten sensitivity or CD were considered as controls.

The fourth and final section of the survey enquired about abdominal discomfort due to 17 different high FODMAP-containing supplements.

2.3. Statistical Analysis

Statistical analysis was performed using SPSS version 22.0 software (SPSS Inc., Chicago, IL, USA). Categorical variables were summarized by descriptive statistics, including total numbers, percentages and odds ratio (OR). Significance was analyzed using the two-tailed Fisher exact test. Continuous variables were summarized by mean and standard deviation (sd), with significant differences between two groups analyzed using the Independent Samples T-test. A p-value of less than 0.05 was considered as statistically significant.

3. Results

A total of 785 adults completed the questionnaire, of whom 66% were recruited in dental practices, 28% at markets and 6% at a university. Two individuals had an established diagnosis of CD and were excluded from further analysis. Mean age at the time of survey was 47 years old (sd: 18 years, range 18–90) with a slight predominance of women (60%). The majority of questionnaires (57%) was completed in the urban region.

A total of 49 individuals (6.2%) indicated symptoms after the ingestion of gluten-containing foods. Such srGS individuals were younger (39 vs. 47 years old, $p = 0.001$), predominantly female (80% vs. 58%, $p < 0.01$) and mostly lived in the urban region (76% vs. 56%, $p < 0.01$) compared with the controls. Although not statistically significant, there was a trend for a higher education level in srGS individuals (49% with a high education level vs. 39%, not statistically significant).

3.1. Characteristics of Self-Reported Gluten Sensitivity

The most frequently reported intestinal symptoms in srGS were bloating, abdominal discomfort and flatulence. Tiredness and headache were the most frequent extra-intestinal symptoms reported, as shown in Figure 2. Especially bread ($n = 32$, 65%), pizza ($n = 15$, 31%) and pasta ($n = 18$, 37%) induced these symptoms. Interestingly, 35% ($n = 17$) of the srGS respondents reported a reduction of clinical signs when consuming spelt bread.

The median duration of symptoms was four years (range 0 months–40 years) at the time of the survey. Most srGS individuals ($n = 16$, 33%) reported symptoms nearly every day after eating gluten, with the onset of symptoms 1 to 6 h after ingestion of a gluten-containing food ($n = 23$, 47%). In most srGS individuals, these symptoms resolved within hours ($n = 29$, 59%). More details are shown in Figure 3.

The prevalence of individuals fulfilling the Rome III criteria for IBS in srGS was 37% vs. 9% in controls ($p < 0.001$). Medical history showed more often anxiety, anemia, chronic headache, IBS and gastro-intestinal reflux disease in srGS individuals. Table 1 shows basic demographic information and medical history. Family medical history was more often positive for CD, thyroid disease and IBS in srGS (Table 2).

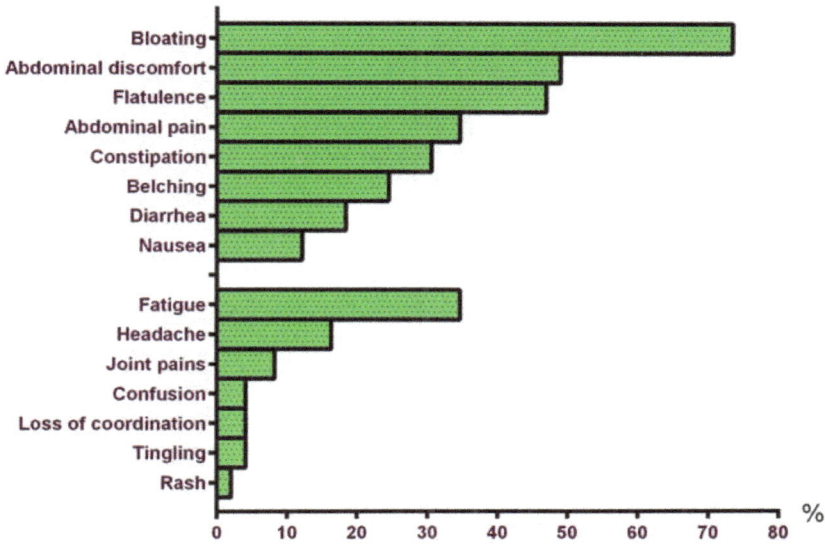

Figure 2. Intestinal and extra-intestinal symptoms in self-reported gluten sensitivity (*n* = 49).

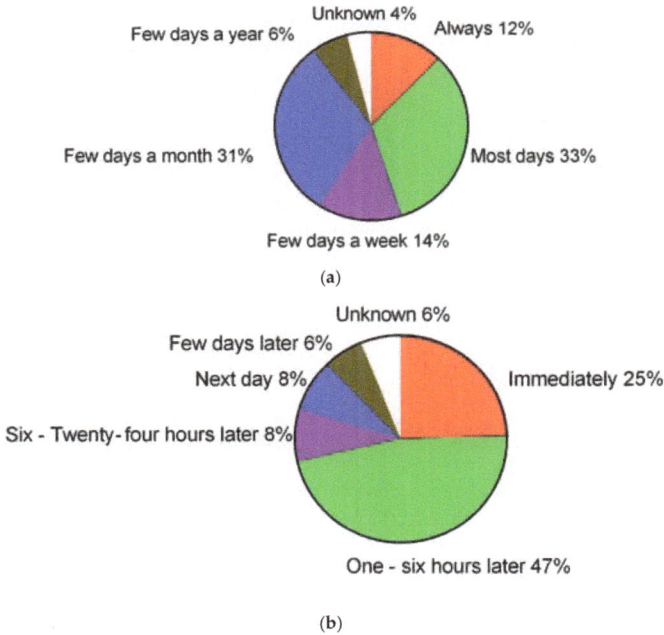

(a)

(b)

Figure 3. *Cont.*

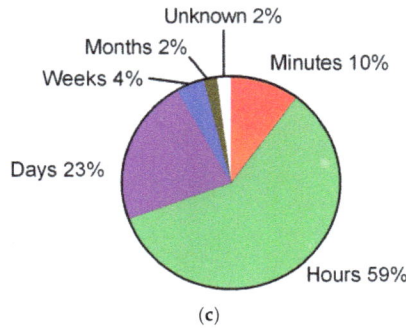

(c)

Figure 3. Frequency (**a**); time of onset (**b**) and duration (**c**) of srGS symptoms.

Table 1. Comparison between self-reported gluten sensitivity individuals and controls: basic demographic information and medical history.

Variables	srGS (*n* = 49) (6.2%)	Controls (*n* = 734) (93.5%)	Odds Ratio (95% CI)	*p*-Value
Mean age ± sd (years)	39 ± 15.1	47 ± 18.3	-	0.001
Sex (% female)	79.6	58.3	2.8 (1.4–5.7)	<0.01
Education level (% high educated)	49.0	39.3	1.5 (0.8–2.7)	NS
Region (% urban)	75.5	55.7	2.5 (1.3–4.8)	<0.01
Rome III criteria for IBS (%)	36.7	9.0	5.9 (3.1–11.1)	<0.001
Anxiety (%)	16.3	3.1	6.0 (2.5–14.3)	<0.001
Depression (%)	14.3	8.3	1.8 (0.8–4.3)	NS
Bipolar disorder (%)	2.0	0.4	5.1 (0.5–49.7)	NS
Schizophrenia (%)	0	0.1	-	NS
Thyroid disease (%)	4.1	4.6	0.9 (0.2–3.8)	NS
Diabetes mellitus (young age onset) (%)	4.1	1.1	3.9 (0.8–18.7)	NS
Anemia (%)	16.3	6.1	3.0 (1.3–6.8)	0.01
Chronic Fatigue (%)	6.1	3.1	2.0 (0.6–7.0)	NS
Fibromyalgia (%)	0	1.2	-	NS
Chronic fatigue syndrome (%)	2.0	0.8	2.5 (0.3–21.4)	NS
Rheumatoid arthritis (%)	4.1	4.0	1.0 (0.2–4.5)	NS
Chronic headache (%)	12.2	3.3	4.1 (1.6–10.6)	<0.01
Nut allergy (%)	2.0	1.8	1.2 (0.1–9.0)	NS
Egg allergy (%)	0	0.5	-	NS
Lactose intolerance (%)	2.0	1.4	1.5 (0.2–12.0)	NS
Inflammatory bowel disease (%)	4.1	1.2	3.4 (0.7–16.3)	NS
Gastro-intestinal reflux disease (%)	18.4	7.8	2.7 (1.2–5.8)	<0.05
Psoriasis (%)	4.1	2.0	2.0 (0.5–9.2)	NS

Table 2. Medical history of relatives.

Variables	srGS (*n* = 49) (6.2%)	Controls (*n* = 734) (93.5%)	Odds Ratio (95% CI)	*p*-Value
Celiac disease in all relatives (%)	8.2	2.5	3.4 (1.1–10.6)	<0.05
Celiac disease in children of srGS individuals (%)	6.1	0.4	15.9 (3.1–80.3)	<0.01
Rheumatoid arthritis (%)	30.6	20.2	1.7 (0.9–3.3)	NS
Diabetes mellitus (young age onset) (%)	14.3	7.6	2.0 (0.9–4.7)	NS
Thyroid disease (%)	20.4	8.9	2.6 (1.3–5.5)	<0.05
Psoriasis (%)	8.2	7.1	1.2 (0.4–3.4)	NS
Inflammatory bowel disease (%)	6.1	2.2	2.9 (0.8–10.4)	NS
Irritable bowel syndrome (%)	26.5	6.7	5.0 (2.5–10.1)	<0.001

Some srGS individuals reported self-initiated dietary changes, of whom two (4%) followed a strict gluten-free diet and 21 (43%) a gluten-restricted diet.

Eight srGS individuals (16%) visited their general practitioner, five (10%) visited a medical specialist, three (6%) visited an alternative healthcare professional, and two (4%) a dietician. The median time before consulting a healthcare professional after onset of the symptoms was two years (range 0 months–32 years). Six individuals (12%) underwent upper endoscopy examination. None of them reported a diagnosis of CD or other diagnosis after upper endoscopy examination.

3.2. Fermentable Oligosaccharides, Disaccharides, Monosaccharides and Polyols (FODMAPs)

Of all srGS individuals, 74% reported abdominal discomfort related to at least one high FODMAP-containing product compared to 22% of the controls (OR 10.0 (95% confidence interval 5.2–19.3), $p < 0.001$) with a predominance of legume, cabbage, onions and leek (Table 3).

Table 3. Comparison between self-reported gluten sensitivity individuals and controls: abdominal discomfort related to FODMAPs.

Variables	Self-Reported Gluten Sensitivity (n = 49) (6.2%)	Controls (n = 734) (93.5%)	Odds Ratio (95% Confidence Interval)	p-Value
Legume (%)	24.5	2.7	11.6 (5.3–25.5)	<0.001
Cabbage (%)	36.7	7.2	7.5 (3.9–14.2)	<0.001
Onion (%)	38.8	10.2	5.6 (3.0–10.4)	<0.001
Leek (%)	32.7	5.3	8.6 (4.4–17.0)	<0.001
Cauliflower (%)	22.4	3.4	8.2 (3.8–17.9)	<0.001
Mushroom (%)	12.2	2.3	5.9 (2.2–15.7)	<0.01
Apple (%)	10.2	2.0	5.4 (1.9–15.7)	<0.01
Cherry (%)	2.0	0.5	3.8 (0.4–34.7)	NS
Sugar-free gum (%)	12.2	2.7	5.0 (1.9–13.0)	<0.01
Plum (%)	10.2	3.3	3.4 (1.2–9.2)	<0.05
Pear (%)	8.2	1.8	4.9 (1.5–15.7)	<0.05
Mango (%)	2.0	0.4	5.1 (0.5–49.7)	NS
Watermelon (%)	4.1	0.3	15.6 (2.1–113.0)	<0.05
Milk (%)	20.4	4.6	5.3 (2.4–11.5)	<0.001
Buttermilk (%)	8.2	2.0	4.3 (1.4–13.4)	<0.05
Yogurt (%)	14.3	3.3	4.9 (2.0–12.1)	<0.01
Custard (%)	18.4	1.8	12.5 (5.0–30.9)	<0.001

4. Discussion

This study confirms that a significant part of the general adult population reports sensitivity to gluten-containing foods. The percentage is substantially less (6.2%) than in a recent comparable UK study (13%) [12]. Second, we showed that self-reported gluten sensitivity (srGS) individuals more frequently reported symptoms upon consumption of products high in FODMAPs. Third, quite surprisingly, we found that only a small number of the srGS individuals visited a doctor or ever consumed a self-initiated strict gluten-free diet (GFD).

Why srGS was found to be less prevalent in The Netherlands compared to the UK is unknown. It may be related to differences of media attention, but data to support this are lacking.

Despite the large growth of the gluten-free market [6] and the popularity of gluten-free products, knowledge about gluten is still low in the general population as described in Australian and UK literature [17,18]. Indeed, in our survey, a high percentage of srGS individuals (35%) reported no symptoms when consuming spelt bread.

In this study, type and onset of symptoms after consumption of gluten were comparable with other non-celiac wheat sensitivity (NCWS) studies [12,15,19,20]. As shown in Table 1, anxiety, chronic headache and gastro-intestinal reflux disease were more common in the srGS group compared with controls. These subjective health complaints are also common symptoms in patients with irritable bowel syndrome (IBS) and self-reported food intolerance in general [21–23].

A significant number of NCWS patients fulfills the Rome III IBS criteria with a strong overlap between NCWS and IBS symptoms [12]. Foods which are reported to be associated with IBS symptoms are commonly rich in gluten, wheat and carbohydrates [23]. Therefore NCWS could be seen as part of IBS with a gluten-free diet as treatment strategy. Although the pathophysiology of IBS is still not well understood, food could affect a variety of physiologic parameters important in IBS such as visceral perception, motility, permeability, microbiota composition, brain-gut interactions, neuro-endocrine function and immune activation [24].

It is well known that stress and anxiety may exacerbate or contribute to gastrointestinal symptoms [25]. Indeed, individuals with srGS often reported an association between increase of abdominal symptoms and stress (84% vs. 48% in the control group, OR 5.7, $p < 0.001$).

The mechanisms by which gluten causes symptoms in individuals without celiac disease (CD) is unknown. There are some indications that NCWS belongs to the group of the gluten-related disorders. The relatively large number of relatives with CD in srGS individuals could indicate a shared (genetic) predisposition, although current literature is not consistent about the relationship between HLA-DQ2 and NCWS [26–28]. Another indication for (mild) immune activation in NCWS comes from a study which showed that serum levels of soluble CD14 and lipopolysaccharide-binding protein as well as antibody reactivity to microbial antigens are elevated in NCWS patients with resolution after a GFD [29].

Whether or not such immune activation is triggered by gluten is not yet established. At this point, it cannot be excluded that other ingredients in grains, including wheat germ agglutinin [30] and amylase-trypsin inhibitors [31], are in fact responsible for these signs of immune activation.

An alternative explanation is that symptoms are not immune mediated, but caused by the result of other mechanisms. One such mechanism is luminal distention of the intestine via a combination of osmotic effects and gas production caused by bacterial fermentation of poorly absorbed short-chain carbohydrates referred to as FODMAPs [32,33]. FODMAPs can be found in a variety of products, including grains. In support of the FODMAP theory, we found that individuals reporting gluten sensitivity more often reported symptoms after consuming products high in FODMAPs and less symptoms after eating spelt bread.

It is remarkable that only a fraction of srGS individuals started a GFD and that only 16% of them had visited their general practitioner due to srGS. This indicates that apparently burden of symptoms was not severe enough to change the diet or might be related to costs and availability of gluten-free products [34].

5. Conclusions

This study confirms that gluten sensitivity is common, especially in younger individuals, females and in urban regions, although the prevalence was lower than in a comparable UK study. The high number of patients reporting symptoms in relation to FODMAPs suggests that FODMAPs are in fact responsible for part of the symptoms.

Supplementary Materials: The following are available online at http://www.mdpi.com/2072-6643/8/11/714/s1.

Acknowledgments: We would thank all participants who completed our questionnaire. We also would like to thank all sites who made it possible to conduct this questionnaire. Especially, we would thank Henk Brand who made it possible to contact all dentists.

Author Contributions: G.B., T.G., C.J.M., D.S.S. and P.N. conceived and designed the questionnaire; T.G. coordinated the survey conducting; T.G. and C.E.I. analyzed the data; T.G. and G.B. wrote the paper and C.J.M., D.S.S., P.N. and C.E.I. reviewed the manuscript.

Conflicts of Interest: D.S.S. has received educational grants for investigator-conceived and -led studies on both Coeliac Disease and Non-Coeliac Gluten Sensitivity from Schaer.

References

1. Cooper, B.T.; Holmes, G.K.; Ferguson, R.; Thompson, R.; Cooke, W.T. Proceedings: Chronic diarrhoea and gluten sensitivity. *Gut* **1976**, *17*, 398. [PubMed]
2. Ellis, A.; Linaker, B.D. Non-coeliac gluten sensitivity? *Lancet* **1978**, *1*, 1358–1359. [CrossRef]

3. Sapone, A.; Bai, J.C.; Ciacci, C.; Dolinsek, J.; Green, P.H.; Hadjivassiliou, M.; Kaukinen, K.; Rostami, K.; Sanders, D.S.; Schumann, M.; et al. Spectrum of gluten-related disorders: Consensus on new nomenclature and classification. *BMC Med.* **2012**, *10*, 13. [CrossRef] [PubMed]

4. Catassi, C.; Elli, L.; Bonaz, B.; Bouma, G.; Carroccio, A.; Castillejo, G.; Cellier, C.; Cristofori, F.; de Magistris, L.; Dolinsek, J.; et al. Diagnosis of non-celiac gluten sensitivity (ncgs): The salerno experts' criteria. *Nutrients* **2015**, *7*, 4966–4977. [CrossRef] [PubMed]

5. The Great Gluten-Free Scam. Available online: http://www.telegraph.co.uk/food-and-drink/news/the-great-gluten-free-scam/ (accessed on 1 September 2016).

6. Foschia, M.; Horstmann, S.; Arendt, E.K.; Zannini, E. Nutritional therapy–facing the gap between coeliac disease and gluten-free food. *Int. J. Food Microbiol.* **2016**. [CrossRef] [PubMed]

7. Longstreth, G.F.; Thompson, W.G.; Chey, W.D.; Houghton, L.A.; Mearin, F.; Spiller, R.C. Functional bowel disorders. *Gastroenterology* **2006**, *130*, 1480–1491. [CrossRef] [PubMed]

8. Di, S.A.; Biagi, F.; Gobbi, P.G.; Corazza, G.R. How I treat enteropathy-associated t-cell lymphoma. *Blood* **2012**, *119*, 2458–2468.

9. Biesiekierski, J.R.; Peters, S.L.; Newnham, E.D.; Rosella, O.; Muir, J.G.; Gibson, P.R. No effects of gluten in patients with self-reported non-celiac gluten sensitivity after dietary reduction of fermentable, poorly absorbed, short-chain carbohydrates. *Gastroenterology* **2013**, *145*, 320–328; e321–e323. [CrossRef] [PubMed]

10. Tanpowpong, P.; Ingham, T.R.; Lampshire, P.K.; Kirchberg, F.F.; Epton, M.J.; Crane, J.; Camargo, C.A., Jr. Coeliac disease and gluten avoidance in new zealand children. *Arch. Dis. Child* **2012**, *97*, 12–16. [CrossRef] [PubMed]

11. DiGiacomo, D.V.; Tennyson, C.A.; Green, P.H.; Demmer, R.T. Prevalence of gluten-free diet adherence among individuals without celiac disease in the USA: Results from the continuous national health and nutrition examination survey 2009–2010. *Scand. J. Gastroenterol.* **2013**, *48*, 921–925. [CrossRef] [PubMed]

12. Aziz, I.; Lewis, N.R.; Hadjivassiliou, M.; Winfield, S.N.; Rugg, N.; Kelsall, A.; Newrick, L.; Sanders, D.S. A UK study assessing the population prevalence of self-reported gluten sensitivity and referral characteristics to secondary care. *Eur. J. Gastroenterol. Hepatol.* **2014**, *26*, 33–39. [CrossRef] [PubMed]

13. Volta, U.; Bardella, M.T.; Calabro, A.; Troncone, R.; Corazza, G.R. An Italian prospective multicenter survey on patients suspected of having non-celiac gluten sensitivity. *BMC Med.* **2014**, *12*, 85. [CrossRef] [PubMed]

14. Castillo, N.E.; Theethira, T.G.; Leffler, D.A. The present and the future in the diagnosis and management of celiac disease. *Gastroenterol. Rep. (Oxf.)* **2015**, *3*, 3–11. [CrossRef] [PubMed]

15. Golley, S.; Corsini, N.; Topping, D.; Morell, M.; Mohr, P. Motivations for avoiding wheat consumption in australia: Results from a population survey. *Public Health Nutr.* **2015**, *18*, 490–499. [CrossRef] [PubMed]

16. Ontiveros, N.; Lopez-Gallardo, J.A.; Vergara-Jimenez, M.J.; Cabrera-Chavez, F. Self-reported prevalence of symptomatic adverse reactions to gluten and adherence to gluten-free diet in an adult mexican population. *Nutrients* **2015**, *7*, 6000–6015. [CrossRef] [PubMed]

17. Wu, J.H.; Neal, B.; Trevena, H.; Crino, M.; Stuart-Smith, W.; Faulkner-Hogg, K.; Yu Louie, J.C.; Dunford, E. Are gluten-free foods healthier than non-gluten-free foods? An evaluation of supermarket products in australia. *Br. J. Nutr.* **2015**, *114*, 448–454. [CrossRef] [PubMed]

18. Aziz, I.; Karajeh, M.A.; Zilkha, J.; Tubman, E.; Fowles, C.; Sanders, D.S. Change in awareness of gluten-related disorders among chefs and the general public in the uk: A 10-year follow-up study. *Eur. J. Gastroenterol. Hepatol.* **2014**, *26*, 1228–1233. [CrossRef] [PubMed]

19. Biesiekierski, J.R.; Newnham, E.D.; Shepherd, S.J.; Muir, J.G.; Gibson, P.R. Characterization of adults with a self-diagnosis of nonceliac gluten sensitivity. *Nutr. Clin. Pract.* **2014**, *29*, 504–509. [CrossRef] [PubMed]

20. Fasano, A.; Sapone, A.; Zevallos, V.; Schuppan, D. Nonceliac gluten sensitivity. *Gastroenterology* **2015**, *148*, 1195–1204. [CrossRef] [PubMed]

21. Young, E.; Stoneham, M.D.; Petruckevitch, A.; Barton, J.; Rona, R. A population study of food intolerance. *Lancet* **1994**, *343*, 1127–1130. [CrossRef]

22. Lind, R.; Arslan, G.; Eriksen, H.R.; Kahrs, G.; Haug, T.T.; Florvaag, E.; Berstad, A. Subjective health complaints and modern health worries in patients with subjective food hypersensitivity. *Dig. Dis. Sci.* **2005**, *50*, 1245–1251. [CrossRef] [PubMed]

23. Volta, U.; Pinto-Sanchez, M.I.; Boschetti, E.; Caio, G.P.; De Giorgio, R.; Verdu, E.F. Dietary triggers in irritable bowel syndrome: Is there a role for gluten. *J. Neurogastroenterol. Motil.* **2016**, *22*, 547–557. [CrossRef] [PubMed]

24. Chey, W.D. Food: The main course to wellness and illness in patients with irritable bowel syndrome. *Am. J. Gastroenterol.* **2016**, *111*, 366–371. [CrossRef] [PubMed]

25. Berstad, A. Functional dyspepsia-a conceptual framework. *Gut* **2000**, *47*, iv3–iv4; discussion iv10. [CrossRef] [PubMed]

26. Volta, U.; Tovoli, F.; Cicola, R.; Parisi, C.; Fabbri, A.; Piscaglia, M.; Fiorini, E.; Caio, G. Serological tests in gluten sensitivity (nonceliac gluten intolerance). *J. Clin. Gastroenterol.* **2012**, *46*, 680–685. [CrossRef] [PubMed]

27. Cecilio, L.A.; Bonatto, M.W. The prevalence of hla dq2 and dq8 in patients with celiac disease, in family and in general population. *Arq. Bras. Cir. Dig* **2015**, *28*, 183–185. [CrossRef] [PubMed]

28. Wahnschaffe, U.; Schulzke, J.D.; Zeitz, M.; Ullrich, R. Predictors of clinical response to gluten-free diet in patients diagnosed with diarrhea-predominant irritable bowel syndrome. *Clin. Gastroenterol. Hepatol.* **2007**, *5*, 844–850; quiz 769. [CrossRef] [PubMed]

29. Uhde, M.; Ajamian, M.; Caio, G.; De Giorgio, R.; Indart, A.; Green, P.H.; Verna, E.C.; Volta, U.; Alaedini, A. Intestinal cell damage and systemic immune activation in individuals reporting sensitivity to wheat in the absence of coeliac disease. *Gut* **2016**. [CrossRef] [PubMed]

30. Miyake, K.; Tanaka, T.; McNeil, P.L. Lectin-based food poisoning: A new mechanism of protein toxicity. *PLoS ONE* **2007**, *2*, e687. [CrossRef] [PubMed]

31. Junker, Y.; Zeissig, S.; Kim, S.J.; Barisani, D.; Wieser, H.; Leffler, D.A.; Zevallos, V.; Libermann, T.A.; Dillon, S.; Freitag, T.L.; et al. Wheat amylase trypsin inhibitors drive intestinal inflammation via activation of toll-like receptor 4. *J. Exp. Med.* **2012**, *209*, 2395–2408. [CrossRef] [PubMed]

32. Gibson, P.R.; Shepherd, S.J. Food choice as a key management strategy for functional gastrointestinal symptoms. *Am. J. Gastroenterol.* **2012**, *107*, 657–666, quiz 667. [CrossRef] [PubMed]

33. Nijeboer, P.; Bontkes, H.J.; Mulder, C.J.; Bouma, G. Non-celiac gluten sensitivity. Is it in the gluten or the grain? *J. Gastrointestin. Liver Dis.* **2013**, *22*, 435–440. [PubMed]

34. Burden, M.; Mooney, P.D.; Blanshard, R.J.; White, W.L.; Cambray-Deakin, D.R.; Sanders, D.S. Cost and availability of gluten-free food in the UK: In store and online. *Postgrad. Med. J.* **2015**, *91*, 622–626. [CrossRef] [PubMed]

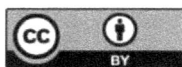

![nutrients logo] **nutrients**

MDPI

Article

Evolution of Gluten Content in Cereal-Based Gluten-Free Products: An Overview from 1998 to 2016

María Ángeles Bustamante, María Pilar Fernández-Gil, Itziar Churruca, Jonatan Miranda, Arrate Lasa, Virginia Navarro and Edurne Simón *

Gluten Analysis Laboratory of the University of the Basque Country, Department of Nutrition and Food Science, University of the Basque Country (UPV/EHU), Vitoria 01006, Spain; marian.bustamante@ehu.es (M.Á.B.); mariadelpilar.fernandez@ehu.es (M.P.F.-G.); itziar.txurruka@ehu.es (I.C.); jonatan.miranda@ehu.es (J.M.); arrate.lasa@ehu.es (A.L.); virginia.navarros@ehu.es (V.N.)
* Correspondence: edurne.simon@ehu.es; Tel.: +34-945-013-069

Received: 28 October 2016; Accepted: 16 December 2016; Published: 3 January 2017

Abstract: The treatment of Celiac disease consists in a strict lifelong gluten-free (GF) diet. As the ingestion of small amounts can have damaging complications, there has been an ongoing discussion regarding the safe threshold for dietary residual gluten. The aim was to analyze the evolution of gluten content in cereal-based GF foodstuffs (n = 3141) from 1998 to 2016 measured by the enzyme-linked immunosorbent assay (ELISA) technique. Eight categories were defined: flours, breakfast cereals/bars, bakery, pasta, breads, dough, snacks, and yeasts, and these were divided into GF labeled-foods (GF-L) or reportedly GF foodstuffs, but not certified (GF-NC). Gluten-detection was decreased over time in line with the evolving European regulations about food information and gluten content claims. This decline started sooner in GF-L products than in GF-NC. As a whole, gluten was detected in 371 samples, with breakfast cereals/bars being the most contaminated group. Snacks and yeasts changed from being high gluten-detected samples to being totally GF over the years. The downside is that, of contaminated samples, those in the low levels of gluten detection range have decreased while flour samples containing over 100 mg/kg gluten have risen in the 2013–2016 period. Obtained data confirm that GF cereal-based foods are becoming safer but gluten control must be maintained.

Keywords: gluten-free; cereal based foodstuff; gluten content evolution; ELISA; European regulation

1. Introduction

The only treatment for Celiac disease (CD) is the exclusion of gluten-containing cereals (e.g., wheat, rye, barley, and other closely-related cereal grains) and their derivatives in a strict lifelong gluten-free (GF) diet, achieving complete remission of symptoms. However, the ingestion of small amounts of gluten (which is called dietary transgression) can have serious and damaging complications [1]. For the majority of the individuals affected, intakes below 10 mg/day are unlikely to cause histological changes, while some authors have found that daily exposure to 50 mg/day is likely to damage intestinal mucosa [2,3].

Maintenance of a reliable gluten-free diet is a challenge, due to the fact that gluten is present in many more forms than just flours, bread, pasta or other cereal derivatives. Firstly, inherently gluten-free grains, such as rice, maize, quinoa, buckwheat, millet, or sorghum can be contaminated with gluten at different steps during their cultivation and processing, such as, crop rotation, milling, transportation, or handling. Furthermore, hidden sources of this protein can be commonly consumed because gluten is also widely used in several types of foodstuff as a thickener, flavour enhancer, emulsifier, filler, and fortification ingredient [4].

Taking the above into account, it has been difficult to establish a secure cutoff for residual gluten amount in GF products. In fact, for many years the standards of the Codex Alimentary Commission (the international organization founded by Food and Agriculture Organization and the World Health Organization) for gluten-free products dated back to 1979. At that time, Codex stated in the GF labelling purposes that products could be labelled gluten-free when total nitrogen content from the protein gluten did not exceed 0.05 g per 100 g of dry food, which was established as 200 mg/kg or ppm [5].

In 2008 The Codex standard for "foods for special dietary use for persons intolerant to gluten" [6] and the European Commission (Commission Regulation (EC) No. 41/2009) [7] introduced compositional and labelling standards that set levels of gluten for foods claiming to be either "gluten-free" (less than 20 mg per 1 kg food or 20 ppm) or "very low gluten" (less than 100 mg per 1 kg food, also expressed as 100 ppm). A similar rule for gluten-free labeling was established by the Food and Drug Administration (FDA) in 2013 [8].

Nowadays, Regulation (EC) No. 41/2009 has been repealed and these levels are supported by the Commission Implementing Regulation (EU) No. 828/2014. This regulation explains that different gluten sensitivity levels vary among people with gluten intolerance over a restricted range and that, on this basis, a food market with different low levels of gluten, always within that range, should be possible. Thus, this new standard allows the inclusion of food information for consumers accompanied by the statements "suitable for people intolerant to gluten" or "suitable for celiac" either for "gluten-free" or for "very low gluten" foods [9]. Nevertheless, considering that individual gluten sensitivity of celiac people is not commonly known, the general recommendation is to consume foodstuffs with the lowest gluten content and, thus, those advisory statements could be misleading among celiac consumers. In fact, the Association of European Celiac Societies (AOECS), only licences the use of the Cross-Grain symbol—quality mark—to manufactured products containing less than 20 mg/kg, that is, "gluten-free".

Although the market demand for GF food products is long-established, in recent years growing consumer need for GF foods has led to an increased development of these products. Therefore, the food industry has responded by improving its offer with new formulas of cereal-based GF foods [10]. To this end, as the removal of gluten from gluten-containing grains presents considerable technical difficulties and economic constraints, some celiac organizations have encouraged manufacturers of gluten-free-rendered foods towards the use of trademarks, such as the above-mentioned Crossed Grain symbol. Producers interested in using these trademarks should follow technical requirements for licensing. These include good manufacturing practices and Hazard Analysis of Critical Control Points (HACCP), thus ensuring the avoidance of gluten contamination during all stages of production, storage, transportation, and handling. Nevertheless, there are food manufacturers that decide not to include any quality mark in the labels of gluten-free products, although these, in fact, appear to be free of gluten based on a review of the list of ingredients contained.

In order to ensure consumer safety, it is necessary to evaluate gluten content in foods for special dietary use as gluten-free foodstuffs. Moreover, regulations like (EU) No. 1169/2011 require the declaration of cereals containing gluten even in unpackaged foodstuffs [11]. The few studies carried out in Europe and the USA have revealed a variety of gluten contamination (from 0.5% to 37% of the samples analyzed had over 20 mg/kg of gluten) [1,12]. Those studies were carried out over particular time-periods, but currently there is no information about the evolution on this prolamin content among the most commonly consumed cereal-based GF products over the years. The objective of this study was to analyze the changes in gluten content of these GF foodstuffs from 1998 to 2016. This overview would provide information for practitioners or CD patients about the reliability of gluten-free labeled products, as well as the potential safety of GF rendered products over the years.

2. Experimental Section

2.1. Food Samples

A number of samples (3141) of cereal-based GF foods sold in Spain were selected for gluten analysis from 1998 to 2016. Sampling was performed according to the production of cereal based GF products by food companies linked to guarantee marks, or by food safety control programs organized by health authorities or celiac associations. In the case of some samples, the same food products made by the same companies were analyzed in different years.

These products were divided into two subgroups: either GF-labelled foods using a quality mark (GF-L) or foods assumed to be this on the basis of gluten-free ingredient list. This second group can be considered as reportedly GF, but not certified, as such (GF-NC).

Depending on the food characteristics, the samples were further sorted by eight categories flours, breakfast cereals/bars, pasta, breads, dough/pastry/pizza, bakery, snacks and yeasts. Although yeasts are not a final product, these samples were included as a regular raw material in bakery foods (Table 1).

Table 1. Food categories of samples used for gluten quantification.

Category	Selected Examples
Flours	starches, baking mixes, all-purpose flours, grains and seeds
Breakfast cereals/bars	corn and other GF cereal pancakes, granola bars, soy/quinoa/almond/rice beverages, corn flakes, rice crisps, rice and quinoa waffle, muesli
Pasta products	macaroni, rices/multigrain/corn pasta, rice, lasagna sheets, semolina, noodles, tagliatelle, pasta with egg, with vegetables, fettuccini, cooked and dry pasta, organic pasta
Breads	baguettes, loaf, sliced or toasted bread, breadcrumbs, breadsticks, white/multi-grains/artisan/rustic bread, pita bread, crackers, wraps, bread rolls, ciabatta, bagels, hamburger buns
Dough/pastry/pizza	all types of pizza, pastry, croquettes, baked dough, wafers, pizza bases, all kind of sandwiches, cooked lasagna
Bakery	all types of cakes, chocolate/fruit/filled cookies, biscuits, muffins, cupcakes, scones, pies, donuts, sweet rolls, croissants, shortbread, sponge cake
Cereal-based snacks	salted/sweet popcorn, tortilla chips, pretzel cereal treats, cheddar/chili corn sticks, rice/corn triangles, fried corn nuts, baked corn snack with flavours (butter, ham, cheese, ketchup), flavour fried potato crisps, flavour rice and corn snack, crunchy/crispy/flavour crackers and bugles
Yeasts	bakery yeast and chemical leavening agents

2.2. Gluten Analysis by ELISA Techniques

Gluten content was studied by enzyme-linked immunosorbent assay (ELISA), as it is the currently accepted technique for gluten detection in foodstuffs [6]. During the period 1998–2016, two different methods have been used. The main differences between them are based on (1) the employment of different specificity antibodies; (2) diverse extraction methods; and (3) different reference materials or standards used for the assay calibration. Both methods have been recommended by organizations, such as Codex Alimentarius and/or AOAC International [13].

From 1998 to 2001, gluten was extracted using 40% aqueous ethanol solution. In this period gluten detection was performed using the commercial ELISA test Transia Plate Gluten (Diffchamb, Lyon, France), approved by AOAC International (method 991.19). This test is based on the anti ω-gliadin antibody (also called, 401.21) [13,14]. The reference material included in the kit was lyophilized gliadin extracted from bread wheat flour.

From 2001 to 2016, analysis were carried out using a RIDASCREEN® Gliadin kit, (R7001, R-Biopharm AG, Darmstadt, Germany), approved by AOAC International (method 2012.01), INGEZIM gluten (R.30.GLU.K.2, Ingenasa, Madrid, Spain) and INGEZIM gluten Quick kit (R.30.GL2.K.2, Ingenasa, Madrid, Spain). All of these are based on the monoclonal secalin antibody R5. This detects gliadin fractions of wheat and corresponding prolamins from rye (secalins) and barley (hordeins), whereas prolamins from oats, maize, and rice are not detected [15]. Using these commercial kits, extraction was, in general, carried out using a 60% aqueous ethanol buffer containing reducing agents such as 2-mercaptoethanol. For those samples containing tannins and polyphenols like chocolate, cocoa, millet, etc., a special extraction procedure, consisting of adding the sample and different proteins in the same quantity, was carried out. When using the Ridascreen kit, skim milk powder (food quality, Nestlé España S.A., Barcelona, Spain) was added to the sample, whereas with Ingezim ones, gelatin from fish skin (SIGMA, St. Louis, MO, USA) plus polyvinylpyrrolidone (PVP) (SIGMA, St. Louis, MO, USA) were used (16.7% PVP in the sum sample and gelatin). In all cases the extraction was then completed following the general extraction procedure.

Prolamin Working Group (PWG) gliadin solutions are included as standards for preparing the calibration curve. This gliadin has been prepared from 40 different European wheat varieties by the European Working Group on Prolamin Analysis and Toxicity [16].

No significant differences were found among the different methods used in terms of false negatives or positives or detected (gluten) content range [17]. During the period from 1998 to 2008 the analyses were carried out according to the kit's manufacturer instructions. The Transia Plate Gluten kit fixed the limit of quantification (LQ) at 10 mg/kg, whereas R5 antibody-based kits fixed the LQ at 5 mg/kg. Furthermore, internal validations were made to assure these assays. Since 2009 all analysis have been carried out using the ENAC (Spanish National Accreditation Body) accredited method 774/LE1626 according to ISO 17025 International Standards (ISO, 2005), which is based on the R5 antibody. The quantitative method was validated in terms of precision (repeatability and reproducibility), accuracy, and LQ. Repeatability (intra-day) showed a relative standard deviation (RSD) of 15%, while reproducibility (inter-day) obtained a RSD of 20%, and accuracy, calculated as recovery, was in the range 67%–115%. The limit of quantification (LQ) was determined at 5 mg/kg.

2.3. Statistical Analysis

Statistical analyses of our results were performed by using the IBM SPSS statistical program 21 (IBM Inc., Armonk, NY, USA). The χ^2 test followed by multiple comparisons (Bonferroni correction) was performed to determine differences in frequencies of categorized variables between groups. *p*-values < 0.05 were accepted as statistically significant.

3. Results

In total, 3141 GF products, analyzed from 1998 to 2016, were divided into eight categories. Among these categories, bakery, flours, and bread were the most frequently analyzed samples (with 905, 564, and 498 sample numbers, respectively). As a whole, gluten was detected in 371 samples (Table A1). Yeasts and breakfast cereals/bars food groups represented the highest proportion of gluten-detected samples with 22.2% (8/36) and 21.5% (73/339), respectively.

A decrease in gluten-detected samples (>20 mg/kg of gluten) was observed over the years (Figure 1). The evolution of gluten-detected products from 1998 revealed that there were three different periods in relation to gluten content. The first period was from 1998 to 2002, the second period from 2003 to 2008, and the last one from 2009 to 2016.

In the 1998–2002 period, the GF market was small and many of the foodstuffs contained gluten traces. In that period, 356 samples were analyzed and a 30% (107/356) contained detectable gluten. By food groups, percentages of contamination samples (>20 mg/kg of gluten) were as follows: breads, 17.5% (7/40; flours, 16.7% (8/48); bakery, 13.2% (16/121); breakfast cereal/bars, 11.3% (8/71); pastry/dough, 10.0% (2/20); pasta, 7.8% (4/51); snacks, 0% (0/4); and yeast, 0% (0/1). Six of forty bread samples analyzed contained more than 100 mg/kg of gluten.

Table 2 shows the evolution of gluten-detected samples from 2003 to 2016, according to three different gluten quantity intervals proposed by Regulation No. 828/2014 (gluten-free ≤20 mg/kg, very low gluten 21–100 mg/kg, and out of labelling >100 mg/kg). In the case of flour group, a progressive diminution in the percentage of gluten-free and very low gluten samples was observed among the detected-gluten samples. Meanwhile the ratio of samples not suitable for celiac people was continuously increasing from 2003 to 2016. Taken as a whole, the same tendency was revealed in all analyzed food groups (Table 2). The percentage of samples whose gluten content was in the range of

5–20 mg/kg from all gluten detected samples was 55% (57/104) in 2003–2005 time period and reduced to 19% (6/31) in 2013–2016 period. By contrast, in the case of samples over 100 mg/kg of gluten the percentages increased from 13% (14/104) to 58% (18/31) for the same time periods.

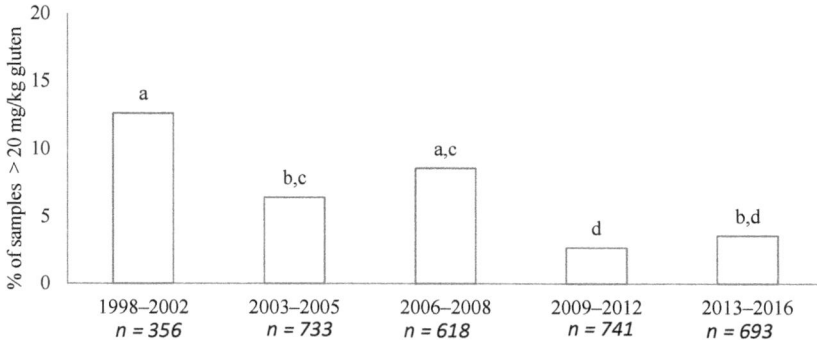

Figure 1. Evolution of gluten-containing samples (>20 mg/kg), sorted by five periods (1998–2002, 2003–2005, 2006–2008, 2009–2012, and 2013–2016). Data are expressed as the percentage of total samples analyzed in each period. Bars not sharing a common letter (a, b, c, d) are significantly different ($p < 0.05$).

Until 2008 the snack and yeast food groups differed from the rest of the groups analyzed, with a higher percentage of samples over 100 mg/kg of gluten (Table 3). From 2008, these two groups dramatically reduced the percentage of samples not suitable for any statement on the product label. Therefore, after 2008, there was no difference between snack and yeast and the rest of the groups. In the 2009–2016 time period, only the flour food group showed a slightly greater percentage of samples not suitable for any label mark (5% (14/276) for flours vs. 1% (2/374) for bakery products) (Table 3). In order to relate the decrease of gluten-positive products in line with the changing of European regulations requiring information to be given about gluten content in foods, a specific analysis of gluten-free-labeled products (GF-L) and reportedly gluten free, but not certified (GF-NC), products was made (Figure 2). Considering that most of the samples analyzed were carried out from 2004 to 2016, this period was selected for the evaluation. The number of products studies for GF-L was 1652, and for GF-NC was 962. As it is indicated in Figure 2, at the start point there was a higher percentage of gluten-positive samples in GF-NC than in GF labeled ones (12.6%, 45/358 vs. 4.9%, 41/817). The comparison revealed differences between GF-L and GF-NC in 2004–2008 and 2008–2014 periods of time, but not in the last two years (Figure 2).

Table 2. Time-period comparison of gluten-detected samples.

Food Group	Gluten Content (mg/kg)	Time Period			
		2003–2005	2006–2008	2009–2012	2013–2016
Flour	5–20	67 (6/9) [a]	37 (11/30) [a,b]	27 (3/11) [a,b]	0 (0/10) [b]
	21–100	22 (2/9)	40 (12/30)	18 (2/11)	20 (2/10)
	>100	11 (1/9) [b]	23 (7/30) [b]	55 (6/11) [a,b]	80 (8/10) [a]
Breakfast cereals/bars	5–20	72 (21/29)	40 (6/15)	33 (1/3)	33 (1/3)
	21–100	24 (7/29)	27 (4/15)	33 (1/3)	33 (1/3)
	>100	4 (1/29)	33 (5/15)	33 (1/3)	33 (1/3)
Bakery	5–20	57 (17/30)	38 (3/8)	67 (6/9)	67 (2/3)
	21–100	37 (11/30)	50 (4/8)	11 (1/9)	33 (1/3)
	>100	7 (2/30)	12 (1/8)	22 (2/9)	0 (0/3)

Table 2. *Cont.*

Food Group	Gluten Content (mg/kg)	Time Period			
		2003–2005	2006–2008	2009–2012	2013–2016
Pastry/dough	5–20	50 (3/6)	0 (0/3)	83 (5/6)	0 (0/1)
	21–100	33 (2/6)	33 (1/3)	17 (1/6)	0 (0/1)
	>100	17 (1/6)	67 (2/3)	0 (0/6)	100 (1/1)
Breads	5–20	100 (4/4)	60 (3/5)	0 (0/1)	27 (3/11)
	21–100	0 (0/4)	20 (1/5)	0 (0/1)	9 (1/11)
	>100	0 (0/4)	20 (1/5)	100 (1/1)	64 (7/11)
Pasta	5–20	24 (4/17) [b]	78 (7/9) [a]	33 (1/3) [a,b]	0 (0/3) [a,b]
	21–100	59 (10/17)	11 (1/9)	0 (0/3)	67 (2/3)
	>100	18 (3/17)	11 (1/9)	67 (2/3)	33 (1/3)
Snacks	5–20	40 (2/5)	40 (8/20)	67 (2/3)	-
	21–100	20 (1/5)	20 (4/20)	33 (1/3)	-
	>100	40 (2/5)	40 (8/20)	0 (0/3)	-
Yeasts	5–20	0 (0/4)	67 (2/3)	-	-
	>100	100 (4/4)	33 (1/3)	-	-
Total	5–20	55 (57/104) [a]	43 (40/93) [a,b]	50 (18/36) [a,b]	19 (6/31) [b]
	21–100	32 (33/104)	29 (27/93)	17 (6/36)	23 (7/31)
	>100	13 (14/104) [c]	28 (26/93) [b,c]	33 (12/36) [a,b]	58 (18/31) [a]

Notes: Data are expressed as percentage of gluten-content interval (5–20, 21–100, and >100 mg/kg) from total gluten-detected samples, analyzed by each period and categorized by food group. The numerical fraction of samples detected for each range, in each food group and in each time period are expressed in brackets. Percentages not sharing a common letter ([a, b, c]) are significantly different ($p < 0.05$).

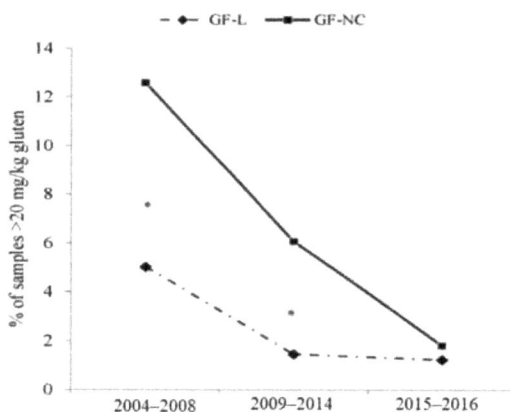

Figure 2. Evolution of gluten-containing samples (>20 mg/kg) sorted by three time periods related to gluten regulation (2004–2008, 2009–2014, and 2015–2016). From the total number of 2614 samples, 1652 were gluten-free-labeled products (GF-L) and 962 reportedly gluten free, but not certified, products (GF-NC). Data are expressed as percentages of the total sample analyzed in each period. Significantly different time period are expressed as * ($p < 0.05$).

Table 3. Comparison by food groups of samples under or over 100 mg of gluten per kg of product before and after 2008 year.

Time Period	Gluten Content (mg/kg)	Food Group							
		Flour	Breakfast Cereals/Bars	Bakery	Pastry/Dough	Breads	Pasta	Snacks	Yeasts
2003–2008	≤100	97 [a,b] (232/240)	97 [a,b] (171/177)	99 [a] (407/410)	97 [a,b] (96/99)	99 [a] (167/168)	97 [a,b] (145/149)	88 [b,c] (74/84)	79 [c] (19/24)
	>100	3 [a,b] (8/240)	3 [a,b] (6/177)	1 [a] (3/410)	3 [a,b] (3/99)	1 [a] (1/168)	3 [a,b] (4/149)	12 [b,c] (10/84)	21 [c] (5/24)
2009–2016	≤100	95 [b] (262/276)	98 [a,b] (89/91)	99 [a] (372/374)	99 [a,b] (172/173)	97 [a,b] (282/290)	97 [a,b] (110/113)	100 [a,b] (106/106)	100 [a,b] (11/11)
	>100	5 [b] (14/276)	2 [a] (2/91)	1 [a] (2/374)	1 [a,b] (1/173)	3 [a,b] (8/290)	3 [a,b] (3/113)	0 [a,b] (0/106)	0 [a,b] (0/11)

Notes: Data are expressed as percentage of gluten content interval (≤100 and >100 mg/kg) from total analyzed samples, categorized by each food group. The numerical fraction of samples detected for each range, in each food group and in each time period are expressed in brackets. Percentages not sharing a common letter [a, b, c] are significantly different ($p < 0.05$).

4. Discussion

According to the Mintel's report the GF product market not only represents one of the most prosperous markets in the field of food and beverages nowadays, but also offers positive perspectives in the near future, with a forecast growth of around 10% [10]. Apart from celiac people, other consumers as a result of cultural- or health-beliefs and dietary habits, are responsible for the growth of the GF food market [18].

For people with CD, the involuntary intake of gluten, apart from dietary transgressions of GFD, is probably one of the major reasons for symptom persistence. This unintentional intake could be for two main reasons: contamination of the foodstuff at some step of the manufacturing process, or inadvertent gluten intake due to misleading nutritional labelling. In order to protect the celiac population's rights several laws have been put into place in the last decade. First, in 1979 the Codex adopted a standard for foods for special dietary use for people intolerant to gluten, which, later, in 2008, was revised and corrected [6]. This document set the definition of gluten-free foods as those containing less than 20 mg/kg. As mentioned, the terms gluten free ($\leq$20 mg/kg) and very low gluten (21–100 mg/kg) are nowadays covered by 2014 legislation relating to GF foods [9]. Consequently, samples with gluten content over 100 mg/kg are not suitable for any statement on the product label.

Bearing this in mind, our results for products sold in Spain confirmed that rules implemented to control gluten content were effective. There was a marked cutoff year, 2008, with a strong reduction of the gluten-positive samples (>20 mg/kg of gluten).

Other studies in Europe have been conducted in order to evaluate the gluten content of GF products. Before the cut-off year, Valdes et al. carried out research where a large miscellaneous group (*n* = 4454 samples) comprising gluten-free foods was analyzed [12]. They found that close to half of the samples contained detectable gluten whereas in that period (1998–2002), we found that nearly one third of the analyzed samples were contaminated (Figure 1). This discrepancy might be justified, at least in part, by the quantification limit (LQ) established because these authors set a lower LQ (3.2 mg/kg) than ours. Furthermore, they found a higher ratio of samples over 20 mg/kg than we did during the period of 1998–2002. It has to be taken into account that they analyzed many flours (rice, maize, oats origin) while we measured processed products. Indeed, in less processed categories such as bread or flours, we found a larger percentage of contaminated samples over 20 mg/kg, data that are closer to those obtained by Valdes et al. [12].

1998–2002 was a confusing time-period, due to the scarce European regulation in terms of gluten control. This allowed a high proportion of gluten contaminated samples in a low diversity GF product market. By contrast, from 2003 onwards, analyses performed by Gibert et al. for Italian, Spanish, German, and Norwegian samples indicated that, out of 205 samples, only one (0.5%) was over the gluten threshold [1]. These data are in the same line as our results obtained in the 2009–2012 period (2.7%), confirming that Codex revision implementation was efficiently followed by Central and Western European countries.

Nevertheless, celiac people cannot completely presume the foodstuffs on offer to be safe. The evolution of analyzed products revealed that, in general, when gluten is detected in samples nowadays, it is detected in higher quantities (<100 mg/kg of gluten) than 10 years ago. Considering that most of the analyzed products have to represent the basis of the diet, due to the fact that they provide carbohydrates and, thus, the main energy source, those gluten-contained products represent a real concern for celiac people.

Additionally, it must be emphasized that before Codex revision (prior to 2008) snacks and yeast could be considered the most risky food for celiac people. Both showed elevated percentages of samples not suitable for people with celiac disease compared to the rest of analyzed food groups (12% for snacks and 21% for yeasts). However, after the revision, no more differences in samples containing more than 100 mg/kg among food groups were observed.

In the case of snacks, one possible explanation for this fact could be related to consumer preferences. A Nielsen global snacking report indicated that, nowadays, the GF aspect of a snack is very important for one-fifth of global respondents [19]. Traditionally maize has been the prime flour source to produce extruded snacks [20], despite the addition of wheat in some formulations. Taking into account the tendencies in snack preferences in recent years, they cannot be discounted as responsible for the gluten-contamination control improvement from 2008. Apparently, something similar could take place for bakery yeasts. Sugars are the source of yeast fermentation and, therefore, of bakery yeast production. Whether the origin of sugars is related to gluten containing cereals (rye, wheat, and barley) or not is a simple decision of yeast manufacturers. It might be said that the 2008 Codex revision made bakery yeast manufacturers aware of the need to reinforce their gluten control, probably changing the sugar source.

In terms of GF cereal products, as mentioned before, two cases apply to a gluten-free claim. On one hand, there are gluten-free foodstuffs produced by manufacturers which include a quality mark, label, or certificate of prolamin content below 20 mg/kg. Alternatively, there are unlabeled products that appeared gluten-free based on scrutiny of their listed ingredients [21]. Our results reveal that there were differences in both, GF labelled (GF-L), and reportedly GF, but not certified products (GF-NC), over time. Specifically during the 2004–2014 time-period, a higher rate of gluten-positive samples was detected in GF-NC samples than in GF labelled ones. However, after 2015 both groups of samples showed a similar range of positives.

After the revision of the Codex standard (2008), and basing on it, the European commission regulated the provision of food information to consumers with No. 1169/2011 [11]. Although this regulation was made in 2011, the deadline for its mandatory complementation was 13 of December 2014. It could be postulated that this brought about the closing of the gap between GF-labeled and GF-NC products in terms of positive samples.

It is worth noting the evolution of not certified GF products from 2004, during which time a constant and noticeable reduction in gluten-positive samples can be observed. Very much in line with this tendency, the literature reflects how research conducted in Europe and published in 2010, 2011, and 2013, detected decreasing ratios of gluten-positives samples (10.5%, 9.7%, and 0.5%, respectively) [1,22,23].

Outside Europe, other countries adopted similar rules in terms of gluten. With compliance date of August 2014, the USA Food and Drug Administration regulated the term GF as did European regulation [8]. Prior to 2014, in the USA, there was reported a high gluten detection in gluten-free grains, seeds, and flours but not in the labelled products (32% vs. 3.6%–5.1%) [21,24,25]. As in our study, there was a clear difference between both kinds of GF products before GF regulation. However, a study published in 2016 revealed that positive samples ratio for GF-NC products went down (4.9% from a total of 101) [26]. In view of the above, it seems that GF rule implementation in the USA was effective as the number of positive samples decreased not only among GF labeled products, but also in GF-NC ones.

As far as we know this is the first study that analyzes the evolution of gluten detection in GF products over a long period of time. Furthermore, data of gluten presence sorted by five ranges provide useful information for food safety authorities, manufactures, practitioners, and other related professionals working on gluten and CD from other countries, who do not set the gluten threshold at 20 mg/kg (Table A1). For instance, Australia and New Zealand, recently, set narrower regulations establishing that "gluten-free" foods must not contain detectable gluten [27]. However, it is necessary to consider that the non-standardized sampling of this research is not representative of the entire Spanish gluten-free cereal retail market. Due to this fact, information about the raw material in origin (rice, corn, quinoa, or others) of all of the samples was not collected. On the other hand, the categorization proposed in this research could not fit with other authors, limiting, at least in part, specific comparison. For instance, some authors include bread in bakery foods [28] and others defined other group, such as a convenience food category [29].

5. Conclusions

In summary, a tendency toward a reduction in the presence of gluten contamination in gluten-free rendered foods over the years has been observed. Our results confirm the effectiveness of European regulation in terms of gluten control for GF foodstuffs. Indeed, the significant drops which have taken place can be linked to European regulations about gluten content in food and, probably, to the involvement of the food industry over the years. In this context, the data obtained in recent years are reassuring and make grain-based foods more reliable products for the celiac population, but strict gluten control should be maintained.

Acknowledgments: This research was supported by a grant from the University of the Basque Country (UPV/EHU) (University-Society US15/06) and a grant from the Basque Government (Proyectos de Investigación Focalizada Agricultura PA15/01). We thank to Ana Corrales and Idoia Larretxi the collaboration during the experiment performance.

Author Contributions: Edurne Simón and María Ángeles Bustamante conceived and designed the experiments; María Ángeles Bustamante, Virginia Navarro and María del Pilar Fernández-Gil performed the experiments; Arrate Lasa and Edurne Simón analyzed the data; Itziar Churruca and Jonatan Miranda contributed materials/analysis tools; Jonatan Miranda wrote the paper.

Conflicts of Interest: The authors declare no conflict of interest.

Appendix A

Table A1. Summary of results obtained in gluten detection analysis from 1998 to 2016.

Food Group	Analyzed Sample Number	Gluten-Detected Samples	Gluten (mg/kg)				
			5–10	11–20	21–100	101–200	>200
Flours	564	75	10	17	21	11	16
Breakfast cereals/bars	339	73	22	22	15	6	8
Bakery	905	87	21	28	24	6	8
Pastry/dough	292	23	7	6	6	0	4
Bread	498	31	5	8	3	4	11
Pasta	313	45	8	13	14	4	6
Cereal based-Snacks	194	29	5	8	6	2	10
Yeasts	36	8	2	1	0	1	4
Total	3141	371	80	103	87	34	67

Notes: Data related to gluten quantification are expressed as number of samples.

References

1. Gibert, A.; Kruizinga, A.G.; Neuhold, S.; Houben, G.F.; Canela, M.A.; Fasano, A.; Catassi, C. Might gluten traces in wheat substitutes pose a risk in patients with celiac disease? A population-based probabilistic approach to risk estimation. *Am. J. Clin. Nutr.* **2013**, *97*, 109–116. [CrossRef] [PubMed]
2. Catassi, C.; Fabiani, E.; Iacono, G.; D'Agate, C.; Francavilla, R.; Biagi, F.; Volta, U.; Accomando, S.; Picarelli, A.; de Vitis, I.; et al. A prospective, double-blind, placebo-controlled trial to establish a safe gluten threshold for patients with celiac disease. *Am. J. Clin. Nutr.* **2007**, *85*, 160–166. [PubMed]
3. Akobeng, A.K.; Thomas, A.G. Systematic review: Tolerable amount of gluten for people with coeliac disease. *Aliment. Pharmacol. Ther.* **2008**, *27*, 1044–1052. [CrossRef] [PubMed]
4. Scherf, K.A.; Poms, R.E. Recent developments in analytical methods for tracing gluten. *J. Cereal Sci.* **2016**, *67*, 112–122. [CrossRef]
5. Codex Alimentarius. CODEX STAN 118-1979: Standard for Foods for Special Dietary Use for Persons Intolerant to Gluten. Available online: http://www.fao.org/fao-who-codexalimentarius/standards/en/ (accessed on 25 October 2016).
6. Codex Alimentarius. CODEX STAN 118-2008: Revised Version Standard for Foods for Special Dietary Use for Persons Intolerant to Gluten. Available online: http://www.fao.org/fao-who-codexalimentarius/standards/en/ (accessed on 25 October 2016).

7. Commission Regulation (EC). No. 41/2009 Concerning the composition and labelling of foodstuffs suitable for people intolerant to gluten. *Off. J. Eur. Union L* **2009**, *1620*, 3–5.
8. U.S. Government Publishing Office. 78 FR 47154-Food Labeling; Gluten-Free Labeling of Foods. Available online: https://www.gpo.gov/fdsys/granule/FR-2013-08-05/2013-18813 (accessed on 25 October 2016).
9. Commission Implementing European Parliament and of the Council. Regulation (EU). No. 828/2014 Requirements for the provision of information to consumers on the absence or reduced presence of gluten in food. *Off. J. Eur. Union L* **2014**, *228*, 5–8.
10. Gluten-free Foods-US-September 2013. Available online: http://store.mintel.com/gluten-free-foods-us-september-2013 (accessed on 25 October 2016).
11. Regulation (EU). No. 1169/2011 of European Parliament and of the Council on the provision of food information to consumers. *Off. J. Eur. Union L* **2011**, *304*, 18–63.
12. Valdés, I.; García, E.; Llorente, M.; Méndez, E. Innovative approach to low-level gluten determination in foods using a novel sandwich enzyme-linked immunosorbent assay protocol. *Eur. J. Gastroenterol. Hepatol.* **2003**, *15*, 465–474. [CrossRef] [PubMed]
13. Skerritt, J.H.; Hill, A.S. Enzyme immunoassay for determination of gluten in foods: Collaborative study. *J. Assoc. Off. Anal. Chem.* **1991**, *74*, 257–264. [PubMed]
14. Skerritt, J.H.; Hill, A.S. Monoclonal antibody sandwich enzyme immunoassays for determination of gluten in foods. *J. Agric. Food. Chem.* **1990**, *38*, 1771–1778. [CrossRef]
15. Méndez, E.; Vela, C.; Immer, U.; Janssen, F.W. Report of a collaborative trial to investigate the performance of the R5 enzyme linked immunoassay to determine gliadin in gluten-free food. *Eur. J. Gastroenterol. Hepatol.* **2005**, *17*, 1053–1063. [CrossRef] [PubMed]
16. Van Eckert, R.; Berghofer, E.; Ciclitira, P.J.; Chirdo, F.; Denery-Papini, S.; Ellis, H.J.; Ferranti, P.; Goodwin, P.; Immer, U.; Mamone, G.; et al. Towards a new gliadin reference material–isolation and characterisation. *J. Cereal. Sci.* **2006**, *43*, 331–341. [CrossRef]
17. Simón, E.; Navarro, V.; Morera, T.; del Barrio, A.S. Comparación de las condiciones analíticas en la determinación de gluten en alimentos. *Nutr. Hosp.* **2002**, *18*, 121.
18. Worosz, M.R.; Wilson, N.L.W. A Cautionary Tale of Purity, Labeling and Product Literacy in the Gluten-Free Market. *J. Consum. Aff.* **2012**, *46*, 288–318. [CrossRef]
19. Snack Attack: What Consumers are Reaching for Around the World. Available online: http://www.nielsen.com/content/dam/nielsenglobal/kr/docs/global-report/2014/Nielsen%20Global%20Snacking%20Report%20September%202014.pdf (accessed on 13 December 2016).
20. Flores-Silva, P.C.; Rodriguez-Ambriz, S.L.; Bello-Pérez, L.A. Gluten-free snacks using plantain-chickpea and maize blend: Chemical composition, starch digestibility, and predicted glycemic index. *J. Food. Sci.* **2015**, *80*, C961–C966. [CrossRef] [PubMed]
21. Thompson, T.; Simpson, S. A comparison of gluten levels in labeled gluten-free and certified gluten-free foods sold in the United States. *Eur. J. Clin. Nutr.* **2015**, *69*, 143–146. [CrossRef] [PubMed]
22. Agakidis, C.; Karagiozoglou-Lampoudi, T.; Kalaitsidou, M.; Papadopoulos, T.; Savvidou, A.; Daskalou, E.; Dimitrios, T. Enzyme-linked immunosorbent assay gliadin assessment in processed food products available for persons with celiac disease: A feasibility study for developing a gluten-free food database. *Nutr. Clin. Pract.* **2011**, *26*, 695–699. [CrossRef] [PubMed]
23. Daniewski, W.; Wojtasik, A.; Kunachowicz, H. Gluten content in special dietary use gluten-free products and other food products. *Rocz. Panstw. Zakl. Hig.* **2010**, *61*, 51–55. [PubMed]
24. Thompson, T.; Grace, T. Gluten content of selected labelled gluten-free foods sold in the US. *Pract. Gastroenterol.* **2013**, *37*, 14–16.
25. Thompson, T.; Lee, A.R.; Grace, T. Gluten Contamination of Grains, Seeds, and Flours in the United States: A Pilot Study. *J. Am. Diet. Assoc.* **2010**, *110*, 937–940. [CrossRef] [PubMed]
26. Thompson, T.; Lyons, T.B.; Jones, A. Allergen advisory statements for wheat: Do they help US consumers with celiac disease make safe food choices? *Eur. J. Clin. Nutr.* **2016**, *70*, 1341–1347. [CrossRef] [PubMed]
27. Federal Register of Legislation. Australia and New Zealand Food Standars Code. Available online: https://www.legislation.gov.au/Details/F2016C00189 (accessed on 25 October 2016).

28. Farage, P.; de Medeiros Nóbrega, Y.K.; Pratesi, R.; Gandolfi, L.; Assunção, P.; Zandonadi, R.P. Gluten contamination in gluten-free bakery products: A risk for coeliac disease patients. *Public Health Nutr.* **2016**. [CrossRef] [PubMed]
29. Missbach, B.; Schwingshackl, L.; Billmann, A.; Mystek, A.; Hickelsberger, M.; Bauer, G.; König, J. Gluten-free food database: The nutritional quality and cost of packaged gluten-free foods. *PeerJ* **2015**, *3*, e1337. [CrossRef] [PubMed]

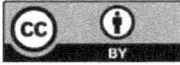

nutrients

MDPI

Review

What Do We Know Now about IgE-Mediated Wheat Allergy in Children?

Grażyna Czaja-Bulsa [1,2,*] and Michał Bulsa [3]

[1] Paediatrics and Paediatric Nursery Unit, Pomeranian Medical University, Żołnierska 48, Szczecin 71-210, Poland
[2] Division of Paediatrics, Gastroenterology and Rheumatology of the "Zdroje" Hospital, Szczecin 70-780, Poland
[3] Chair and Department of Pathology, Pomeranian Medical University, Unii Lubelskiej 1, Szczecin 71-252, Poland; michal.bulsa@gmail.com
* Correspondence address: grazyna.bulsa@wp.pl; Tel.: +48-604-48-44-49

Received: 30 October 2016; Accepted: 27 December 2016; Published: 4 January 2017

Abstract: IgE-mediated wheat allergy is a gluten-related disorder. Wheat is one of the five most common food allergens in children. However, the natural history of IgE-mediated wheat allergy has seldom been described in the research literature. This study presents the current state of knowledge about the IgE-mediated wheat allergy in children.

Keywords: wheat allergy; specific immunoglobulin E; children; gluten-related disorders

1. Introduction

Wild wheat grains (*Triticum aestivum*) were consumed by people in America as early as 11,000 years BC (before Christ). Table 1 shows the centuries of utilization of wheat by people.

Table 1. History of wheat cultivation and consumption.

Years	Event
11,000 years BC	Wild wheat grains were consumed by people in America.
7800 years BC	The first records of wheat cultivation began in fertile lands of Southwest (Palestine) and Middle Asia (Mesopotamia); people living in farming settlements grew wheat and barley.
400 years BC	The type of wheat that could be used for baking bread or pastries was first cultivated in China.
100 years BC	The first bread prepared with the use of the brewer's yeast was baked in France.

Today almost a half of the calories consumed by the human population worldwide come from cereals, with wheat being the most popular grain in Europe and the Americas. Its use is so widespread that people suffering from gluten-related disorders have great difficulty in avoiding it. Flour and bran are used in the production of bread, muesli, breakfast cereals, pasta, bulgur, couscous, and pastries. Being a binding agent, wheat is added to cold cuts, desserts, ice cream, and cream. Starch is used for coating pills, pralines, and roasted coffee grains, as well as in cosmetic, paper, and chemical industries.

2. Wheat-Related Allergic Disorders

Depending on the routes of entry, wheat-related allergic disorders are classified into: food allergies, respiratory allergies, and skin allergies (Figure 1) [1]. The allergy classifications also consider celiac disease (CD) as a wheat-related allergic disorder. However, CD is, rather, an autoimmune disease and in most countries it is treated according to gastroenterological protocols. Food allergies triggered by wheat consumption are divided to IgE-dependent wheat allergy (WA) and IgE-non-dependent WA [1]. One of the WA syndromes is also wheat-dependent, exercise-induced anaphylaxis (WDEIA). In the latest EAACI (European Academy of Allergy and Clinical Immunology) classification it has been recognized as an independent form of wheat allergy [1].

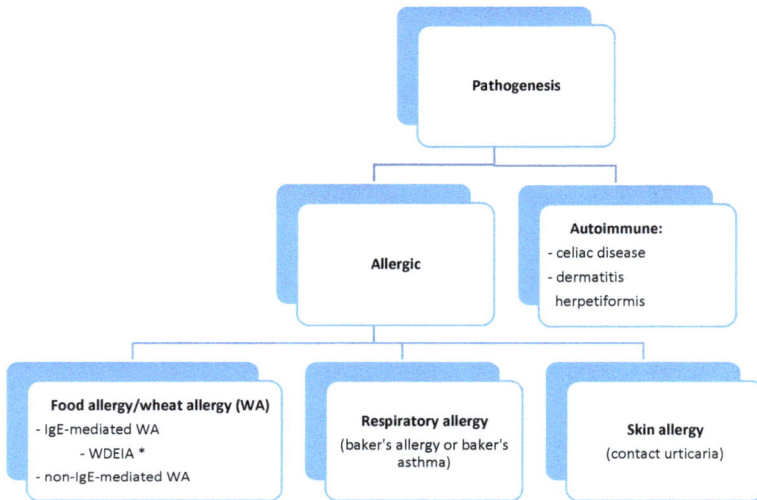

Figure 1. Classification of wheat-related allergic diseases. * WDEIA—wheat-dependent exercise-induced anaphylaxis.

WA is also one of the gluten-related disorders, the classification of which was published in 2012 (Figure 2) [2]. It is important to note that although WA belongs to this group, all of its forms stem solely from the adverse effect of wheat proteins (including gluten proteins). Therefore, the treatment is based on the elimination of wheat grains only. The allergy induced by proteins contained in other gluten grains is less common and has not been included in the classification discussed herein.

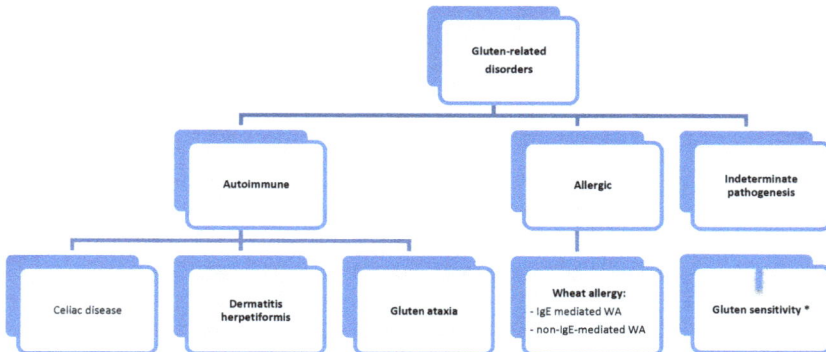

Figure 2. Classification of gluten-related disorders. * Gluten sensitivity (GS) = non-celiac gluten sensitivity (NCGS).

3. Prevalence of IgE-Mediated Wheat Allergy

Wheat is one of the five most common foods that trigger allergic reactions in children. In Germany, Japan, and Finland it has been reported as the third most common allergen, after milk and egg [3]. WA prevalence, both in children and adults, is usually approximately 1% (0.4%–4%), depending on age and region [3–6]. In patients with food allergies, WA is diagnosed in 11%–20% of children and in 25% of adults [7]. Taking into account all gluten-related disorders, it has been estimated that about 3% of the human population suffers from wheat intolerance (1% WA, 1% celiac disease, 1% non-celiac gluten sensitivity) [4,5,8].

4. Clinical Picture of IgE-Mediated Wheat Allergy

WA prevails chiefly in children with a family history of atopy. Almost all of the juvenile WA patients are diagnosed with allergies to other foods and other allergic disorders, most commonly atopic dermatitis (78%–87%). Half of patients suffer from asthma (48%–67%) and/or allergic rhinitis (34%–62%) [9,10]. The majority of children are allergic to cow's milk (80%), chicken egg white (56%–72%), fish (28%), soya (24%–50%), and peanuts (29%–50%) [9–13].

The WA clinical picture depends on age [10]. Symptoms develop within minutes to 1–2 h after the ingestion of wheat. In young children gastroenterological symptoms prevail, such as vomiting, diarrhea or, rarely, abdomen pains. In about 40% of children skin symptoms are observed in a form of urticaria, erythema, angioedema, pruritus, or worsening atopic dermatitis [9,10,12,13]. Intestinal symptoms recede with age; therefore, older children suffer mostly from dermatitis, which is accompanied by respiratory disorders (wheeze, stridor, persistent cough, hoarse voice, respiratory distress, nasal congestion) and, in the most severe cases, anaphylaxis. In teenagers and adults the most severe forms of allergy prevail, such as anaphylaxis symptoms (in 45%–50%), which is typical of wheat allergy. Intestinal and skin symptoms are less common in these age groups [1,9,10,12].

WA is usually diagnosed in young children, but it is rarely seen in infants, despite the fact that wheat proteins pass into breast milk, which was proven by Linn et al. in 1996 [14]. In our study on 50 children with WA, the disease was diagnosed in 32% of infants. Three of them were fed exclusively on their mother's milk [10]. In 1981, Rudd et al. described a case of an infant with anaphylactic shock after consuming semolina pudding [15].

WA can be accompanied by allergies to other cereals, most often to rye and/or corn [12].

5. Development of Tolerance to IgE-Mediated Wheat Allergy

The prognosis of WA tolerance is not as poor as it is in the case of allergies to peanuts, shellfish, or fish that usually continue into adulthood. It is similar to the tolerance prognosis in children allergic to milk or egg. WA will prevail to maturity in about 10% of patients, with the most severe clinical forms of the disorder [9–11]. In our study the age median of the tolerance was seven years (3–16 years). Fifty-two percent of patients developed the tolerance by the age of eight years, 66% of them by the age of 12, and 76% by the age of 16 [10]. Other researchers have reported similar results [11].

Similarly to other food allergies, the progress of tolerance can be assessed by means of the wheat IgE titers determined repeatedly during the elimination diet. When wheat IgE concentration increases, tolerance is unlikely to develop quickly. Conversely, it is likely to occur when the wheat IgE titers decline steadily. Moreover, such a procedure allows the determination of the maximum wheat IgE concentration. The higher the titers, the older the patient at the time when the tolerance develops. In our studies the tolerance age median was 3.5 years when the maximum wheat IgE concentrations were below 19.9 kU/L. When it was within the range of 20–49.9 kU/L, the median rose to seven years. It reached 16 years of age when the concentrations exceeded 50 kU/L [10].

6. Wheat-Dependent, Exercise-Induced Anaphylaxis—A Rare Form of Wheat Allergy

WDEIA is a rare syndrome [16]. It is typically diagnosed in adults and sporadically in older children. It is clinically characterized by anaphylactic reactions (hives, Quincke's edema, shock) occurring 10–60 min after exercise following the ingestion of wheat 10 min to four hours earlier. The amount of ingested wheat and the intensity of exercise can vary substantially. The rω-5 gliadin is the major WDEIA allergen—it is found in all the patients. The serum concentrations of rω-5 gliadin-specific IgE are correlated with the severity of the WDEIA clinical response. IgE serum concentrations for the rω-5 gliadin higher than 0.89 kU/L confirm the WDEIA diagnosis (sensitivity 78%, specificity 96%), while the sIgE sensitivity for whole wheat extract and gluten is low (48% and 56%, respectively) [17].

7. Wheat Grain Proteins

All of the wheat-induced diseases are caused by wheat proteins which constitute 10%–18% of the grain mass, depending on the strain. The main component (70%) of the wheat grain is starch.

Depending on their dissolving agent, the wheat grain proteins are categorized into four main fractions: albumins (15%), globulins (7%), gliadins (33%), and glutenins (45%). Albumins are soluble in water; globulins, in salt solutions; gliadins, in alcohol; and while glutenins, in dilute acid and alkali. Albumins and globulins are structural proteins that contain many enzymes. Gliadins and glutenins are prolamins and are referred to as gluten. They are storage proteins.

The wheat proteins that are regarded today as the WA major allergens will be discussed in detail in the next chapter. Wheat proteins triggering CD symptoms belong to gliadins. Wheat proteins responsible for non-celiac-gluten sensitivity (NCGS) have not been identified yet. One of the proteins under the researchers' examination is a group of amylase-trypsin inhibitors (ATIs) that do not belong to glutens (JunkerY et al., 2012) [18].

8. Major Allergens of IgE-Mediated Wheat Allergy

In the serum of patients with IgE-mediated wheat allergy numerous IgE antibodies are found that bind with proteins of all of the wheat grain fractions, most commonly with gliadins. However, in different examinations, they are not the same proteins and, therefore, they cannot be regarded as the major allergens in children with WA [19,20]. A protein can be regarded as the major allergen when IgE antibodies specific for this protein are found in a considerable number of children with WA.

The list of the World Health Organization includes 27 wheat allergens [21]. Clinical relevance of many of them has not been determined yet.

The best-understood allergenic molecule of WA is rω-5 gliadin (Tri a 19) [16,22,23]. The rω-5 gliadin-specific IgEs are present in all patients with WDEIA, in 80% of children with anaphylaxis symptoms after wheat ingestion, and in 20%–30% of children with WA and atopic eczema [20,24–28].

The second allergenic molecule of WA, for which commercial tests are available, is a non-specific lipid transfer protein (Tri a 14) (nsLTP). Antibodies signaling the presence of the IgE specific to Tri a 14 are found in WA children and in patients with WDEIA. They are not very sensitive. It is now thought that they do not exhibit cross-reactivity with grass pollen, although there is not enough data to exclude this. Their assessment may help in differentiating wheat sensitization from pollen allergy, which is vital in patients with high levels of grass pollen-specific IgE [1].

In everyday allergological practice the possibility of swift and simple exclusion of cross-reactions is very important. Wheat is highly cross-reactive with other cereals; mainly rye and barley [20]. It has been shown that prolamins, like gamma-70 and gamma-35 secalins in rye, as well as gamma-3 hordein in barley, cross-react with rω-5 gliadin [29]. These three cereals contain several other proteins that are highly cross-reactive. It has also been confirmed that there is high sequence identity (>80%) among many other proteins, such as alpha-purothionins from wheat, rye, and barley [30]. Positive SPTs and elevated assays of IgE specific to whole wheat extract are common among atopic patients.

Up to 65% of the patients with grass pollen allergy have false positive results when tested for wheat extract, i.e., they do not report any health problems after the ingestion of wheat [31]. If the medical history of patients with positive SPT results and with IgE specific to whole wheat extract does not rule out negative reactions to wheat, it is necessary to perform a wheat challenge test, which is rather time consuming. Such a test will be positive in barely 20% of the patients and such a low probability of positive allergy incidence in allergic individuals is reported only in WA.

Today, intense studies are conducted on some wheat protein components: glutenins with low and high molecular weight (LMW-glutenins and HMW-glutenins), α-, β-, and γ-gliadins, as well as non-specific lipid transport protein Tri a 14 [32,33]. However, none have reached a high specificity and sensitivity to become a gold standard in the diagnosis of WA and, therefore, the precise diagnosis still relies on standardized challenges which must be done under medical supervision [1,31,33].

9. Diagnosis of IgE-Mediated Wheat Allergy

The WA diagnosis is difficult because not all of the major wheat grain allergens are recognized. Similarly, to any other allergy, the gold standard of WA diagnosis remains the oral food challenge. It is usually performed in its open form, as the majority of the observed adverse reactions is of the objective nature. The patient is given whole wheat starting from small doses of wheat-specific protein (1–50 mg) followed by increasingly larger hourly doses (digestion of wheat can be slower than egg or milk), ending with a cumulative dose of up to 0.5–1 g of wheat protein [1]. Additionally, double-blind placebo-controlled protocols of WA have been published both for children and adults [28,34]. WA is diagnosed when the challenge test results are positive and the symptoms appear up to two hours after ingestion.

In the next stage, allergological tests should be performed to confirm the elevated levels of wheat allergen-specific IgE. The first are skin tests (SPTs) to wheat flour. Generally, commercial wheat extract is used, the specificity of which is very low [1]. Some allergologists prepare an in-house wheat flour solution, but its specificity is also very low. It can be improved by additional testing to ω-5 gliadin or other gliadins, but these solutions are not routinely available and are mainly used in scientific research.

Another step is the determination of serum concentrations of allergen-specific IgE to whole wheat extract. They are commercially available but their specificity is low despite high sensitivity [1,33].

Solutions used for skin tests to wheat flour and for the assessment of allergen-specific IgE to whole wheat extract consist of the mixture of grain albumins and globulins and, thus, do not contain the insoluble major wheat allergens, i.e., prolamins. This is why the utility of these tests in WA diagnosis is lower than in allergies to other foods, such as milk, egg, or peanuts [35]. Moreover, their concentration is not correlated with the severity of clinical reactions after wheat ingestion.

Gluten-specific IgE can also be assessed. Since the commercial test contains wheat gluten proteins, it is positive only in the case of a wheat allergy and negative in the case of allergies to other gluten-containing cereals. It is not known if it includes major wheat allergens. Gluten-specific IgE assays are positive in two thirds of children with WA [10].

Currently, there are commercial tests for the IgE specific to two known allergenic molecules of wheat: Tri a 14 non-specific lipid transfer protein and Tri a 19 rω-5-gliadin [1]. Their importance to the WA diagnosis has been discussed in the section "Major Allergens in IgE-Mediated Wheat Allergy" of this paper.

It is characteristic of children who had WA, and have developed a tolerance to wheat, that in most of them (approximately 80%) SPTs to wheat continue to be positive and IgE specific to whole wheat extract and gluten-specific IgE remain elevated, which is rare in other food allergies [9,10]. For the majority of food allergens, tolerance development is accompanied by negative SPTs and normalized specific IgE levels. In our studies, at the time of tolerance development, the levels of IgE specific to whole wheat extract ranged between 0.35–23.9 kU/L (median: 3.0 kU/L) [10]. In that group of patients, at the time of WA diagnosis, the levels of IgE specific to whole wheat extract had been between 2.2 kU/L and 39.3 kU/L (median: 8.42 kU/L). This is why the size of SPT and the levels of

IgE specific to whole wheat extract are not useful in differentiating between the periods of allergy and tolerance. It should be stressed, however, that in individual children who have developed tolerance to wheat the SPT values and IgE specific to whole wheat extract and gluten are lower than when WA was diagnosed.

10. Treatment of IgE-Mediated Wheat Allergy

It is worth emphasizing that even though IgE-mediated wheat allergy belongs to gluten-dependent disorders, it is induced solely by wheat proteins, thus being treated by a wheat-free diet. The remaining gluten cereals, such as rye, barley, and oats are well tolerated by most patients and should not be eliminated from their diet. In WA children, oat allergy is very rare. Rye and barley allergies are slightly more common.

It is believed that different species of wheat have the same allergenicity, therefore, it is not recommended for the patients with severe WA to try different forms of wheat. There are no studies describing changes in allergenicity of wheat during processing [1].

Moreover, it is not recommended to routinely administer a gluten-free diet to WA patients. Gluten-free products made from rice or corn flour, tapioca, millet, or sorghum, are usually well tolerated by WA patients. However, such products often contain wheat starch as the main ingredient which can be insufficiently purified of wheat proteins to be safe for WA patients. The gluten-free products dedicated to CD patients can contain no more than 20 mg of gluten proteins per 1 kg.

Since 2009 the packaging of all products sold in the European Union must inform consumers about the wheat content.

In 2013 the case was reported of two children with anaphylaxis after wheat ingestion who had developed prior tolerance to pressure-cooked whole wheat. The process of pressure-cooking changes the structure of the wheat husk. It is not known, however, if it damages the structure of the allergens [36]. No other cases of such a two-stage process of tolerance to wheat have been reported so far.

The research literature has provided the first report on the oral immunotherapy administered to older children with anaphylaxis triggered by wheat ingestion. After two years, the therapy resulted in the desensitization in 61% of the patients [37]. Further studies are necessary to evaluate the effectiveness of this type of WA treatment [1].

In the USA the rω-5 gliadin-free variety of wheat has been produced [38].

11. Prophylaxis against IgE-Mediated Wheat Allergy

It is presently believed that the time when foods are introduced into the infants' diet is relevant to their tolerance. For half of the century, from 1955 to 2005, Europe, America, and Australia used nutrition charts for infants where the delayed introduction of strong allergens was strictly recommended. It is a general opinion that those schemes were responsible for the increased incidence of allergies in that period of time. Today, it is recommended to introduce foods containing strong allergens into the infants' diets as early as between the 17th and 26th weeks of life.

The initial exposure to wheat grains delayed until after six months of age may increase the risk of wheat allergy [39]. So far only one prospective study has been published (EAT study) which assesses the effects of introducing wheat (and other allergens) after the third vs. the sixth month of life on the incidence of WA in three year olds. The study was inconclusive because in neither group had WA been diagnosed [40].

In recent years the results of two extensive studies (Celiprev, Prevent CD) have been published that indicate that the time of introducing wheat into the diet of infants at high risk of celiac disease has no effect on the CD prevalence [41,42]. In spring 2016, ESPGHAN issued recommendations to introduce wheat into the infant diet between the 4th and 12th months of life.

Author Contributions: Grażyna Czaja-Bulsa—conceptualized and designed the study, coordinated and supervised publication collection, drafted the initial manuscript, and approved the final manuscript as submitted. Michał Bulsa—conceptualized the study, supervised publication collection, carried out the analyses, drafted the initial manuscript and approved the final manuscript as submitted.

Conflicts of Interest: The authors declare no conflict of interest.

References

1. Mäkelä, M. Wheat allergy. In *EAACI Molecular Allergology User's Guide*, 1st ed.; Matricardi, P.M., Kleine-Tebbe, J., Hoffmann, H., Rudolf, V., Ollert, M., Eds.; European Academy of Allergy and Clinical Immunology: Viena, Austria, 2016; pp. 213–223.
2. Sapone, A.; Bai, J.; Ciacci, C.; Dolinsek, J.; Green, P.H.; Hadjivassiliou, M.; Kaukinen, K.; Rostami, K.; Sanders, D.S.; Schumann, M.; et al. Spectrum of gluten disorders: Consensus on new nomenclature and classification. *BMC Med.* **2012**, *10*, 13. [CrossRef] [PubMed]
3. Longo, G.; Berti, I.; Burks, A.W.; Krauss, B.; Brabie, E. IgE-mediated food allergy in children. *Lancet* **2013**, *382*, 1656–1664. [CrossRef]
4. Nwaru, B.I.; Hickstein, L.; Panesar, S.S.; Roberts, G.; Muraro, A.; Sheikh, A. on behalf of The EAACI Food Allergy and Anaphyllaxis Guidelines Group. Prevelence of common food allergies in Europe. In *Food Allergy and Anaphylaxis Guidelines*, 1st ed.; Muraro, A., Roberts, G., Eds.; European Academy of Allergy and Clinical Immunology (EAACI): Zurich, Switzerland, 2014; pp. 23–45.
5. Zuidmeer, L.; Goldhahn, K.; Rona, R.J.; Gislason, D.; Madsen, C.; Summers, C.; Sodergren, E.; Dahlstrom, J.; Lindner, T.; Sigurdardottir, S.T.; et al. The prevalence of plant food allergies: A systematic review. *J. Allergy Clin. Immunol.* **2008**, *121*, 1210–1218. [CrossRef] [PubMed]
6. Ostblom, E.; Lilja, G.; Pershagen, G.; van Hage, M.; Wickman, M. Phenotypes of food hypersensitivity and development of allergic diseases during the first 8 years of life. *Clin. Exp. Allergy* **2008**, *38*, 1325–1332. [CrossRef] [PubMed]
7. Sicherer, S.H.; Morrow, E.H.; Sampson, H.A. Dose-response in double-blind, placebo-controlled oral food challenges in children with atopic dermatitis. *J. Allergy Clin. Immunol.* **2004**, *114*, 144–149. [CrossRef] [PubMed]
8. Catassi, C.; Gatti, S.; Fasano, A. The new epidemiology of celiac disease. *J. Pediatr. Gastroenterol. Nutr.* **2014**, *59*, S7–S9. [CrossRef] [PubMed]
9. Keet, C.A.; Matsui, E.C.; Dhillon, G.; Lenehan, P.; Paterakis, M.; Wood, R.A. The natural history of wheat allergy. *Ann. Allergy Asthma Immunol.* **2009**, *102*, 410–415. [CrossRef]
10. Czaja-Bulsa, G.; Bulsa, M. The natural history of IgE mediated wheat allergy in children with dominant gastrointestinal symptoms. *Allergy Asthma Clin. Immunol.* **2014**, *10*, 12. [CrossRef] [PubMed]
11. Kotaniemi-Syrjänen, A.; Palosuo, K.; Jartti, T.; Kuitunen, M.; Pelkonen, A.S.; Mäkelaä, M.J. The prognosis of wheat hypersensitivity in children. *Pediatr. Allergy Immunol.* **2010**, *21*, e421–e428. [CrossRef] [PubMed]
12. Mansouri, M.; Pourpak, Z.; Mozafari, H.; Abdollah Gorji, F.; Shokouhi Shoormasti, R. Follow-up of the wheat allergy in children; consequences and outgrowing the allergy. *Iran. J. Allergy Asthma Immunol.* **2012**, *11*, 157–163. [PubMed]
13. Christensen, M.J.; Eller, E.; Mortz, C.H.; Bindslev-Jensen, C. Patterns of suspected wheat-related allergy: A retrospective single-centre case note review in 156 patients. *Clin. Transl. Allergy* **2014**, *4*, 39. [CrossRef] [PubMed]
14. Linna, O. Specific IgE antibodies to uningested cereals. *Allergy* **1996**, *51*, 849–850. [CrossRef] [PubMed]
15. Rudd, P.; Manuel, P.; Walker-Smith, J. Anaphylactic shock in an infant after feeding with a wheat rusk. A transient phenomenon. *Postgrad Med. J.* **1981**, *57*, 794–795. [CrossRef] [PubMed]
16. Matsuo, H.; Dahlström, J.; Tanaka, A.; Kohno, K.; Takahashi, H.; Furumura, M.; Morita, E. Sensitivity and specificity of recombinant omega-5 gliadin-specific IgE measurement for the diagnosis of wheat-dependent exercise-induced anaphylaxis. *Allergy* **2008**, *63*, 233–236. [CrossRef] [PubMed]
17. Borres, M.P.; Ebisawa, M.; Eigenmann, P.A. Us of allergen components begins a new era in pediatric allergology. *Pediatr. Allergy Immunol.* **2011**, *22*, 454–461. [CrossRef] [PubMed]

18. Junker, Y.; Zeissinq, S.; Kim, S.J.; Barisani, D.; Wieser, H.; Leffler, D.A.; Zevallos, V.; Libermann, T.A.; Dillon, S.; Freitaq, T.L.; et al. Wheat amylase trypsin inhibitors drive intestinal inflammation via activation of toll-like receptor 4. *J. Exp. Med.* **2012**, *209*, 2395–2408. [CrossRef] [PubMed]
19. Tatham, A.S.; Shewry, P.R. Allergens in wheat and related cereals. *Clin. Exp. Allergy* **2008**, *38*, 1721–1726.
20. Nilsson, N.; Sjolander, S.; Baar, A.; Berthold, M.; Pahr, S.; Vrtala, S.; Valenta, R.; Morita, E.; Hedlin, G.; Borres, M.P.; et al. Wheat allergy in children evaluated with challenge and IgE antibodies to wheat components. *Pediatr. Allergy Immunol.* **2015**, *26*, 119–125. [CrossRef] [PubMed]
21. Allergen Nomenclature WHO/International Union of Immunological Societes Allergen Nomenclature Sub-Committee. Allergen Nomenclature. Available online: www.allergen.org (accessed on 30 June 2016).
22. Shibata, R.; Nishima, S.; Tanaka, A.; Borres, M.P.; Morita, E. Usefulness of specific IgE antibodies to ω-5 gliadin in the diagnosis and follow-up of Japanse children with wheat allergy. *Ann. Allergy Asthma Immunol.* **2011**, *107*, 337–343. [CrossRef] [PubMed]
23. Ebisawa, M.; Shibata, R.; Sato, S.; Borres, M.P.; Ito, K. Clinical utility of IgE antibodies to ω-5 gliadin in the diagnosis of wheat allergy: A pediatric multicenter challenge study. *Int. Arch. Allergy Immunol.* **2011**, *158*, 71–76. [CrossRef] [PubMed]
24. Park, H.J.; Kim, J.H.; Kim, J.E.; Jin, H.J.; Choi, G.S.; Ye, Y.M.; Park, H.S. Diagnostic value of the serum-specific IgE ratio of ω-5 gliadin to wheat in adult patients with wheat-induced anaphylaxis. *Int. Arch. Allergy Immunol.* **2011**, *157*, 147–150. [CrossRef] [PubMed]
25. Calamelli, E.; Ricci, G. Wheat allergy in a pediatric population from the Mediterranean area. *Pediatr. Allergy Immunol.* **2015**, *26*, 681–682. [CrossRef] [PubMed]
26. Palosuo, K.; Varjonen, E.; Kekki, O.M.; Klemola, T.; Kalkkinen, N.; Alenius, H.; Reunala, T. Wheat omega-5 gliadin is a major allergen in children with immediate allergy to ingested wheat. *J. Allergy Clin. Immunol.* **2001**, *108*, 634–638. [CrossRef] [PubMed]
27. Mäkelä, M.J.; Eriksson, C.; Kotaniemi-Syrjänen, A.; Palosuo, K.; Marsh, J.; Borres, M.; Kuitunen, M.; Pelkonen, A.S. Wheat allergy in children—New tools for diagnostics. *Clin. Exp. Allergy* **2014**, *44*, 1420–1430. [CrossRef] [PubMed]
28. Ito, K.; Futamura, M.; Borres, M.P.; Takaoka, Y.; Dahlstrom, J.; Sakamoto, T.; Tanaka, A.; Kohno, K.; Matsuo, H.; Morita, E. IgE antibodies to ω-5 gliadin associate with immediate symptoms on oral wheat challenge in Japanese children. *Allergy* **2008**, *63*, 1536–1542. [CrossRef] [PubMed]
29. Palosuo, K.; Alenius, H.; Varjonen, E.; Kalkkinen, N.; Reunala, T. Rye gamma-70 and gamma-35 secalins and brley gamma-3 hordein cross-react with omega-5 gliadin, a major allergen in wheat-dependent, exercise-induced anaphylaxis. *Clin. Exp. Allergy* **2014**, *69*, 1316–1323. [CrossRef] [PubMed]
30. Pahr, S.; Constantin, C.; Papadopoulos, N.G.; Giavi, S.; Mäkelä, M.; Pelkonem, A.; Ebner, C.; Mari, A.; Scheiblhofer, S.; Thalhamer, J.; et al. α-Purothonin, a new wheat allergen associated with severe allergy. *J. Allergy Clin. Immunol.* **2013**, *132*, 1000–1003. [CrossRef] [PubMed]
31. Jones, S.M.; Magnolfi, C.F.; Cooke, S.K.; Sampson, H.A. Immunologic cross-reactivity among cereal grains and grasses in children with food hypersensitivity. *J. Allergy Clin. Immunol.* **1995**, *96*, 341–351. [CrossRef]
32. Constatntin, C.; Quirce, S.; Poorafshar, M.; Touraev, A.; Niggemann, B.; Mari, A.; Ebner, C.; Akerström, H.; Heberle-Bors, E.; Nystrand, M.; et al. Micro-arrayed wheat seed and grass pollen allergens for component-resolved diagnosis. *Allergy* **2009**, *64*, 1030–1037. [CrossRef] [PubMed]
33. Cianferoni, A. Wheat allergy: Diagnosis and management. *J. Asthma Allergy* **2016**, *9*, 13–25. [CrossRef] [PubMed]
34. Scibilia, J.; Pastorello, E.A.; Zisa, G.; Ottolenghi, A.; Bindslev-Jensen, C.; Pravettoni, V.; Scovena, E.; Robino, A.; Ortolani, C. Wheat allergy: A double-blind, placebo-controlled study in adults. *J. Allergy Clin. Immunol.* **2006**, *117*, 433–439. [CrossRef] [PubMed]
35. Sampson, H.A. Utility of food-specific IgE concentrations in predicting symptomatic food allergy. *J. Allergy Clin. Immunol.* **2001**, *107*, 891–896. [CrossRef] [PubMed]
36. Turner, P.J.; Wong, M.; Varese, N.; Rolland, J.M.; O'Hehir, R.E.; Campbell, D.E. Tolerance to wheat in whole-grain cereal biscuit in wheat-allergic children. *J. Allergy Clin. Immunol.* **2013**, *3*, 920–923. [CrossRef] [PubMed]
37. Sato, S.; Utsunomiya, T.; Imai, T.; Yanagida, N. Wheat oral immunotherapy for wheat-induced anaphylaxis. *J. Allergy Clin. Immunol.* **2015**, *4*, 1131–1133. [CrossRef] [PubMed]

38. Altenbach, S.B.; Allen, P.V. Transformation of the US bread wheat 'Butte 86' and silencing of omega-5 gliadin genes. *GM Crops* **2011**, *2*, 66–73. [CrossRef] [PubMed]
39. Poole, J.A.; Barriga, K.; Leung, D.Y.; Hoffman, M.; Eisenbarth, G.S.; Rewers, M.; Norris, J.M. Timing of initial exposure to cereal grains and the risk of wheat allergy. *Pediatrics* **2006**, *117*, 2175–2182. [CrossRef] [PubMed]
40. Perkin, M.R.; Lack, G. Introducing allergenic foods in infants. *N. Engl. J. Med.* **2016**, *25*, 375.
41. Lionetti, E.; Castellaneta, S.; Francavilla, R.; Pulvirenti, A.; Tonutti, E.; Arnarri, S.; Barbato, M.; Barbera, C.; Barera, G.; Bellantoni, A.; et al. Introduction of gluten, HLA status, and the risk of celiac disease in children. *N. Engl. J. Med.* **2014**, *371*, 1295–1303. [CrossRef] [PubMed]
42. Szajewska, H.; Shamir, R.; Mearin, L.; Ribes-Koninckx, C.; Catassi, C.; Domellöf, M.; Fewtrell, M.S.; Husby, S.; Papadopoulou, A.; Vandenplas, Y.; et al. Gluten introduction and the risk of coeliac disease: A position paper by the European society for pediatric gastroenterology, hepatology, and nutrition. *J. Pediatr. Gastroenterol. Nutr.* **2016**, *62*, 507–513. [CrossRef] [PubMed]

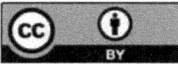

nutrients

MDPI

Article

Content Validation and Semantic Evaluation of a Check-List Elaborated for the Prevention of Gluten Cross-Contamination in Food Services

Priscila Farage [1,*], Renata Puppin Zandonadi [1], Verônica Cortez Ginani [1], Lenora Gandolfi [2], Riccardo Pratesi [2] and Yanna Karla de Medeiros Nóbrega [2]

[1] Department of Nutrition, Faculty of Health Sciences, University of Brasilia (UnB), Campus Darcy Ribeiro, Asa Norte, Brasilia DF 70910-900, Brazil; renatapz@yahoo.com.br (R.P.Z.); vcginani@gmail.com (V.C.G.)
[2] Faculty of Medicine, University of Brasilia (UnB), Campus Darcy Ribeiro, Asa Norte, Brasilia DF 70910-900, Brazil; lenoragandolfi1@gmail.com (L.G.); pratesiunb@gmail.com (R.P.); yannanobrega@gmail.com (Y.K.d.M.N.)
* Correspondence: pri_farage@hotmail.com; Tel.: +55-61-9818-70144

Received: 15 November 2016; Accepted: 26 December 2016; Published: 6 January 2017

Abstract: Conditions associated to the consumption of gluten have emerged as a major health care concern and the treatment consists on a lifelong gluten-free diet. Providing safe food for these individuals includes adapting to safety procedures within the food chain and preventing gluten cross-contamination in gluten-free food. However, a gluten cross-contamination prevention protocol or check-list has not yet been validated. Therefore, the aim of this study was to perform the content validation and semantic evaluation of a check-list elaborated for the prevention of gluten cross-contamination in food services. The preliminary version of the check-list was elaborated based on the Brazilian resolution for food safety *Collegiate Board Resolution 216* (RDC 216) and *Collegiate Board Resolution 275* (RDC 275), the *standard 22000* from the International Organization for Standardization (ISO 22000) and the Canadian Celiac Association *Gluten-Free Certification Program* documents. Seven experts with experience in the area participated in the check-list validation and semantic evaluation. The criteria used for the approval of the items, as to their importance for the prevention of gluten cross-contamination and clarity of the wording, was the achievement of a minimal of 80% of agreement between the experts (W-values $\geq$ 0.8). Moreover, items should have a mean $\geq$4 in the evaluation of importance (Likert scale from 1 to 5) and clarity (Likert scale from 0 to 5) in order to be maintained in the instrument. The final version of the check-list was composed of 84 items, divided into 12 sections. After being redesigned and re-evaluated, the items were considered important and comprehensive by the experts (both with W-values $\geq$ 0.89). The check-list developed was validated with respect to content and approved in the semantic evaluation.

Keywords: gluten; gluten contamination; food safety; celiac disease; gluten related disorders

1. Introduction

Recently, there has been a growing demand for gluten-free products in the world population. The global market of these products approached $2.5 billion (US) in sales in 2010. It seems that the number of individuals embracing a gluten-free diet (GFD) is much higher than the projected number of celiac disease (CD) patients. This finding can be explained by the existence of Gluten Related Disorders (GRD) other than CD, which is now clear. The GRD include three main forms of gluten reactions: allergic (wheat allergy), autoimmune (CD, dermatitis herpetiformis, and gluten ataxia), and possibly immune-mediated (gluten sensitivity) [1].

Despite differences in pathological mechanisms, clinical manifestations, and epidemiology, the treatment for all GRD consists of excluding gluten-containing cereals and sub-products from the diet. Combined, these conditions affect many individuals who consequently need to follow the GFD. CD accounts for around 1% of the general population. In regards to wheat allergy, different prevalence rates have been found in studies around the world, varying from 0.4% in adults to as high as 9% in children [1]. The prevalence of gluten sensitivity is not clearly defined yet. However, indirect evidence suggests that it is slightly more common than CD [2].

According to Codex Alimentarius, "gluten-free foods" (GFF) are those in which the gluten level does not exceed 20 ppm (mg/kg) in total [3]. In a systematic review, Akobeng et al. (2008) [4] investigated the threshold amount of gluten that could be tolerated by people with CD and found that there is a variation among individuals. Although there was no evidence to suggest a single definitive threshold, they found that a daily gluten intake of less than 10 mg was unlikely to cause significant histological abnormalities in celiac patients [4]. As to the other GRD, further studies are necessary to clarify whether the spectrum of toxic cereals, the gluten threshold, and the disease duration are the same as in CD, since their natural history, particularly of gluten sensitivity, is still unclear [1].

Following the GFD is a difficult task for GRD patients due to the presence of gluten in a wide range of products. Moreover, gluten may be found in supposedly gluten-free products as a consequence of cross-contamination, which leads to the involuntary and unconscious consumption of it [5].

Cross-contamination might occur because of shared production areas, kitchenware not properly sanitized, and inadequate procedures by restaurant staff [6]. In most countries there is not a consistent monitoring process to assess gluten content in supposedly GFF in order to guarantee safe products for CD and other GRD patients [7]. Moreover, studies have revealed gluten-contamination in both industrial products and food services preparations [8–10], which represents a problem for these patients since maintaining gluten in the diet triggers symptoms and health problems such as gastrointestinal manifestations and other related conditions [1].

Therefore, eating out may be considered a health risk for GRD individuals [11] and the need to follow the GFD may compromise social activities and influence quality of life [12]. Thus, in order to contribute to a better quality of life for GRD patients, it is important to establish viable and effective strategies to prevent contamination and enable the safe production of gluten-free food [11].

The development of an instrument for the verification of non-conformities in loco that are related to the occurrence of cross-contamination seems like an interesting approach in order to control the production process and provide safe food for GRD patients considering the paucity of studies that investigate possible strategies to prevent gluten cross-contamination in food services.

In a study conducted in Italy, the Hazard Analysis and Critical Control Point system (HACCP) was used for the elaboration of a plan to prevent gluten contamination in a school cafeteria, and the results showed the effectiveness of this plan in the reduction of contamination [13]. In Brazil, Bicudo (2010) [14] elaborated and implemented the standard operating procedures (SOPs) for items related to accidental gluten cross-contamination in a bakery. In this study, a checklist was first applied followed by the elaboration of corrective measures for problems found. The association of the SOPs together with the corrective measures based on good manufacturing practices was effective in controlling gluten contamination in the study site [14].

Most studies on food safety discuss issues related to microbiological contamination, however, it is important that food services adapt to food preparation practices in order to produce safe special diets, such as the GFD.

There are specific regulations on gluten-free labelling in the context of gluten intolerance worldwide. Most of them are based on the Codex Alimentarius Standard 118-1979 and recommend following good manufacturing practices for the prevention of gluten cross-contamination, ranging from country to country. The European Union, United States, and Canada follow the limits proposed by Codex for GFF (20 ppm). In Argentina, the threshold set for GFF is 10 ppm. In Australia and

New Zealand, legislation is stricter and states that to be considered "gluten-free", food must not contain detectable gluten [7,15,16]. However, it must be emphasized that, in food services, this is rarely regulated and monitored.

For the development of an instrument for data collection, the phenomena of interest must be translated into concepts that can be measured, observed, or recorded. Without proper methods for data collection, the validity of the questionnaire conclusions is questionable. Thus, it is very important to consider some points during the process, such as, an extensive review of literature on the theme, experience of the researcher on the subject, care and monitoring of the formulation of each question/item regarding clarity, consistency, relevance, and impartiality; evaluation of the instrument by experts in the field of knowledge, and the testing to verify whether the instrument is useful in order to obtain the desired information [17].

The validation of an instrument consists of a methodological procedure to evaluate its quality, which is related to the capacity of the instrument to accurately measure what it is intended to measure [17]. The content validity refers to the representativeness and relevance of the instrument questions. The content validation can be analyzed by a panel composed of professionals and researchers recognized in their area [18]. The expert panel consensus helps defining the instrument items which should be maintained, revised, or excluded and its application is increasing in several areas [19].

Another important procedure to obtain a satisfactory instrument is to perform the semantic evaluation, which measures the comprehension of the instrument items by the judges and helps to evaluate the need to rewrite the questions in order to achieve a better understanding of the instrument [20].

This study aimed to perform the content validation and semantic evaluation of an instrument (check-list) elaborated for the prevention and control of gluten cross-contamination in food services.

2. Methods

2.1. Development of the Instrument

The instrument (check-list) was elaborated based on extensive literature review and experience of the researchers on the matter. The following documents were used to design the preliminary version of the check-list: the Brazilian resolutions for food safety *Collegiate Board Resolution 216* (RDC 216) and *Collegiate Board Resolution 275* (RDC 275), the international *standard 22000* from the International Organization for Standardization (ISO 22000), and the documents from the *Gluten-Free Certification Program*, of the Canadian Celiac Association [21–24].

Topics and items from the resolutions RDC 216 and RDC 275 and the ISO 22000 standard were carefully evaluated and those thought to be relevant to the prevention of gluten cross-contamination were chosen and adapted for the initial version of the check-list, even though these documents do not specifically address the prevention of gluten cross-contamination. However, the premise of a functional gluten contamination control system is based on prerequisites programs implemented in the establishment, attending minimally to the good manufacturing practices, as proposed by the Codex [3].

Important topics of the *Gluten-Free Certification Program*, Canada, were also selected to compose the check-list and adapted to contemplate the reality of food services. The preliminary version was composed of 136 items divided into 13 major sections, listed below:

- Identification/information of the establishment
- Building and facilities
- Equipment, furniture, and kitchenware
- Food service employees
- Food production and transport
- Distribution

- Documentation
- Responsibility and authority
- Coordinator of the food safety team
- Internal communication
- Flow charts
- Traceability
- Treatment of potentially unsafe products

All of the items had a "Yes/No/Not Applicable" type of answer, such as the check-list presented in the RDC 275, except for the items of the "Identification/information of the establishment" section, which contains open questions to characterize the establishment (name of the place, address, owner, among others).

2.2. Pilot Test (Subjective Evaluation)

For the content validation, a total of 11 experts with a PhD and known experience in instruments of quality control for food services and/or gluten and CD were invited to participate. A total of seven experts were available for the study. The experts received the necessary information and guidance on the check-list method of evaluation. The check-list was sent by e-mail.

At first, experts were asked to express their opinion on the preliminary version of the instrument and evaluate the overall questionnaire, considering aspects such as the content, clarity, type, and consistency of the items. Experts were also asked to suggest any modification, exclusion, or inclusion of items they judged relevant and to freely comment on any subject regarding the instrument. This was characterized as a qualitative analysis stage.

2.3. Content Validation

The Delphi method was used, with some adaptations, for the content validation. This method is based on obtaining the opinions of experts in order to achieve a consensus on a specific subject. The Delphi method is currently employed in several areas in situations where new ideas are being created. It is a method in which, through collegial communication ordered by individual responses, often conducted by questionnaires, we seek the consensus of a group [19].

The Monkey Survey@ platform was used to create a questionnaire for the application of the content validation of the check-list. On the first page of the questionnaire there was an orientation letter specifying the evaluation criteria for the check-list items. Experts were asked to evaluate each item considering its importance for the prevention of gluten cross-contamination using a Likert scale, as follows: (1) "I totally disagree with the item"; (2) "I partially disagree with the item"; (3) "I neither agree nor disagree with the item"; (4) "I partially disagree with the item"; and (5) "I fully agree with the item".

The Monkey Survey@ platform was also used to provide feedback to the experts in regards to the evaluations performed by other experts and final results of the analysis. Two stages of evaluation were performed in the content validation process. For the items which did not receive approval in the first stage, the means resulting from the experts' opinions were presented to each one of them. After being informed about the other experts' opinions, the experts were asked to review their analysis and decide whether or not they would confirm previous answers. This procedure was performed in order to obtain consensus among the experts. All seven experts participated in this phase.

2.4. Semantic Evaluation

The semantic evaluation of the check-list was performed simultaneously with the content validation, using the same questionnaire in the Monkey Survey@ platform. Experts were asked to evaluate each item in regards to its clarity, considering their level of understanding of the item. For that purpose, the Likert scale was used, as follows: (0) "I did not understand it at all"; (1) "I understood it a little"; (2) "I somewhat understood it"; (3) "I understood almost everything, but I had some questions"; (4) "I understood almost everything"; (5) "I understood it perfectly and had no questions". According to Conti et al. (2010) [20], answers from 0 to 3 indicate insufficient understanding and a new version of the item is required [20].

In cases of poor understanding of the item or unsuitable language, experts were also asked to suggest changes. These commentaries were used to create new versions of the items for further evaluation. Three stages of evaluation were performed in the semantic evaluation process. Six experts participated in the last stage.

2.5. Data Analysis

For data analysis, all answers obtained with the questionnaire were compiled using the Microsoft Excel 97-2003 software.

The mean grade for the evaluation of importance and clarity of each item was calculated considering the answers provided by the seven experts, except for the last stage of the semantic evaluation, in which six experts participated. The degree of agreement among the experts for the evaluation of importance and clarity of the items was evaluated through the Kendall (W) coefficient of concordance, which ranges from 0 to 1. High W-values (W $\geq$ 0.66) indicate that the experts applied the same standards of evaluation as opposed to Low W-values, which suggest disagreement among the experts [17].

The criteria established for the approval of the item was a minimal of 80% of agreement between the experts (W-values $\geq$ 0.8). Moreover, items should have a mean $\geq$4 for the evaluation of importance (content validation) and clarity (semantic evaluation) in order to be maintained in the instrument. Items not considered important for the prevention of gluten-cross contamination in food services were excluded from the instrument. Items considered unclear were rewritten in a different manner and subject to further evaluation by the experts.

Suggestions made by the experts were considered and incorporated into the final version of the instrument.

3. Results

Considering the suggestions made by the experts in the pilot test, a new version of the check-list was created, consisting of 88 items, divided into 12 sections. The "Traceability" section was not considered applicable for the food service environment and it was removed from the check-list. This new version was then submitted to an objective evaluation. At this point, the first stage of the content validation and the semantic evaluation was performed. In total, two stages of evaluation were necessary in order to obtain agreement among the experts for the content validation and three stages were necessary for the semantic evaluation.

The summary of stages and exclusion or corrections of items of the whole validation process are displayed in Figure 1.

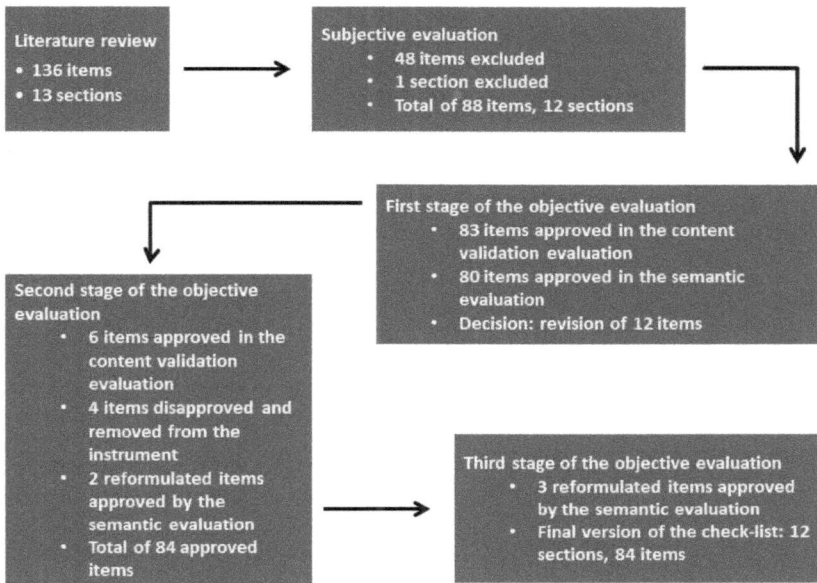

Figure 1. Stages of the content validation and semantic evaluation processes.

3.1. First Stage: Content Validation and Semantic Evaluation

In the first evaluation of the content validation process, a total of 83 items (94.3%) were approved, that is, there was a minimal of 80% of agreement between the experts (W-values $\geq$ 0.8) and the items displayed a mean $\geq$4 in the evaluation of importance. The remaining five items without approval in this stage were: 1.6.2 (regarding goods lift for gluten-free food), 1.8.1 (regarding washbasins and soap supply in the production area), 1.12.1 (regarding the proper layout for food production), 8.5 (regarding the report on effectiveness and adequacy of the control of gluten contamination by the coordinator of the food safety team), and 9.8 (regarding information about relevant issues from outside concerned parties).

As to the semantic evaluation, a total of 80 items (90.9%) were considered sufficiently understandable (these items received grades "4" or "5" in the Likert scale) and thus were approved without needing to adjust the wording.

The mean grades and W-values for each section, considering the means of all items, for the content validation and semantic evaluation are presented in Table 1.

Despite being approved in regards to the content validation in stage 1, items 9.7 (regarding information about customer requirements, sectoral requirements, and others), 9.9 (regarding information about customer complaints indicating food safety hazards associated with the product), 9.10 (regarding information about other conditions which might impact the gluten contamination control), 9.11 (regarding update of the gluten contamination control system), and 9.12 (regarding the inclusion of relevant information for critical analysis in the system) were not considered clear enough by the experts in the semantic evaluation.

Moreover, some experts suggested the removal of some of those items and made comments about the lack of understanding of the purpose of the item in the check-list and how to verify what it proposed regarding food service practices. They also mentioned that some of those items were too subjective and/or repetitive. Therefore, researchers considered it important to resubmit these items to the evaluation of importance in the instrument, through a new evaluation of content, before rewriting the items and submitting them to a new semantic evaluation.

Thus, a total of 12 items were subject to further evaluation in stage 2.

Table 1. Experts evaluation of the check-list—mean grades and Kendall coefficient of concordance of the check-list sections.

Section of the Check-List	Content Validation (Mean Grade ± SD *)	Content Validation (W-Value)	Semantic Evaluation (Mean Grade ± SD *)	Semantic Evaluation (W-Value)
Building and facilities	4.74 ± 0.30	0.96	4.76 ± 0.15	0.92
Equipment, furniture and kitchenware	4.79 ± 0.25	0.97	4.83 ± 0.17	0.96
Food service employees	4.81 ± 0.20	0.98	4.79 ± 0.20	0.93
Food production and transport	4.79 ± 0.21	0.96	4.87 ± 0.17	0.98
Distribution	4.86 ± 0.14	0.94	5.00 ± 0.00	1.00
Documentation	4.82 ± 0.27	0.96	4.75 ± 0.32	0.96
Responsibility and authority	4.86 ± 0.00	1.00	5.00 ± 0.00	1.00
Coordinator of the food security team	4.57 ± 0.26	0.89	5.00 ± 0.00	1.00
Internal communication	4.78 ± 0.23	0.92	4.71 ± 0.29	0.94
Flow charts	4.86 ± 0.14	1.00	4.71 ± 0.14	0.90
Treatment of potentially unsafe products	4.52 ± 0.24	0.90	4.76 ± 0.20	0.95

* Standard Deviation.

3.2. Second Stage: Content Validation and Semantic Evaluation

In this stage, items 1.6.2, 1.8.1, 1.12.1, 8.5, 9.7, 9.8, 9.9, 9.10, 9.11, and 9.12 were submitted once more to the content validation. For that purpose, the means of grades attributed by the experts in the previous stage were presented to them in order for them to check whether they wanted to maintain the grade that was previously assigned to the item or whether they wanted to reconsider taking into consideration the opinion of the other experts. A sum of comments made by the experts was also presented for them to help achieve a consensus.

At this point, six of these items (60%)—1.6.2, 1.8.1, 1.12.1, 9.9, 9.10, and 9.11—were considered important by the experts and thus maintained in the check-list. The other four items—8.5, 9.7, 9.8, and 9.12—were removed from the check-list (mean grade < 4).

Items 1.6.1 (regarding ramps and workbenches) and 1.11.1 (regarding containers for the collection of waste within the facility) were not considered sufficiently understandable in stage 1. These items were reformulated considering comments and suggestions made by the experts in stage 1 and subject to semantic evaluation. Both of them were approved in this new version.

Since items 9.9, 9.10, and 9.11 were reassessed by the experts as to their importance for the prevention of gluten cross-contamination and received grades >4, they were kept in the check-list. However, they had not been approved as to their clarity in the first stage of the semantic evaluation. Therefore, these items were subject to a new stage of semantic evaluation.

3.3. Third Stage: Semantic Evaluation

At this point, only three items—9.9, 9.10, and 9.11—needed further evaluation, in regards to their clarity. The items were reformulated based on previous comments and suggestions by the experts. In this stage, one expert was not available to participate and the mean grades were calculated based on the other six experts' opinions. The new versions of the items were approved in this stage and the process of content validation and semantic evaluation was accomplished. It is important to mention that the content validation and semantic evaluation were performed in Portuguese, the original version of the instrument. However, the complete check-list (Appendix A) was translated into English in order to facilitate the readers' understanding. It can be found in the appendix section.

4. Discussion

Gluten contamination in supposedly gluten-free food is a very concerning issue. As the study by Hollon et al. (2013) [25] showed, gluten traces may impair histological and clinical recovery of patients, even leading to an incorrect diagnosis of refractory celiac disease (RCD), which would result in the unnecessary use of corticosteroids or immunotherapy with potential adverse health effects [25].

The most common cause of non-response in the treatment for CD is related to the failure to adhere to the GFD [25], including unintentional consumption of gluten by means of contaminated food. This fact highlights the importance of providing safe food for CD patients.

In the process of development and validation of an instrument, it is very important to use rigorous methods [17]. In this study, the Delphi technique was chosen. It allows the implementation of an experts panel in order to perform the content validation, facilitating the achievement of consensus on the experts' opinions [26].

As in the study by Ceniccola et al. (2014) [26], the Delphi technique was used to guide the stages of the experts' evaluations, making them interact with the research group through structured rounds. As mentioned earlier, this was performed using the Survey Monkey® platform, which enables the provision of feedback to the experts. The feedback is proposed in the Delphi technique as it helps to assure a more organized interaction with the experts [26].

The appropriate selection of the experts is also a critical point to obtain solid results and it is based on the experience and the knowledge of the participants in a certain area, besides the willingness to collaborate with the study. There is no consensus in the literature in regards to the number of experts to perform the validation process [19,27–30]. Nevertheless, Pasquali (1999) [28] considers that a minimum of six experts is necessary to reach a consensus, although this number may vary according to the type of the instrument [28]. In this study, a total of seven experts participated.

The obtaining of a validated check-list for the control of gluten contamination is of urgent need for food services. In Brazil, hygienic-sanitary control in food production has been improving in recent years. The rules defined in resolutions on the subject have proved to be effective, since a lot of studies have shown the reduction of outbreaks of foodborne diseases [31]. However, there is a lack of studies on the development of quality control instruments for the prevention of gluten cross-contamination. Despite the fact that the Brazilian legislation sets the obligatoriness when including a statement regarding the presence or absence of gluten in the label of industrial products, it does not address the production of gluten-free food in food services [8].

In this study, a check-list was elaborated and evaluated with the purpose of providing an appropriate tool to assist in the gluten-free food production system and ensuring the right to safe food for GRD patients. The final check-list was carefully revised and all items included were considered important and comprehensive by the experts (both with agreement by Kendall coefficient ≥0.89).

The check-list created presents strong points, since it was submitted to the evaluation of experts on the area, who were free to make any comments which they deemed relevant to improve the instrument. Moreover, the semantic evaluation process helps to ensure that the items are clear and comprehensive as to the language and writing.

As a study by Araújo et al. (2011) [32] revealed, individuals who follow a GFD ingest food with gluten because of lack of alternatives and/or information in food found in public places [32]. Having a meal in a restaurant creates a problem for those individuals because of the lack of knowledge by the restaurant staff concerning the correct procedures to prevent contamination and provide safe food [33]. In a study conducted in Brazil, Laporte et al. (2011) [34] interviewed restaurant chefs regarding their knowledge about CD and only 30% of the participants referred knowing the disease [34].

Machado et al. (2013) assessed adherence to the GFD by structural interviews with CD patients and the results were compared to their IgA anti-transglutaminase antibodies' levels. The serological tests showed that 56.5% of the individuals did not follow the GFD. However, 60.9% referred complete elimination of gluten from the diet. Among those, 35.7% presented a positive result in the serological test, which possibly indicates involuntary diet transgression [35].

This fact compromises social activities which ultimately impair quality of life [5]. Thus, viable and effective strategies to prevent contamination must be developed, including quality control audits to assure that established protocols are being followed. This has already been accomplished for the control of microbiological contamination and there is an urgent need to enable the same for the control of gluten cross-contamination.

Although there are other available check-lists for the control of gluten contamination, this study brings a novelty that is the validation of a specific tool for food services. Moreover, the use of the Delphi method allows for the ability to have a great volume of information; better reflection on the subject and more elaborated answers due to the use of questionnaires; elimination of influences of judgment that could interfere with the quality of the answers due to the anonymity of the technique; and the possibility of incorporating new ideas raised by experts in the area [19]. The semantic evaluation performed also makes this check-list an interesting tool since it helps to assure proper understanding of the items, which is crucial for the correct evaluation of conformities/non-conformities situations in loco and ultimately might impact the safety of the food produced in certain establishments.

This study is part of a larger study currently in progress. The check-list will be applied in food services where samples will be collected for the evaluation of gluten contamination. Data obtained will be submitted to statistical analysis to determine which items/sections are in fact related to the contamination and which trigger higher chances of generating contaminated food. Thus, in this second phase, it will be possible to evaluate the removal of unnecessary items from the check-list—which will make the check-list shorter and more practical—and also provide different grades to each item/section which will culminate in a score for classifying the establishment as to its risk of providing contaminated food.

The proposed check-list is attractive for its practicality and low cost. Moreover, it can be used for identifying inappropriate routines and allowing the correction of non-conformities to ensure safe food for those who need to engage a GFD.

5. Conclusions

The instrument (check-list) developed for the verification of non-conformities related to gluten-contamination in food services was validated with respect to content, after careful revision of its items. After it was redesigned, the items were considered important and comprehensive by the experts (both with agreement by Kendall coefficient ≥0.89).

However, it is important to highlight that future studies are necessary to assess other properties of the instrument, such as reliability using the criteria of reproducibility which aims at verifying the proportion of agreement among the responses when the instrument is applied in the same location and circumstances by different professionals.

Further studies are also necessary in order to test this instrument in food services and evaluate its effectiveness in contributing to the prevention of gluten cross-contamination. Strategies such as this are very important to improve the access to safe food by GRD patients and ultimately contribute to greater quality of life.

Acknowledgments: The authors acknowledge the important contribution of the experts involved in the content validation and semantic evaluation processes. The research received funding from the "Fundação de Apoio à Pesquisa do Distrito Federal—FAP/DF" (Edital 03/2015—0193.000982/2015) and "Laboratório Interdisciplinar de Biociências da Universidade de Brasília".

Author Contributions: Priscila Farage: conception and design of the study; acquisition, analysis and interpretation of data; drafting of the manuscript. Renata Zandonadi: conception and design of the study; analysis and interpretation of data; supervision; drafting and critical revision of the manuscript. Verônica Cortez Ginani: conception and design of the study; supervision; critical revision of the manuscript. Lenora Gandolfi: conception and design of the study; supervision; critical revision of the manuscript. Riccardo Pratesi: conception and design of the study; supervision; critical revision of the manuscript. Yanna Karla de Medeiros Nóbrega: conception and design of the study; supervision; critical revision of the manuscript.

Conflicts of Interest: The authors declare no conflict of interest.

Appendix A

Check-List for the Verification of Non-Conformities Related to Gluten-Contamination in Food Services

Legend:			
Y—Yes	N—No	NA—Not Applicable	OBS—Observation

Number:	Year:		
Company identification:			
Company name:			
Trading name:			
Health license:	State/municipal registration:		
National record of legalized person/individual registration:	Phone:	Fax:	
E-mail:			
Address:			
Neighborhood:	City:	State:	Zip code:
Activity branch:	Monthly output:		
Number of employees:	Number of shifts:		
Products' categories:			
Category description:			
Technical manager:	Academic background of the technical manager:		
Is there an employee responsible for the good manufacturing practices in the establishment? ( ) Yes ( ) No	Academic background of the employee responsible for the good manufacturing practices: ( ) training course ( ) technical course. Which? ( ) college degree. On what?		

Legal representative/owner of the establishment:				
Items	Y	N	NA	OBS
1. Building and Facilities				
1.1. floor				
1.1.1. Floor material that allows easy and proper sanitation (smooth, drained with slope, waterproof).				
1.1.2. Floor in proper conservation (free of defects, cracks, holes, and others).				
1.2. Ceiling				
1.2.1. Ceiling easy to clean waterproof with smooth finishing.				
1.3. Walls				
1.3.1. Smooth finishing walls, impermeable and easy to clean at suitable height for all operations.				
1.3.2. Wall in proper conservation (free from cracks and peeling).				
1.4. Doors				
1.4.1. Smooth surface doors, adjusted to the jambs and without coating faults in order to reduce the risk of contamination coming from the external area.				

1.5.	**Windows and other openings**				
	1.5.1.	Smooth surface windows, adjusted to the jambs and without coating faults in order to reduce the risk of contamination coming from the external area.			
1.6.	**Stairs, service elevators, goods lift, and auxiliary structures**				
	1.6.1.	In case of ramps and workbenches used to support both gluten-free and gluten-containing food, a hygienic procedure is performed between the use of this surface for gluten-containing and gluten-free food.			
	1.6.2.	There is a goods lift exclusive for the use of gluten-free food.			
1.7.	**Toilets and dressing rooms for employees**				
	1.7.1.	Toilets equipped with washbasins and products intended for personal hygiene: antiseptic odorless liquid soap or odorless liquid soap and antiseptic, non-recycled paper towel or other safe and hygienic drying system, collectors with lid and without manual activation.			
1.8.	**Washbasins in the production area**				
	1.8.1.	Existence of washbasins in the production area with running water, in appropriate positions in relation to the production and service flow, with sufficient number to suit the entire production area, preferably equipped with automatic stopcock, antiseptic odorless liquid soap or odorless liquid soap and antiseptic, non-recycled paper towels or other hygienic and safe drying system and paper collectors without manual activation.			
1.9.	**Ventilation and air conditioning**				
	1.9.1.	Artificially air-conditioned environments, without fans, without generating airflow and absence of natural airflow from the production area of gluten-containing food to the production area of gluten-free food, avoiding an environment with particles in suspension.			
1.10.	**Cleaning of the facilities**				
	1.10.1.	Facilities kept under appropriate hygienic-sanitary conditions, that is, without the presence of accumulation of residues, with proof by means of registration in specific spreadsheets, updated and with information consistent with what is being observed.			
	1.10.2.	Utensils used for the cleaning of facilities distinct from those used for the cleaning of equipment that come into contact with food, with hygiene products and utensils exclusive for the use in the production area of gluten-free food.			
1.11.	**Waste management**				
	1.11.1.	Containers for the collection of waste inside the establishment which are easily sanitized (i.e., without cracks that allow dirt to accumulate and are difficult to access by cleaning utensils) and transported (i.e., can be easily moved by those responsible for the procedure); emptied whenever its content reaches 2/3 of its capacity and constantly sanitized, showing no evidence of accumulated dirt; use of appropriate garbage bags.			
	1.11.2.	Waste removed from the gluten-containing food production area does not pass through the production area of gluten-free food.			

1.12. Layout					
1.12.1.	Layout suitable for the productive process: number, capacity, and distribution of dependencies according to the branch of activity, production volume, and expedition.				
1.12.2.	Areas for receiving and depositing ingredients distinct from the areas of production, storage, and expedition of the final product.				
1.12.3.	Gluten-free ingredients warehouse identified and in a different space from that of gluten-containing ingredients.				
1.12.4.	Area of production of gluten-free food identified and in a separate space from that of the production area of gluten-containing food.				
2. Equipment, furniture, and kitchenware					
2.1. Equipment					
2.1.1.	Equipment arranged in a way that allows easy access and proper cleaning.				
2.1.2.	Equipment with contact surfaces which are smooth, undamaged, waterproof, and easy to clean.				
2.1.3.	Production line equipment (mixers, processors, blenders, toasters, etc.) identified and exclusive to the production of gluten-free food.				
2.1.4.	Food preservation equipment (refrigerators, freezers, cold rooms) exclusive for gluten-free products or, when not possible, the disposal of products is done in separate spots and/or with some kind of physical separation between gluten-free and gluten-containing products.				
2.1.5.	Thermal processing equipment (ovens) exclusive for gluten-free food or, when of common use, not used for baking gluten-free and gluten-containing food simultaneously.				
2.1.6.	Thermal processing equipment (fryers, hot plate for tapiocas, pancakes, and others) exclusive for gluten-free food.				
2.2. Furniture (tables, workbenches, window displays, shelves)					
2.2.1.	Furniture designed for easy cleaning (smooth, without wrinkles and cracks, and of a waterproof material).				
2.2.2.	Existence of specific furniture for the production of gluten-free food or existence of a proper cleaning process between the use of the furniture for gluten-containing and gluten-free food proved by an updated registration worksheet with information consistent with what is being observed.				
2.3. Kitchenware					
2.3.1.	Kitchenware of material, size, and shape that allow easy cleaning.				
2.3.2.	General kitchenware (pans, spoons, knives, cutlery, etc.) exclusive for gluten-free food, stored in an appropriate and identified place, in organized manner, and protected against contamination by gluten or, when not exclusive, properly sanitized prior to the usage and preparation of gluten-free food.				
2.3.3.	Difficult to clean kitchenware (sieves, pastry brush, graters, etc.) exclusive for the production of gluten-free food.				

2.4. Cleaning of equipment, machinery, furniture, and kitchenware				
2.4.1.	Equipment, machinery, furniture, and kitchenware kept in proper hygienic-sanitary conditions, that is, without the presence or accumulation of residues, with proof by means of registration in specific spreadsheets, updated, and with information consistent with what is observed.			
2.4.2.	Availability of cleaning products required to perform the operation and dilution, contact time, and form of use/application according to the instructions recommended by the manufacturer.			
2.4.3.	Availability and suitability of all necessary utensils to carry out the cleaning operation with those in good condition.			
2.4.4.	Whenever gluten-free food is handled, cleaning of equipment, machinery, furniture, and kitchenware that are of common use for gluten-free and gluten-containing foods is performed properly.			
2.4.5.	Use of an exclusive sponge or similar to sanitize all kitchenware, equipment, and surfaces that will come into contact with gluten-free food.			
2.4.6.	Dishwasher usage: crockery used for gluten-containing and gluten-free food sanitized at different moments.			
3. Food service employees				
3.1. Clothing				
3.1.1.	Employees display proper personal cleanliness: body cleanliness, clean hands, short nails, clean uniforms.			
3.1.2.	Employees use a uniform exclusive for handling gluten-free food or a uniform which has not been previously used to handle food with gluten, without having been washed afterwards.			
3.2. Hygienic habits				
3.2.1.	There is guidance (posters) for proper hand hygiene, which includes appropriate moments and procedures, accessible to employees and followed correctly.			
3.2.2.	Employees do not handle gluten-containing and gluten-free foods simultaneously or engage in any act that could lead to cross-contamination, such as eating during food preparation.			
3.3. Employees training program and supervision				
3.3.1.	Existence of a proper and continuous training program related to the production of gluten-free food and registration of these trainings.			
3.3.2.	Existence of supervision of the procedures to avoid gluten contamination by a properly trained supervisor.			
4. Food production and transport				
4.1. Raw materials, ingredients, and package				
4.1.1.	Raw materials, ingredients, and packaging are inspected at the reception, observing if the labels of the raw material and ingredients meet the specific legislation for gluten. Potential sources of gluten are identified and controlled upon reception.			
4.1.2.	Defrosting of gluten-free food held in a separate location from gluten-containing food and without getting in touch with utensils and equipment where gluten-containing food is stored or held in locations that are cleaned before procedure.			

4.2.	Selection of recipes and ingredients and food preparation				
	4.2.1.	The selection of recipes and ingredients and the manufacturing technical cards are accurately followed for gluten-free food, with the label of all ingredients being checked at the time of preparation.				
	4.2.2.	Water or oil previously used in the preparation of gluten-containing food is not reused at the preparation of gluten-free food.				
	4.2.3.	Ingredients are not of common use for the production of gluten-free and gluten-containing food (e.g., margarine). All products intended for the preparation of gluten-free food are identified.				
4.3.	Production flow				
	4.3.1.	The reception of gluten-free products occurs in a separated space from other products or carried out at a different moment.				
	4.3.2.	Segregation or separation of procedures such as production scheduling or specific/exclusive lines for gluten-free food, with an ordered flow without crossing between gluten-free and gluten-containing food.				
4.4.	Labeling and storage of final product and/or semi-prepared products				
	4.4.1.	Final and/or semi-finished products (products that will be used in the elaboration of pasta, fillings, sauces, etc.), packaged in a suitable container (known composition of the container material—gluten-free), intact and exclusive for gluten-free food.				
	4.4.2.	Labeling statements with visible identification and in accordance with current legislation regarding the presence or absence of gluten.				
	4.4.3.	Products with and without gluten stored separately by a physical barrier or proper distance, in order to avoid contact between them.				
4.5.	Transportation of the final product				
	4.5.1.	Transportation maintains the integrity of food.				
	4.5.2.	The vehicle does not simultaneously carry gluten-containing and gluten-free food or it does carry these products simultaneously, but with due care of separation by physical barrier or proper distance between them (use of sealed containers, of impermeable material).				
5.	Distribution				
5.1.	At the distribution of food, employees follow procedures to eliminate the risk of gluten contamination, through hand hygiene, use of protective utensils, and disposable gloves and others whenever there is previous contact with gluten-containing food.				
5.2.	Separate disposal, at different distribution counters. Preparation according to the presence/absence of gluten.				
5.3.	Preparation identified with labels or other visible method according to its gluten content.				
5.4.	Kitchenware used for serving food exclusive for gluten-free preparation and identified with different colors.				
5.5.	Monitoring of the preparation identification plates in regards to the presence/absence of gluten at the moment of distribution.				

6. Documentation				
6.1. Manual of good practices				
6.1.1. Operations carried out at the facility are in accordance with an on-site Good Practices Manual that meets the legal requirements in regards to content and updating.				
6.2. Proper hygienization of furniture and facilities in order to prevent gluten contamination				
6.2.1. Existence of Standard operating procedures established for this item, which are being fulfilled.				
6.3. Proper hygienization of surfaces, equipment, and kitchenware in order to prevent gluten contamination				
6.3.1. Existence of SOPs established for this item, which are being fulfilled.				
6.4. Food recall program				
6.4.1. Existence of SOPs established for this item, which is being fulfilled.				
7. Responsibility and authority				
7.1. Responsibilities and authorities are defined and communicated within the organization to ensure effective operation and maintenance of the gluten contamination control.				
8. Coordinator of the food safety team				
8.1. Top management has a Gluten Contamination Control Team Coordinator.				
8.2. The designated Coordinator has the responsibility and authority to administer the Gluten Contamination Control Team and to organize their work.				
8.3. The designated Coordinator has the responsibility and authority to ensure relevant training and education of all members of the gluten contamination control team.				
8.4. The designated Coordinator has the responsibility and authority to ensure that the gluten contamination control system is established, implemented, maintained, and updated.				
9. Methods for comunication in the gluten contamination control				
9.1. The organization ensures that the team is informed in proper time of changes of raw materials, ingredients, and services.				
9.2. The organization ensures that the team is informed in proper time of changes in production systems and equipment.				
9.3. The organization ensures that the team is informed in proper time of changes in production facilities, location of equipment, and surroundings.				
9.4. The organization ensures that the team is informed in proper time of changes in cleaning and sanitation programs.				
9.5. The organization ensures that the team is informed in proper time of changes in levels of staff qualification and/or designation of responsibilities and authorities.				
9.6. The organization ensures that the team is informed in proper time of changes in knowledge regarding gluten contamination and control measures.				
9.9. The organization ensures that the team is informed as soon as possible in the event of a consumer complaint indicating a possible risk of gluten contamination in the food.				
9.10. The organization ensures that the team is informed in proper time of any circumstances or occurrences not covered in the previous items that may have an impact on the control of gluten contamination.				
9.11. The team ensures that any information relevant to the control of gluten contamination is always updated in the system by the responsible party and passed on to the rest of the employees.				

10. Flow charts				
10.1. Flowcharts are prepared for categories of products or processes (implemented) by the gluten contamination control system.				
10.2. Flowcharts are clear, precise, and sufficiently detailed.				
10.3. Flowcharts are checked on site by the gluten contamination control team and verification records are kept.				
11. Treatment of potentially unsafe products				
11.1. The organization treats non-compliant products preventing them from entering the food production chain or attesting the presence of gluten on the label of such foods in case of possible contamination.				
11.2. All food produced that may have been affected by a nonconformity situation is kept under the control of the organization until it has been evaluated.				
11.3. The organization notifies interested parties when products that are no longer under the organization's control are subsequently determined to be unsafe (contaminated with gluten), initiating the recall process.				

References

1. Sapone, A.; Bai, J.C.; Ciacci, C.; Dolinsek, J.; Green, P.H.; Hadjivassiliou, M.; Kaukinen, K.; Rostami, K.; Sanders, D.S.; Schumann, M.; et al. Spectrum of gluten-related disorders: Consensus on new nomenclature and classification. *BMC Med.* **2012**, *10*, 1–12. [CrossRef] [PubMed]
2. Catassi, C. Gluten sensitivity. *Ann. Nutr. Metab.* **2015**, *67* (Suppl. 2), 16–26. [CrossRef] [PubMed]
3. Codex Alimentarius Commission. *Draft Revised Standard for Foods for Special Dietary Use for Persons Intolerant to Gluten, Joint FAO/WHO Food Standards Program, 30ty Session, ALINORM08/31/26 Appendix III*; Food and Agriculture Organization/World Health Organization: Geneva, Switerland, 2008.
4. Akobeng, A.K.; Thomas, A.G. Systematic review: Tolerable amount of gluten for people with coeliac disease. *Aliment. Pharmacol. Ther.* **2008**, *27*, 1044–1052. [CrossRef] [PubMed]
5. Farage, P.; Zandonadi, R.P. The Gluten-Free Diet: Difficulties Celiac Disease Patients have to Face Daily. *Austin J. Nutri. Food Sci.* **2014**, *2*, 1–8.
6. Araújo, H.M.C.; Araújo, W.M.C.; Botelho, R.B.A.; Zandonadi, R.P. Doença celíaca, hábitos e práticas alimentares e qualidade de vida. *Rev. Nutr.* **2010**, *23*, 467–474. [CrossRef]
7. Diaz-Amigo, C.; Popping, B. Gluten and gluten-free: Issues and considerations of labeling regulations, detection methods, and assay validation. *J. AOAC Int.* **2012**, *95*, 337–348. [CrossRef] [PubMed]
8. Oliveira, O.M.V.; Zandonadi, R.P.; Gandolfi, L.; de Almeida, R.C.; Almeida, L.M.; Pratesi, R. Evaluation of the presence of gluten in beans served at self-service restaurants: A problem for celiac disease carriers. *J. Culin. Sci. Technol.* **2014**, *12*, 22–33. [CrossRef]
9. Silva, R.P.; Lordello, M.L.L.; Nishitokukado, I.; Ortiz-Agostinho, C.L.; Santos, F.M.; Leite, A.Z.; Sipahi, A.M. Detection and quantification of gluten in processed food by ELISA in Brazil. *Gastroenterology* **2010**, *138*, S306.
10. Laureano, A.M. Análise da Presença de Glúten em Alimentos Rotulados como Livres de Glúten Através de Ensaio Imunoenzimático e de Fitas Imunocromatográficas. Master's Thesis, Federal University of Rio Grande do Sul, Porto Alegre, Brazil, 23 May 2010.
11. Farage, P.; de Medeiros Nóbrega, Y.K.; Pratesi, R.; Gandolfi, L.; Assunção, P.; Zandonadi, R.P. Gluten contamination in gluten-free bakery products: A risk for coeliac disease patients. *Public Health Nutr.* **2016**. [CrossRef] [PubMed]
12. Biagetti, C.; Naspi, G.; Catassi, C. Health-related quality of life in children with celiac disease: A study based on the critical incident technique. *Nutrients* **2013**, *5*, 4476–4485. [CrossRef] [PubMed]
13. Petruzzelli, A.; Foglini, M.; Paolini, F.; Framboas, M.; Serena Altissimi, M.; Naceur Haouet, M.; Mangili, P.; Osimani, A.; Clementi, F.; Cenci, T.; et al. Evaluation of the quality of foods for special diets produced in a school catering facility within a HACCP-based approach: A case study. *Int. J. Environ. Health Res.* **2013**, *24*, 73–81. [CrossRef] [PubMed]
14. Bicudo, M.O.P. Avaliação da Presença de Glúten em Produtos Panificados para Celíacos—Estudo de caso. Master's Thesis, Federal University of Paraná, Curitiba, Brazil, 2010.

15. Health Canada. Health Canada's Position on Gluten-Free Claims. 2012. Available online: http://www.hc-sc. gc.ca/fn-an/securit/allerg/cel-coe/gluten-position-eng.php (accessed on 10 February 2016).
16. Código Alimentario Argentino. Resolución Conjunta 131/2011. Available online: http://www. alimentosargentinos.gob.ar/contenido/marco/CAA/ModificacionesCAA.html (accessed on 10 February 2016).
17. Lima, T.C. Content validation of an instrument to characterize people over 50 years of age living with Human Immunodeficiency Virus/Acquired Immunodeficiency Syndrome. *Acta Paul. Enfer.* **2012**, *25*, 4–10. [CrossRef]
18. Polit, D.F.; Beck, C.T. *Nursing Research: Principles and Methods*, 7th ed.; Lippincott Willians and Wilkings: Philadelphia, PA, USA, 2004.
19. Wendisch, C. Avaliação da Qualidade de Unidades de Alimentação e Nutrição (UAN) Hospitalares: Construção de um Instrumento. Master's Thesis, Osvaldo Cruz Foundation, Sergio Arouca National School of Public Health, Rio de Janeiro, Brazil, 10 October 2010.
20. Conti, M.A.; Scagliusi, F.; de Oliveira Queiroz, G.K.; Hearst, N.; Cordás, T.A. Adaptação transcultural: tradução e validação de conteúdo para o idioma português do modelo da Tripartite Influence Scale de insatisfação corporal. *Cad Saúde Pública* **2010**, *26*, 503–513. [CrossRef] [PubMed]
21. Brasil Ministério da Saúde. *Agência Nacional de Vigilância Sanitária. Resolução RDC n° 216, de 15 de Setembro de 2004*; Diário Oficial da República Federativa do Brasil: Brasília, Brazil, 2004.
22. Brasil Ministério da Saúde. *Agência Nacional de Vigilância Sanitária. Resolução RDC n° 275, de 21 de Outubro de 2002*; Diário Oficial da República Federativa do Brasil: Brasília, Brazil, 2003.
23. International Organization for Standardization (ISO). *ISO 22000. Food Safety Management Systems and Requirements for Any Organization in the Food Chain*; ISO: Geneva, Switzerland, 2005.
24. Canadian Celiac Association. *Standards and Policies Respecting the Certification of Gluten-Free Products under the Gluten-Free Certification Program*; Canadian Celiac Association: Mississauga, ON, Canada, 2011.
25. Hollon, J.R.; Cureton, P.A.; Martin, M.L.; Leonard Puppa, E.L.; Fasano, A. Trace gluten contamination may play a role in mucosal and clinical recovery in a subgroup of diet-adherent non-responsive celiac disease patients. *BMC Gastroenterol.* **2013**, *13*, 1–9. [CrossRef] [PubMed]
26. Ceniccola, G.D.; Araújo, W.M.C.; Akutsu, R. Development of a tool for quality control audits in hospital enteral nutrition. *Nutr. Hosp.* **2014**, *29*, 102–120.
27. Reichenheim, M.E.; Moraes, C.L. Operacionalização de adaptação transcultural de instrumentos de aferição usados em epidemiologia. *Rev. Saúde Pública* **2007**, *41*, 665–673. [CrossRef] [PubMed]
28. Pasquali, L. Testes referentes ao construto: Teoria e modelo da construção. In *Instrumentos Psicológicos: Manual Prático de Elaboração*; Labpam: Brasília, Brazil, 1999.
29. Pasquali, L. Psicometria. *Rev. Esc. Enferm. USP* **2009**, *43*, 992–999. [CrossRef]
30. Alexandre, N.M.C.; Coluci, M.Z.O. Validade de conteúdo nos processos de construção e adaptação de instrumentos de medidas. *Ciência Saúde Coletiva* **2011**, *16*, 3061–3068. [CrossRef] [PubMed]
31. Saccol, A.L.F.; Stangarlin, L.; Hecktheuer, L.H. *Instrumentos de Apoio para Implantação das boas Práticas em Empresas Alimentícias*, 1st ed.; Editora Rubio: Rio de Janeiro, Brasil, 2012.
32. Araújo, H.M.C.; Araújo, W.M.C. Coeliac disease. Following the diet and eating habits of participating individuals in the Federal District, Brazil. *Appetite* **2011**, *57*, 105–109. [CrossRef] [PubMed]
33. Karajeh, M.A.; Hurlstone, D.P.; Patel, T.M.; Sanders, D.S. Chefs' knowledge of coeliac disease (compared to the public): A questionnaire survey from the United Kingdom. *Clin. Nutr.* **2005**, *24*, 206–210. [CrossRef] [PubMed]
34. Laporte, L.; Zandonadi, R.P. Conhecimento dos chefes de cozinha acerca da doença celíaca. *Aliment. Nutr.* **2011**, *22*, 465–470.
35. Machado, J.; Ganolfi, L.; de Almeida, R.C.; Almeida, L.M.; Zandonadi, R.P.; Pratesi, R. Gluten-free dietary compliance in Brazilian celiac patients: questionnaire versus serological test. *Nutr. Clín. Diet. Hosp.* **2013**, *33*, 46–49.

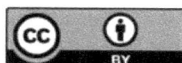

nutrients

MDPI

Review

Biomarkers to Monitor Gluten-Free Diet Compliance in Celiac Patients

María de Lourdes Moreno [1], Alfonso Rodríguez-Herrera [2], Carolina Sousa [1] and Isabel Comino [1,*]

[1] Departamento de Microbiología y Parasitología, Facultad de Farmacia, Universidad de Sevilla, c/Profesor García González 2, 41012 Sevilla, Spain; lmoreno@us.es (M.d.L.M); csoumar@us.es (C.S.)

[2] Unidad de Gastroenterología y Nutrición, Instituto Hispalense de Pediatría, 41013 Sevilla, Spain; alfonsorodriguez@ihppediatria.com

* Correspondence: icomino@us.es; Tel.: +34-954-556-452

Received: 31 October 2016; Accepted: 27 December 2016; Published: 6 January 2017

Abstract: Gluten-free diet (GFD) is the only treatment for celiac disease (CD). There is a general consensus that strict GFD adherence in CD patients leads to full clinical and histological remission accompanied by improvement in quality of life and reduced long-term complications. Despite the importance of monitoring the GFD, there are no clear guidelines for assessing the outcome or for exploring its adherence. Available methods are insufficiently accurate to identify occasional gluten exposure that may cause intestinal mucosal damage. Serological tests are highly sensitive and specific for diagnosis, but do not predict recovery and are not useful for follow-up. The use of serial endoscopies, it is invasive and impractical for frequent monitoring, and dietary interview can be subjective. Therefore, the detection of gluten immunogenic peptides (GIP) in feces and urine have been proposed as new non-invasive biomarkers to detect gluten intake and verify GFD compliance in CD patients. These simple immunoassays in human samples could overcome some key unresolved scientific and clinical problems in CD management. It is a significant advance that opens up new possibilities for the clinicians to evaluate the CD treatment, GFD compliance, and improvement in the quality of life of CD patients.

Keywords: celiac disease; gluten-free diet; gluten immunogenic peptides; feces; urine

1. Introduction

Gluten is a complex mixture of water insoluble proteins from wheat, barley, rye, and oats that are damaging to celiac patients. The term gluten includes prolamins (gliadins in wheat) and glutelins (glutenins in wheat). The prolamins, a complex group of alcohol-soluble proteins, constitute the major seed proteins in cereals and comprise about 50% of the proteins in mature cereal grain. Other gluten proteins showing that analogous immunogenic properties are present also in barley (hordeins), rye (secalins), oats (avenins), and other-closely related grains [1–3]. These proteins are rich in proline and glutamine residues, making them resistant to gastrointestinal digestion and encouraging the deamination by tissue transglutaminase (tTG).

Celiac disease (CD) is an immune-mediated systemic disorder elicited by ingestion of gluten in genetically-susceptible individuals. It affects around 1% of the population and it is based on a variable combination of intestinal and extraintestinal signs and symptoms, celiac specific antibodies, HLA-DQ2/DQ8 haplotypes, and enteropathy.

To date, the mainstay of CD is a lifelong strict gluten-free diet (GFD). There is a general consensus that strict GFD adherence in CD patient results in complete histological and clinical remission and an improvement in the quality of life and reduced long-term complications [4–6]. Thereby, the strict adherence to GFD leads to significant improvement in bone density [7–10] and the normalization of vitamins (e.g., vitamin B12 among others) and minerals, although sometimes supplements may be necessary to achieve optimum levels [11].

The gluten content in food is regulated by the Codex Alimentarius [12]. This regulation (CODEX STAN 118—1979, revised in 2008) states that gluten-free foods are those in which the total levels of gluten are ≤20 ppm [3]. Gluten-free cereals, such as rice, buckwheat, corn, and millet, can replace gluten-containing cereals. Some legumes, such as amaranth, quinoa, and soybean, are especially convenient due to their high protein content and quality. Moreover, non-processed food as fish, meat, poultry, egg, vegetables, and fruit are recommended to promote GFD adherence and secure the nutritional value of the diet [13].

Although conceptually simple, dietary changes are substantial and have a profound effect on a patient's life. Indeed, there are barriers related with GFD, such as availability, cost, and safety of gluten-free foods, or gluten cross-contamination [14,15]. Estimated compliance rates vary considerably (17%–80%), depending on factors such as the patient's age or the age at diagnosis of CD, among others [16–19]. The poor dietary adherence has shown to be negative to promote other autoimmune disease [20,21], fertility problems [22–24], and increased risk of bone fracture [25] or lymphoma [26,27]. Furthermore, after adoption of the GFD, 4%–30% of CD patients reported persisting symptoms and are considered to be affected by nonresponsive CD (NRCD) [6]. However, only 10% of these NRCD patients have refractory CD (RCD), being inadvertent or deliberate gluten exposure the most frequent cause of NRCD [28].

Additionally, in the last decade CD research is changing rapidly as gluten-related disorders have gradually emerged as an epidemiologically-relevant phenomenon with a global prevalence. Such disorders include, besides CD, wheat allergy, which affects 0.2%–0.5% of the population [29], and non-celiac gluten sensitivity (NCGS), a pathology in which gluten ingestion results in symptomatic and morphological manifestations in the absence of CD and wheat allergy [30], with highly variable incidence from 0.6% to 6% [31]. It has become more complex both the differential diagnosis and monitoring of patients since the requirements of adherence to GFD vary in each of the disorders. Moreover, this also makes more noticeable the dilemma of how to measure dietary transgressions. Although the importance of monitoring the GFD, there are no clear guidelines for assessing the outcome or for exploring its adherence. In addition, there is no consensus on the frequency of monitoring or the suitable measurements for evaluating compliance and outcome [32]. A variety of surrogate markers are available to assess the GFD compliance including clinical assessment of symptoms, patient self-report about the level of adherence, dietary history, evaluation carried out by a professional nutritionist, small-bowel biopsy, or serologic screening tests. Nevertheless, the lack of standardized and accurate indicators of GFD adherence is a significant problem both in the clinic and in research.

In order to evaluate the recent literature relating to CD and the monitoring of GFD, a search of scientific literature was conducted for recent publications on GFD compliance and CD. Based on these updates, the aim of this paper is to show and discuss the current concepts on the available tools to follow-up patients on GFD.

The search was conducted in PubMed MEDLINE and SCOPUS databases. The following search terms were used: "celiac disease and gluten-free diet", "follow-up celiac disease", "monitoring gluten-free diet", and "management celiac disease". The keywords "symptoms and celiac disease", "biopsy and celiac disease", "serological test and celiac disease", "questionnaire and celiac disease", "dietary interview and celiac disease", "feces and celiac disease", and "urine and celiac disease" were also used.

2. Monitoring of Gluten-Free Diet Compliance

2.1. Symptom Assessment

Follow-up of initial symptoms or the manifestations of newly-developed ones serve to check the improvement and evolution of CD. Intestinal bowel symptoms have been reported as common in CD patients not adherent to GFD (odds ratios 2.69; 95% confidence intervals 0.75–9.56) according to a meta-analysis of seven studies, including more than 3000 subjects [33]. Although seemingly intuitive, clinical response could not be a single method for monitoring adherence to the GFD as a large number of celiac patients are asymptomatic or minimally symptomatic at presentation and in these cases it would not be feasible to use clinical response as an indicator of mucosal healing and GFD compliance [34]. A controlled study examining the effects of gluten challenge found that symptoms were absent in 22% of celiac patients, despite the presence of significant villous atrophy in the small bowel biopsy [35].

2.2. Validated Surveys and Dietary Interviews

The dietitian or dedicated physician is responsible for dietetic review. In addition to a number of questionnaires evaluating food frequency and self-reported GFD adherence, there is a visual analogue score scale which consists of an unmarked line with the anchor sentences 'I never adhere to my diet' and 'I always adhere to my diet' at each end [36–41]. Nonetheless, no quality control or standard is available for dietetic review due to local diets and habits targeting a specific structured interview related to the quality of the diet. To date, there is a lack of studies on GFD review outcomes in different countries, and there is no evidence that a proper review can replace other tools (e.g., biopsy) to predict mucosal damage. Moreover, individuals tend to inaccurately report their adherence level, whether intentionally or not, so that dietetic review could be subjective and not identify involuntary infringements [42,43].

2.3. Biopsies

Biopsies are a key component for diagnosis, and sometimes it is also necessary for monitoring. During upper intestinal endoscopy at least one biopsy samples should be taken from the bulb and, at least four biopsies, from the second or third portion of the duodenum. Typical features of CD include an increase of intraepithelial lymphocytes (IELs), elongation of the crypts, and partial to total villous atrophy. Therefore, a complete description of the orientation, number of IELs, the presence or not of normal villi or degree of atrophy and crypt elongation, and grading according to the Marsh-Oberhuber classification must appear in the pathology report [44]. The original Marsh classification [45] based on normal mucosa (Marsh 0) to the appearance of lymphocytic infiltration (Marsh 1), crypt hyperplasia (Marsh 2), and different levels of villous atrophy (Marsh 3a–c) results may be subjective. In the last years the modifications made by Oberhuber [46], Corazza and Villanacci [47], Ensari et al. [48], Villanacci [49], or by Ensari [50] have been proposed as more objective and practical. Both classifications made by Corazza and Villanacci [47] and by Ensari [48] are practical and have proven to be useful with good specificity and sensitivity, discriminating latent CD from patients with normal mucosa and identifying those at an early stage. Moreover, Villanacci [51] points out the advantage of including the term of "microscopic enteritis" as a separate histopathology diagnosis. Peña [52] provided a very useful tabbed comparison between different classifications, allowing for compilation and analysis of data for public health.

Classifications based on objective quantitative morphological parameters, such as measurements of height-to-crypt-depth ratio and inflammatory variables, such as the density of IELs with a proper protocol, have been welcome. Taavela et al. [53] evaluated these quantitative morphological and inflammatory variables in the assessment of different degrees of damage to provide cut-off values to be employed in routine clinical practice in CD. The subtyping of the IELs by histological and immunological research and the utilization of flow cytometry and/or immunohistochemistry to the study of IELs have been pointed out to be of paramount importance in the diagnosis and follow-up of CD [54–56]. The ratio of the upper normal limit of IELs in the proximal small intestine used as a criterion of the Marsh-Oberhuber classification for gluten sensitivity was established in 40 IELs per 100 epithelial cells (EC) [57]. However, recent studies have observed the upper normal limit in the proximal small intestine to be as low as 20 IEL/100 EC at the tips of five villi on hematoxylin-eosin stained sections and 25 IEL/100 EC with immunohistochemistry by using more thinly cut sections of 3 μm and 4 μm and CD3 immunohistochemistry [58].

Despite the use of endoscopies to collect biopsies and assess mucosal healing being the gold standard, it is an invasive, expensive, and impractical procedure for frequent monitoring of disease activity or severity [59]. There are a proportion of cases difficult to monitor and evaluate with biopsy because they have mild histological changes or there is a lack of concordance between serology and histology. Therefore, the idea of re-assessing the emphasis on the biopsy as a gold standard in the follow up of CD, in light of available less invasive tests, is a welcoming one. It has been reported that complete recovery of duodenal mucosa extends over one year, with IELs frequent even 2–5 years after celiac diagnosis [60]. Some experts do not routinely perform a follow-up biopsy in asymptomatic patients with negative serology and good adherence [61]. However, inflammation of the intestinal mucosa can occur long before the development of clinical signs or a rise in antibody titers following a gluten challenge. On the other hand, in NRCD patients with absence of clinical response to a strict GFD should prompt repeat biopsy and additional investigations [62]. Therefore, there is no consensus on the role of follow-up biopsies [18,44].

2.4. Serological Tests

Anti-gliadin antibodies (AGA) were the first to be used as screening tool for the disease [63]. Since that time, serologic testing advanced from an adjunctive aid in diagnosis to an integral component of diagnosis, management, and clinical research. Highly sensitive and specific tests, including tTG, endomysial antibodies (EMA), and deamidated gliadin peptide (DGP) antibodies, have been identified in optimizing diagnostics and screening studies [44]. Indeed, for all individuals in whom CD is being considered, serological blood testing should be the initial step in evaluation [62,64]. Despite these advances and the overall laudable test performance of EMA, tTG, and DGP for CD diagnosis, current testing still is subject to a number of important limitations that are important for both clinicians and researchers to recognize. One of the most practical issues currently faced by clinicians is the diversity of available testing platforms, many of which have different cutoff levels, dynamic ranges, and overall test performance. This issue, which has gone largely unaddressed, can be a major impediment to both patient care and research when values are not comparable between providers or between studies. Furthermore, monitoring disease activity in treated CD patients remains a challenge [64]. Although the CD antibody tests show a high accuracy for selecting patients needing a diagnostic biopsy, these tests do not seem to be reliable after diagnosis as the autoantibody titers do not correlate well with histological findings or symptoms in CD patients on a GFD [34,65–70]. This may be due to their long half-life and the fact that these titers reflect the immune response rather than direct intestinal damage. IgA- and IgG-class tests can often take 6–24 months to decrease after the antigen source has been eliminated from the diet. In addition, it is important to note that serological tests are not adequate enough to show positive results in patients submitted to small or infrequent exposures to gluten [61].

2.5. Other Markers

Other studies suggested as suitable diet monitoring markers the permeability test, fecal calprotectine, REG Iα or, recently, plasma total alkylresorcinols [71–74]. However, several studies have reported these tests not being only specific to CD but also of limited efficacy in the diagnosis of uncomplicated CD [75–77]. Two other markers are intestinal-fatty acid binding protein (I-FABP), a marker reflecting enterocyte damage, and citrulline, a marker for functional enterocyte mass [64], but they are not specific for CD, so they do not discriminate between a celiac relapse or other gastrointestinal disorders in the patient.

Autoantibodies against pancreatic secretory-granule membrane glycoprotein 2 (GP2), especially of IgA isotype, have been demonstrated in patients with Crohn's disease and, recently, also with CD. In CD patients with anti-GP2 antibody positivity, this marker could be used as indicator for intestinal inflammation and for follow-up. However, CD should be differentiated from Crohn's disease by parallel testing of CD-specific EMA or anti-tTG [78,79].

Recently, Ryan et al. [80] reviewed the metabolomics associated to the diagnosis and prognosis in CD as a significant potential tool. The identification of three main components (malabsorption, energy metabolism, and alterations of gut microbiota) in matrices, such as sera, urine, and feces, has been of particular interest in the metabolome of CD. Different compounds related to malabsorption (decreased levels of amino acids, lipids, pyruvate, and choline in the sera of celiac patients), other components were related to energy metabolism (higher levels of glucose and 3-hydroxybutyric acid in sera) and, thirdly, those related to alterations of gut microbiota and/or intestinal permeability as higher levels of indoxyl sulfate, meta-[hydroxyphenyl] propionic acid, and phenylacetylglycine in urines [81,82].

2.6. Detection of Gluten Immunogenic Peptides (GIP)

The above tests to monitoring GFD compliance only evaluate the consequences of GFD transgressions. Moreover, they are unable to detect occasional gluten exposure that may impede total gut mucosa recovery in the celiac patient [34,65–67,83–88]. In this respect, it is noted that a diet with zero gluten intake is impossible due to its ubiquity; thus, a minimal level of gluten contamination is present in the daily diet. In fact, total daily gluten consumption that could be critical for most CD patients is of <50 mg gluten [89], and some patients need as little as 10 mg of daily gluten to promote development of intestinal mucosal abnormalities [90]. Therefore, there is a need for accurate, non-invasive tools for managing patients to show gluten intake and avoid the harmful aftermaths.

CD is triggered by the certain gluten immunogenic peptides (GIP) are resistant to gastrointestinal digestion and can interact with the immune system of patients with CD to trigger an autoimmune response against tTG and other antigens. Shan et al. [91] showed by in vitro and in vivo studies in rats and humans that a 33-mer peptide from α2-gliadin is stable toward breakdown by all gastric, pancreatic, and intestinal brush border membrane endoproteases. This peptide was identified as the primary initiator of the inflammatory response to gluten in patients with CD [91]. Toward the assessment of toxicity and GIP in foods for celiac patients, G12 and A1 monoclonal antibodies (moAbs) were obtained against 33-mer peptides. The reactivity of these antibodies was correlated with the potential immunotoxicity of the proteins analyzed and they proved to be useful in studies about the enzymatic detoxification of gluten [92,93]. These antibodies displayed a great sensitivity to toxic peptides (besides the 33-mer peptide) from wheat, rye, barley, and varieties of oats [92,93]. A sandwich enzyme-linked immunosorbent assay (ELISA) based on G12 and A1 moAbs gave very promising results for gluten analysis across a range of samples. This method had a limit of detection of 0.6 ppm gluten, 1/3 of the concentration obtained by other methods described to date. Similarly, a rapid test for the detection of gluten in solid food, drinks, and on surfaces using G12 moAb lateral flow devices (LFD) or dipsticks [94,95], as well as a competitive ELISA method were also developed for the detection of toxic gluten peptides in hydrolyzed foods [94,96]. More interesting, G12 immunodepletion experiments with hydrolyzed gliadin from beers showed that this moAb recognize those with the highest immunoactivity for celiac patients, this is a significant advance in the detection of the inmunoactive gluten content in the gluteome [97]. Based on these methodologies, new tools have been proposed for monitoring the GFD by determining GIP in human samples.

2.6.1. Feces

Immunoassays with G12 moAb showed that >30% of the inmunoreactive gliadin peptides persisted intact after hydrolysis during in vitro simulated gastrointestinal digestion [98]. Based on these findings, Comino et al. [98] described a novel method to monitor the GFD by detection of GIP in feces by using the G12 antibody [99]. This study supports the resistance of the 33-mer to in vitro peptic-tryptic-chymotryptic hydrolysis; and, most significantly, it was shown that toxic epitopes of gluten are measurable by moAbs in the feces of normal subjects and CD patients receiving a gluten-containing diet. The resistance of gluten peptides to gastrointestinal digestion, in particular peptides related to the immunotoxic 33-mer peptide, ensures that an important part of the ingested gluten is eliminated in feces. Consequently, the recovery of measurable levels of the immunotoxic fraction in feces suggests that gluten has passed through the digestive tract and, therefore, that gluten has been ingested. GIP were detected in the feces of healthy individuals and CD patients receiving gluten-containing diets, and GIP disappeared when a GFD was introduced [100]. With diets that contained variable quantities of gluten, GIP excretion was proportional to the amount ingested. These tests could also detect differences when, being in GFD, subjects were challenged with known amounts of oral gluten [98].

A recent study has shown the clinical usefulness of this new method of measuring fecal GIP as a marker of adherence to GFD [43]. A multicenter clinical trial prospectively examined the compliance to the GFD of both celiac children and adults. Furthermore, the response rate to GFD was evaluated by dietary questionnaire, celiac serology, and clinical response. Correlations between fecal GIP and traditional methods to monitoring the GFD were investigated. The majority (85.7%) of celiac children between zero and three years of age had feces negative for GIP, with only 14.3% showing levels above the limit of quantification. The proportion of celiac patients with feces positive for GIP increased to 27.8% in children between four and 12 years of age. Among those $\geq$13 years old, the proportion rose up to 39.2% with positive GIP. When further stratified by gender, adherence to the GFD was found to be closely related to the patient's gender in certain age groups. More males $\geq$13-years old had positive GIP feces compared with females in the same age group (60% vs. 31.5%, $p = 0.034$), indicating higher numbers of dietary transgressions among males than in their female peers (Figure 1). Although no overall significant differences between the percentage of GIP-positive feces in celiac patients and the duration of the GFD were observed, the patients who had been on the GFD for a longer period of time showed higher rates of noncompliance. No significant association was found between GIP levels in celiac patients and history of CD in their first- or second-degree relatives.

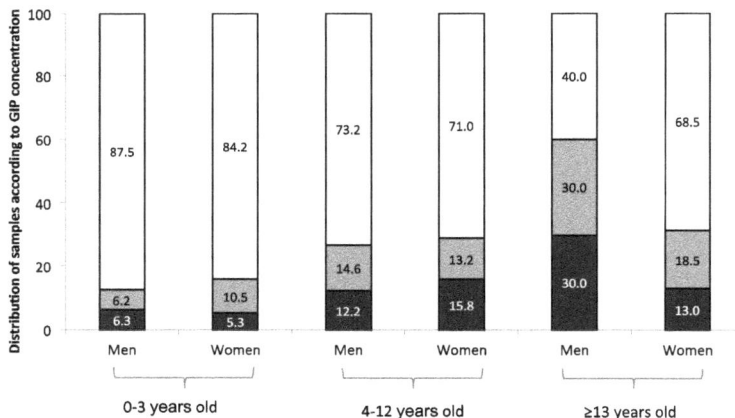

Figure 1. Percentage distribution of celiac patients by GIP content in feces by age and sex. GIP, gluten immunogenic peptides. GIP positive (>0.30 µg GIP/g feces, black bar), weak positive (0.16–0.30 µg GIP/g feces, grey bar), and negative (<0.16 µg GIP/g feces, white bar).

Comino et al. [43] also showed no association between fecal GIP and dietary questionnaires or anti-tTG antibodies. However, association was detected between GIP and anti-DGP antibodies, although 46 of the 53 GIP feces-positive patients were negative for anti-DGP. Detection of gluten peptides in feces reveals limitations of traditional methods for monitoring GFD in celiac patients. Fecal GIP analysis is an accurate and noninvasive method that enables a direct and quantitative assessment of gluten exposure early after ingestion. Therefore, these methods could aid in the diagnosis and clinical management of NRCD and RCD [43].

2.6.2. Urine

A proportional fraction of the GIP absorbed in the gastrointestinal tract makes it to the circulation and is excreted in urine [101,102]. The methodology proposed by Moreno et al. [103] based on urine gluten testing may be useful in clinical practice as a monitoring tool to follow-up the compliance of GFD. Clinical assays in urine based on LFD are used in many diseases. Coupling a reader to the LFD in urine of CD patients could provide a quantitative measurement of dietary infringement, providing significant advantages in the management of GFD. A positive correlation between the amount of ingested gluten and GIP detected in human urine samples has been demonstrated [103]. It has been determined in urine the low intake of gluten in processed bread, >25 mg corresponding to the lower limit to exert damage to most celiac patients. GIP were detected in urine samples 6–48 h after gluten intake. The methodology demonstrated the high level of noncompliance in patients with CD who had supposedly consumed long-term GFD through the presence of GIP (48% and 45% in adults and children, respectively). These results were consistent with reports showing that ~30%–50% continue with mucosal atrophy in CD patients despite following a GFD [5,104–106]. More interestingly, a direct correlation was demonstrated between the absence of GIP in urine and healing of the gut intestinal epithelium (Figure 2). Furthermore, 100% of the adult patients with higher damage in the epithelia (Marsh II/III), according to the histological analysis, had GIP in urine. In accordance with other above-mentioned studies [34,67,85], this study confirmed the poor correlation of serological tests with mucosal healing, as well as the shortcomings of the dietary history questionnaires to assess GFD compliance.

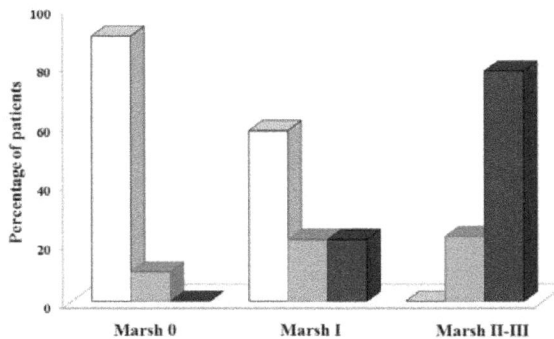

Figure 2. Presence of GIP in urine of adult CD patients and correlation with their small bowel histology. Severity of mucosal lesion (Marsh I–III) and histological appearance determined by the Marsh scale. GIP negative (white bar), absence of GIP in urine; GIP weak positive (grey bar), visual presence of GIP not quantifiable in urine (>LDT < QL); GIP positive (black bar), presence of GIP visible and quantifiable in urine (>QL). $p = 0.0007$ (Fisher's exact test). Values are expressed as the percentage of patients. CD, celiac disease; GIP, gluten immunogenic peptides; LDT, limit of technique detection; QL, quantification limit. Modified according to Moreno et al. [103].

The development of point-of care devices for an accurate, simple, and efficient GFD monitoring motived the creation of the highly-sensitive surface plasmon resonance biosensor for the detection of GIP in urine [107]. The easy-to-handle samples, such as urine and user-friendly biosensors could be suitable for the portable and simple devices for the GFD compliance of celiac patients. Soler et al. [107] demonstrated that the sensing methodology enables rapid and label-free quantification of the GIP in urine by using G12 moAb, reaching a limit of detection of 0.33 ng/mL. This study also clearly differed gluten consumers from non-consumers by measuring several urine samples from both healthy (normal diet) and celiac subjects (GFD). Therefore, biosensors offer significant advantages over conventional techniques enabling biochemical analysis with excellent reproducibility and high sensitivity in a matter of minutes.

3. Conclusions and Future Directions

It is often difficult to evaluate compliance with GFD. Persistent gluten exposure is usually unintentional. Exposure may occur no matter how careful a patient is, due to cross-contamination or simple lack of knowledge regarding the diet. Serum markers for CD play an important role in CD management (mostly tTG); however, the evidence suggests that it is not sensitive enough to detect occasional significant dietary transgressions that impede mucosa healing. There is no agreement on the role of follow-up biopsies and it is an invasive procedure, expensive and impractical for frequent monitoring of this disease. Moreover, an issue to address is the lack of studies comparing diagnostic efficacy of biomarkers with histology in patient follow-up. Notwithstanding, the need for non-invasive approaches to monitor CD is certainly warranted. Some studies related to metabolomics and other recent markers can measure the consequences of dietary transgressions, but they cannot show direct gluten intake, and they are not specific for CD. The incorporation of simple immunological assays based on GIP analysis in human samples could resolve some scientific and clinical problems in CD management such as (i) detection of inadvertent lapses after appearance of acute symptoms; (ii) in celiac patients, with or without symptoms, and patients with non-celiac gluten sensitivity; (iii) non-compliance of the GFD before any anatomic damage; (iv) to prove gluten intake during CD diagnosis; (v) examining the adherence to the GFD in the initial period after diagnosis when patients are less familiar with this diet; and (vi) the accurate diagnosis and management of the diet in NRCD and RCD. Therefore, these tests may prevent a potentially invasive and extensive medical analysis to assess the cause of the ongoing symptoms of celiac patients.

Acknowledgments: IC was supported by the Contrato de Acceso al Sistema Español de Ciencia, Tecnología e Innovación para el Desarrollo del Programa Propio de I + D + i from the Universidad de Sevilla. MLM was supported by the Contrato Postdoctoral associated to Proyecto de Investigación de Excelencia from the Junta de Andalucía. This work was supported by grants from Ministerio de Ciencia, Economía y Competitividad (AGL2013-48946-C3-2-R) and FEDER funds, Corporación Tecnológica de Andalucía (Junta de Andalucía), Agencia IDEA and Asociación de Celíacos y Sensibles al gluten de Madrid (Spain).

Author Contributions: All authors contributed to the preparation of this review article.

Conflicts of Interest: The authors declare no conflict of interest.

References

1. Jabri, B.; Sollid, L.M. Mechanisms of disease: Immunopathogenesis of celiac disease. *Nat. Clin. Pract. Gastroenterol. Hepatol.* **2006**, *3*, 516–525. [CrossRef] [PubMed]
2. Makharia, G.K.; Catassi, C.; Goh, K.L.; Mulder, C.J. Celiac disease. *Gastroenterol. Res. Pract.* **2012**, *2012*, 758560. [CrossRef] [PubMed]
3. Ludvigsson, J.F.; Leffler, D.A.; Bai, J.C.; Biagi, F.; Fasano, A.; Green, P.H.; Hadjivassiliou, M.; Kaukinen, K.; Kelly, C.P.; Leonard, J.N.; et al. The Oslo definitions for coeliac disease and related terms. *Gut* **2013**, *62*, 43–52. [CrossRef] [PubMed]
4. Bernardo, D.; Peña, A.S. Developing strategies to improve the quality of life of patients with gluten intolerance in patients with and without coeliac disease. *Eur. J. Intern. Med.* **2012**, *23*, 6–8. [CrossRef] [PubMed]
5. Hall, N.J.; Rubin, G.P.; Charnock, A. Intentional and inadvertent non-adherence in adult coeliac disease. A cross-sectional survey. *Appetite* **2013**, *68*, 56–62. [CrossRef] [PubMed]
6. Ludvigsson, J.F.; Bai, J.C.; Biagi, F.; Card, T.R.; Ciacci, C.; Ciclitira, P.J.; Green, P.H.R.; Hadjivassiliou, M.; Holdoway, A.; van Heel, D.A.; et al. BSG Coeliac Disease Guidelines Development Group and British Society of Gastroenterology. Diagnosis and management of adult coeliac disease: Guidelines from the British Society of Gastroenterology. *Gut* **2014**, *63*, 1210–1228. [CrossRef] [PubMed]

7. Bai, J.C.; Gonzalez, D.; Mautalen, C.; Mazure, R.; Pedreira, S.; Vazquez, H.; Smecuol, E.; Siccardi, A.; Cataldi, M.; Niveloni, S.; et al. Long-term eff ect of gluten restriction on bone mineral density of patients with coeliac disease. *Aliment. Pharmacol. Ther.* **1997**, *11*, 157–164. [CrossRef] [PubMed]
8. Jafri, M.R.; Nordstrom, C.W.; Murray, J.A.; Van Dyke, C.T.; Dierkhising, R.A.; Zinsmeister, A.R.; Melton, L.J. Long-term fracture risk in patients with celiac disease: A population-based study in Olmsted County, Minnesota. *Dig. Dis. Sci.* **2008**, *53*, 964–971. [CrossRef] [PubMed]
9. Sanchez, M.I.; Mohaidle, A.; Baistrocchi, A.; Matoso, D.; Vázquez, H.; González, A.; Mazure, R.; Maffei, E.; Ferrari, G.; Smecuol, E.; et al. Risk of fracture in celiac disease: Gender, dietary compliance, or both? *World J. Gastroenterol.* **2011**, *17*, 3035–3042. [CrossRef] [PubMed]
10. Dickey, W. Low serum vitamin B12 is common in coeliac disease and is not due to autoimmune gastritis. *Eur. J. Gastroenterol. Hepatol.* **2002**, *14*, 425–427. [CrossRef] [PubMed]
11. Halfdanarson, T.R.; Kumar, N.; Hogan, W.J.; Murray, J.A. Copper deficiency in celiac disease. *J. Clin. Gastroenterol.* **2009**, *43*, 162–164. [CrossRef] [PubMed]
12. Codex Alimentarius, International Food Standars. Standard for Foods for Special Dietary Use for Persons Intolerant to Gluten CODEX STAN 118-1979. Available online: http://www.codexalimentarius.net (accessed on 2 January 2017).
13. Peña, A.; Bernardo, D. Immunogenetic pathogenesis of celiac disease and non-celiac gluten sensitivity. *Curr. Gastroenterol. Rep.* **2016**, *18*, 36.
14. See, J.A.; Kaukinen, K.; Makharia, G.K.; Gibson, P.R.; Murray, J.A. Practical insights into gluten-free diets. *Nat. Rev. Gastroenterol. Hepatol.* **2015**, *12*, 580–591. [CrossRef] [PubMed]
15. Vriezinga, S.L.; Schweizer, J.J.; Koning, F.; Mearin, M.L. Coeliac disease and gluten-related disorders in childhood. *Nat. Rev. Gastroenterol. Hepatol.* **2015**, *12*, 527–536. [CrossRef] [PubMed]
16. Ciacci, C.; Cirillo, M.; Cavallaro, R.; CiacMazzaccaci, G. Long-term follow-up of celiac adults on gluten-free diet: Prevalence and correlates of intestinal damage. *Digestion* **2002**, *66*, 178–185. [CrossRef] [PubMed]
17. Högberg, L.; Grodzinsky, E.; Stenhammar, L. Better dietary compliance in patients with coeliac disease diagnosed in early childhood. *Scand. J. Gastroenterol.* **2003**, *38*, 751–754. [PubMed]
18. Pietzak, M.M. Follow-up of patients with celiac disease: Achieving compliance with treatment. *Gastroenterology* **2005**, *128*, 135–141. [CrossRef]
19. Herman, M.L.; Rubio-Tapia, A.; Lahr, B.D.; Larson, J.J.; Dyke, V.C.T.; Murray, J.A. Patients with celiac disease are not followed up adequately. *Clin. Gastroenterol. Hepatol.* **2012**, *10*, 893–899. [CrossRef] [PubMed]
20. Ventura, A.; Magazzù, G.; Greco, L. Duration of exposure to gluten and risk for autoimmune disorders in patients with celiac disease. SIGEP study group for autoimmune disorders in celiac disease. *Gastroenterology* **1999**, *117*, 297–303. [CrossRef] [PubMed]
21. Corrao, G.; Corazza, G.R.; Bagnardi, V.; Brusco, G.; Ciacci, C.; Cottone, M.; Guidetti, C.S.; Usai, P.; Cesari, P.; Pelli, M.A.; et al. Mortality in patients with coeliac disease and their relatives: A cohort study. *Lancet* **2001**, *358*, 356–361. [CrossRef]
22. Rampertab, S.D.; Fleischauer, A.; Neugut, A.I.; Green, P.H.R. Risk of duodenal adenoma in celiac disease. *Scand. J. Gastroenterol.* **2003**, *38*, 831–833. [PubMed]
23. Ludvigsson, J.F.; Montgomery, S.M.; Ekbom, A. Celiac disease and risk of adverse fetal outcome: A population-based cohort study. *Gastroenterology* **2005**, *129*, 454–463. [CrossRef] [PubMed]
24. Khashan, A.S.; Henriksen, T.B.; McNamee, R.; Mortensen, P.B.; McCarthy, F.P.; Kenny, L.C. Parental celiac disease and offspring sex ratio. *Epidemiology* **2010**, *21*, 913–914. [CrossRef] [PubMed]
25. Lebwohl, B.; Granath, F.; Ekbom, A.; Montgomery, S.M.; Murray, J.A.; Rubio-Tapia, A.; Green, P.H.; Ludvigsson, J.F. Mucosal healing and mortality in coeliac disease. *Aliment. Pharmacol. Ther.* **2013**, *37*, 332–339. [CrossRef] [PubMed]
26. Silano, M.; Volta, U.; De Vincenzi, A.; Dessì, M.; De Vincenzi, M. Collaborating Centers of the Italian Registry of the Complications of Coeliac Disease. Effect of a gluten-free diet on the risk of enteropathy-associated T-cell lymphoma in celiac disease. *Digest Dis. Sci.* **2008**, *53*, 972–976. [CrossRef] [PubMed]
27. Olén, O.; Askling, J.; Ludvigsson, J.F.; Hildebrand, H.; Ekbom, A.; Smedby, K.E. Coeliac disease characteristics, compliance to a gluten free diet and risk of lymphoma by subtype. *Digest Liver Dis.* **2011**, *43*, 862–868. [CrossRef] [PubMed]
28. Leffler, D.A.; Dennis, M.; Hyett, B.; Kelly, E.; Schuppan, D.; Kelly, C.P. Etiologies and predictors of diagnosis in nonresponsive celiac disease. *Clin. Gastroenterol. Hepatol.* **2007**, *5*, 445–450. [CrossRef] [PubMed]

29. Zuidmeer, L.; Goldhahn, K.; Rona, R.J.; Gislason, D.; Madsen, C.; Summers, C.; Sodergren, E.; Dahlstrom, J.; Lindner, T.; Sigurdardottir, S.T.; et al. The prevalence of plant food allergies: A systematic review. *J. Allergy Clin. Immunol.* **2008**, *121*, 1210–1218. [CrossRef] [PubMed]

30. Sapone, A.; Bai, J.C.; Ciacci, C.; Dolinsek, J.; Green, P.H.; Hadjivassiliou, M.; Kaukinen, K.; Rostami, K.; Sanders, D.S.; Schumann, M.; et al. Spectrum of gluten-related disorders: Consensus on new nomenclature and classification. *BMC Med.* **2012**, *7*, 10–13. [CrossRef] [PubMed]

31. Volta, U.; Caio, G.; De Giorgio, R.; Henriksen, C.; Skodje, G.; Lundin, K.E. Non-celiac gluten sensitivity: A work-in-progress entity in the spectrum of wheat-related disorders. *Best Pract. Res. Clin. Gastroenterol.* **2015**, *29*, 477–491. [CrossRef] [PubMed]

32. Bai, J.C.; Fried, M.; Corazza, G.R.; Schuppan, D.; Farthing, M.; Catassi, C.; Greco, L.; Cohen, H.; Ciacci, C.; Eliakim, R.; et al. World Gastroenterology Organisation Global Guidelines on Celiac Disease. *J. Clin. Gastroenterol.* **2013**, *47*, 121–126. [CrossRef] [PubMed]

33. Sainsbury, A.; Sanders, D.S.; Ford, A.C. Prevalence of irritable bowel syndrome-type symptoms in patients with celiac disease: A meta-analysis. *Clin. Gastroenterol. Hepatol.* **2013**, *11*, 359–365. [CrossRef] [PubMed]

34. Sharkey, L.M.; Corbett, G.; Currie E Lee, J.; Sweeney, N.; Woodward, J.M. Optimising delivery of care in coeliac disease -comparison of the benefits of repeat biopsy and serological follow-up. *Aliment. Pharmacol. Ther.* **2013**, *38*, 1278–1291. [CrossRef] [PubMed]

35. Lähdeaho, M.L.; Mäki, M.; Laurila, K.; Huhtala, H.; Kaukinen, K. Small-bowel mucosal changes and antibody responses after low- and moderate-dose gluten challenge in celiac disease. *BMC Gastroenterol.* **2011**, *11*, 129. [CrossRef] [PubMed]

36. Ciacci, C.; D'Agate, C.; De Rosa, A.; Franzese, C.; Errichiello, S.; Gasperi, V.; Pardi, A.; Quagliata, D.; Visentini, S.; Greco, L. Self-rated quality of life in celiac disease. *Dig. Dis. Sci.* **2003**, *48*, 2216–2220. [CrossRef] [PubMed]

37. Edwards George, J.B.; Leffler, D.A.; Dennis, M.D.; Franko, D.L.; Blom-Hoffman, J.; Kelly, C.P. Psychological correlates of gluten-free diet adherence in adults with celiac disease. *J. Clin. Gastroenterol.* **2009**, *43*, 301–306. [CrossRef] [PubMed]

38. Hopman, E.G.; Koopman, H.M.; Wit, J.M.; Mearin, M.L. Dietary compliance and health-related quality of life in patients with coeliac disease. *Eur. J. Gastroenterol. Hepatol.* **2009**, *21*, 1056–1061. [CrossRef] [PubMed]

39. Leffler, D.A.; Dennis, M.; Edwards George, J.B.; Jamma, S.; Magge, S.; Cook, E.F.; Schuppan, D.; Kelly, C.P. A simple validated gluten-free diet adherence survey for adults with celiac disease. *Clin. Gastroenterol. Hepatol.* **2009**, *7*, 530–536. [CrossRef]

40. Chauhan, J.C.; Kumar, P.; Dutta, A.K.; Basu, S.; Kumar, A. Assessment of dietary compliance to gluten free diet and psychosocial problems in Indian children with celiac disease. *Indian J. Pediatr.* **2010**, *77*, 649–654. [CrossRef] [PubMed]

41. Sainsbury, K.; Mullan, B. Measuring beliefs about gluten free diet adherence in adult coeliac disease using the theory of planned behaviour. *Appetite* **2011**, *56*, 476–483. [CrossRef] [PubMed]

42. Leffler, D.; Schuppan, D.; Pallav, K.; Najarian, R.; Goldsmith, J.D.; Hansen, J.; Kabbani, T.; Dennis, M.; Kelly, C.P. Kinetics of the histological, serological and symptomatic responses to gluten challenge in adults with coeliac disease. *Gut* **2013**, *62*, 996–1004. [CrossRef] [PubMed]

43. Comino, I.; Fernández-Bañares, F.; Esteve, M.; Ortigosa, L.; Castillejo, G.; Fambuena, B.; Ribes-Koninckx, C.; Sierra, C.; Rodríguez-Herrera, A.; Salazar, J.C.; et al. Fecal gluten peptides reveal limitations of serological tests and food questionnaires for monitoring gluten-free diet in celiac disease patients. *Am. J. Gastroenterol.* **2016**, *111*, 1456–1465. [CrossRef] [PubMed]

44. Husby, S.; Koletzko, S.; Korponay-Szabó, I.R.; Mearin, M.L.; Phillips, A.; Shamir, R.; Troncone, R.; Giersiepen, K.; Branski, D.; Catassi, C.; et al. ESPGHAN Working Group on Coeliac Disease Diagnosis; ESPGHAN Gastroenterology Committee; European Society for Pediatric Gastroenterology, Hepatology, and Nutrition. European society for pediatric gastroenterology, hepatology, and nutrition guidelines for the diagnosis of coeliac disease. *J. Pediatr. Gastroenterol. Nutr.* **2012**, *54*, 136–160. [PubMed]

45. Marsh, M.N. Gluten, major histocompatibility complex, and the small intestine. A molecular and immunobiologic approach to the spectrum of gluten sensitivity ('celiac sprue'). *Gastroenterology* **1992**, *102*, 330–354. [CrossRef]

46. Oberhuber, G.; Granditsch, G.; Vogelsang, H. The histopathology of coeliac disease: Time for a standardised report scheme for pathologist. *Eur. J. Gastroenterol. Hepatol.* **1999**, *11*, 1185–1194. [CrossRef] [PubMed]

47. Corazza, G.R.; Villanacci, V. Coeliac disease some considerations on the histological diagnosis. *J. Clin. Pathol.* **2005**, *58*, 573–574. [CrossRef] [PubMed]

48. Ensari, A. Gluten-sensitive enteropathy (celiac disease): Controversies in diagnosis and classification. *Arch. Pathol. Lab. Med.* **2010**, *134*, 826–836. [PubMed]

49. Villanacci, V. What is the best histopathological classification for celiac disease? Does it matter? A letter of comment to the review of Amado Salvador Pena; a new proposal. *Gastroenterol. Hepatol. Bed Bench* **2015**, *8*, 306–308. [PubMed]

50. Ensari, A. Coeliac disease: To classify or not to classify-that is the question! *Gastroenterol. Hepatol. Bed Bench* **2016**, *9*, 73–74. [PubMed]

51. Villanacci, V. The histological classification of biopsy in celiac disease: Time for a change. *Dig. Liver Dis.* **2015**, *47*, 2–3. [CrossRef] [PubMed]

52. Peña, A.S. What is the best histopathological classification for celiac disease? Does it matter? *Gastroenterol. Hepatol. Bed Bench* **2015**, *8*, 239–243. [PubMed]

53. Taavela, J.; Kurppa, K.; Collin, P.; Lähdeaho, M.L.; Salmi, T.; Saavalainen, P.; Haimila, K.; Huhtala, H.; Laurila, K.; Sievänen, H.; et al. Degree of damage to the small bowel and serum antibody titers correlate with clinical presentation of patients with celiac disease. *Clin. Gastroenterol. Hepatol.* **2013**, *11*, 166–171. [CrossRef] [PubMed]

54. Peña, A.S. Counting Intraepithelial Lymphocytes. Immunohistochemistry and flow cytometer are necessary new steps in the diagnosis of celiac disease. *Int. J. Celiac Dis.* **2016**, *4*, 7–8. [CrossRef]

55. De Andres, A.; Camarero, C.; Roy, G. Distal duodenum versus duodenal bulb: Intraepithelial lymphocytes have something to say in celiac disease diagnosis. *Dig. Dis. Sci.* **2015**, *60*, 1004–1009. [CrossRef] [PubMed]

56. Sanchez-Munoz, L.B.; Santon, A.; Cano, A.; Lopez, A.; Almeida, J.; Orfao, A.; Escribano, L.; Roy, G. Flow cytometric analysis of intestinal intraepithelial lymphocytes in the diagnosis of refractory celiac sprue. *Eur. J. Gastroenterol. Hepatol.* **2008**, *20*, 478–487. [CrossRef] [PubMed]

57. Antonioli, D. Coeliac disease: A progress report. *Mod. Pathol.* **2003**, *6*, 342–346. [CrossRef] [PubMed]

58. Siriweera, E.H.; Qi, Z.; Yong, J.L.C. Validity of intraepithelial lymphocyte count in the diagnosis of celiac disease: A histopathological study. *Int. J. Celiac Dis.* **2015**, *3*, 156–158. [CrossRef]

59. Buchanan, R.; Dennis, S.; Gendel, S.; Acheson, D.; Assimon, S.A.; Beru, N.; Bolger, P.; Carlson, D.; Carvajal, R.; Copp, C.; et al. Approaches to establish thresholds for major food allergens and for gluten in food. *J. Food Prot.* **2008**, *71*, 1043–1088. [PubMed]

60. Tuire, I.; Marja-Leena, L.; Teea, S.; Katri, H.; Jukka, P.; Päivi, S.; Heini, H.; Markku, M.; Pekka, C.; Katri, K. Persistent duodenal intraepithelial lymphocytosis despite a long-term strict gluten-free diet in celiac disease. *Am. J. Gastroenterol.* **2012**, *107*, 1563–1569. [CrossRef] [PubMed]

61. Rashid, M. Serologic testing in celiac disease. *Can. Fam. Phys.* **2016**, *62*, 38–43.

62. Rubio-Tapia, A.; Hill, I.D.; Kelly, C.P.; Calderwood, A.H.; Murray, J.A. American College of Gastroenterology. ACG clinical guidelines: Diagnosis and management of celiac disease. *Am. J. Gastroenterol.* **2013**, *108*, 656–676. [CrossRef] [PubMed]

63. Berger, E.; Buergin-Wolff, A.; Freudenberg, E. Diagnostic value of the demonstration of gliadin antibodies in celiac disease. *Klin. Wochenschr.* **1964**, *42*, 788–790. [CrossRef] [PubMed]

64. Adriaanse, M.; Leffler, D.A. Serum markers in the clinical management of celiac disease. *Dig. Dis.* **2015**, *33*, 236–243. [CrossRef] [PubMed]

65. Kaukinen, K.; Peräaho, M.; Lindfors, K.; Partanen, J.; Woolley, N.; Pikkarainen, P.; Karvonen, A.L.; Laasanen, T.; Sievänen, H.; Mäki, M.; et al. Persistent small bowel mucosal villous atrophy without symptoms in coeliac disease. *Aliment. Pharmacol. Ther.* **2007**, *25*, 1237–1245. [CrossRef] [PubMed]

66. Kaukinen, K.; Sulkanen, S.; Mäki, M.; Collin, P. IgA-class transglutaminase antibodies in evaluating the efficacy of gluten-free diet in coeliac disease. *Eur. J. Gastroenterol. Hepatol.* **2002**, *14*, 311–315. [CrossRef] [PubMed]

67. Tursi, A.; Brandimarte, G.; Giorgetti, G.M. Lack of usefulness of anti-transglutaminase antibodies in assessing histologic recovery after gluten-free diet in celiac disease. *J. Clin. Gastroenterol.* **2003**, *37*, 387–391. [CrossRef] [PubMed]

68. Bardella, M.T.; Velio, P.M.; Cesana, B.M.; Prampolini, L.; Casella, G.; Di Bella, C.; Lanzini, A.; Gambarotti, M.; Bassotti, G.; Villanacci, V. Coeliac disease: A histological follow-up study. *Histopathology* **2007**, *50*, 465–471. [CrossRef] [PubMed]

69. Lanzini, A.; Lanzarotto, F.; Villanacci, V.; Mora, A.; Bertolazzi, S.; Turini, D.; Carella, G.; Malagoli, A.; Ferrante, G.; Cesana, B.M.; et al. Complete recovery of intestinal mucosa occurs very rarely in adult coeliac patients despite adherence to gluten-free diet. *Aliment. Pharmacol. Ther.* **2009**, *29*, 1299–1308. [CrossRef] [PubMed]

70. Rubio-Tapia, A.; Rahim, M.W.; See, J.A.; Lahr, B.D.; Wu, T.T.; Murray, J.A. Mucosal recovery and mortality in adults with celiac disease after treatment with a gluten-free diet. *Am. J. Gastroenterol.* **2010**, *105*, 1412–1420. [CrossRef] [PubMed]

71. Duerksen, D.R.; Wilhelm-Boyles, C.; Parry, D.M. Intestinal permeability in long-term follow-up of patients with celiac disease on a gluten-free diet. *Dig. Dis. Sci.* **2005**, *50*, 785–790. [CrossRef] [PubMed]

72. Ertekin, V.; Selimoğlu, M.A.; Turgut, A.; Bakan, N. Fecal calprotectin concentration in celiac disease. *J. Clin. Gastroenterol.* **2010**, *44*, 544–546. [CrossRef] [PubMed]

73. Planas, R.; Pujol-Autonell, I.; Ruiz, E.; Montraveta, M.; Cabre, E.; Lucas-Martin, A.; Pujol-Borrell, R.; Martinez-Caceres, E.; Vives-Pi, M. Regenerating gene Iα is a biomarker for diagnosis and monitoring of celiac disease: A preliminary study. *Transl. Res.* **2011**, *158*, 140–145. [CrossRef] [PubMed]

74. Lind, M.V.; Madsen, M.L.; Rumessen, J.J.; Vestergaard, H.; Gøbel, R.J.; Hansen, T.; Lauritzen, L.; Pedersen, O.B.; Kristensen, M.; Ross, A.B. Plasma alkylresorcinols reflect gluten intake and distinguish between gluten-rich and gluten-poor diets in a population at risk of metabolic syndrome. *J. Nutr.* **2016**, *146*, 1991–1998. [CrossRef] [PubMed]

75. Balamtekın, N.; Baysoy, G.; Uslu, N.; Orhan, D.; Akçören, Z.; Özen, H.; Gürakan, F.; Saltik-Temızel, İ.N.; Yüce, A. Fecal calprotectin concentration is increased in children with celiac disease: Relation with histopathological findings. *Turk. J. Gastroenterol.* **2012**, *23*, 503–508. [CrossRef] [PubMed]

76. Capone, P.; Rispo, A.; Imperatore, N.; Caporaso, N.; Tortora, N. Fecal calprotectin in coeliac disease. *World J. Gastroenterol.* **2014**, *20*, 611–612. [CrossRef] [PubMed]

77. Duerksen, D.R.; Wilhelm-Boyles, C.; Veitch, R.; Kryszak, D.; Parry, D.M. A comparison of antibody testing, permeability testing, and zonulin levels with small-bowel biopsy in celiac disease patients on a gluten-free diet. *Dig. Dis. Sci.* **2010**, *55*, 1026–1031. [CrossRef] [PubMed]

78. Laass, M.W.; Röber, N.; Range, U.; Noß, L.; Roggenbuck, D.; Conrad, K. Loss and gain of tolerance to pancreatic glycoprotein 2 in celiac disease. *PLoS ONE* **2015**, *10*, e0128104. [CrossRef] [PubMed]

79. Roggenbuck, D.; Vermeire, S.; Hoffman, I.; Reinhold, D.; Schierack, P.; Goihl, A.; von Arnim, U.; De Hertogh, G.; Polymeros, D.; Bogdanos, D.P.; et al. Evidence of Crohn's disease-related anti-glycoprotein 2 antibodies in patients with celiac disease. *Clin. Chem. Lab. Med.* **2015**, *53*, 1349–1357. [CrossRef] [PubMed]

80. Ryan, D.; Newnham, E.D.; Prenzler, P.D.; Gibson, P.R. Metabolomics as a tool for diagnosis and monitoring in coeliac disease. *Metabolomics* **2015**, *11*, 980–990. [CrossRef]

81. Bertini, I.; Calalbro, A.; De Carli, V.; Luchinat, C.; Nepi, S.; Porfirio, B.; Renzi, D.; Saccenti, E.; Tenori, L. The metabonomic signature of celiac disease. *J. Proteome Res.* **2009**, *8*, 170–177. [CrossRef] [PubMed]

82. Bernini, P.; Bertini, I.; Calabro, A.; la Marca, G.; Lami, G.; Luchinat, C.; Renzi, D.; Tenori, L. Are patients with potential celiac disease really potential? The answer of metabonomics. *J. Proteome Res.* **2011**, *10*, 714–721. [CrossRef] [PubMed]

83. Tursi, A.; Brandimarte, G.; Giorgetti, G.M.; Elisei, W.; Inchingolo, C.D.; Monardo, E.; Aiello, F. Endoscopic and histological findings in the duodenum of adults with celiac disease before and after changing to a gluten-free diet: A 2-year prospective study. *Endoscopy* **2006**, *38*, 702–707. [CrossRef] [PubMed]

84. Biagi, F.; Campanella, J.; Martucci, S.; Pezzimenti, D.; Ciclitira, P.J.; Ellis, H.J.; Corazza, G.R. A milligram of gluten a day keeps the mucosal recovery away: A case report. *Nutr. Rev.* **2004**, *62*, 360–363. [CrossRef] [PubMed]

85. Rashtak, S.; Ettore, M.W.; Homburger, H.A.; Murray, J.A. Comparative usefulness of deamidated gliadin antibodies in the diagnosis of celiac disease. *Clin. Gastroenterol. Hepatol.* **2008**, *6*, 426–432. [CrossRef] [PubMed]

86. Dipper, C.R.; Maitra, S.; Thomas, R.; Lamb, C.A.; McLean-Tooke, A.P.; Ward, R.; Smith, D.; Spickett, G.; Mansfield, J.C. Anti-tissue transglutaminase antibodies in the follow-up of adult coeliac disease. *Aliment. Pharmacol. Ther.* **2009**, *30*, 236–244. [CrossRef] [PubMed]

87. Vives-Pi, M.; Takasawa, S.; Pujol-Autonell, I.; Planas, R.; Cabre, E.; Ojanguren, I.; Montraveta, M.; Santos, A.L.; Ruiz-Ortiz, E. Biomarkers for diagnosis and monitoring of celiac disease. *J. Clin. Gastroenterol.* **2013**, *47*, 308–313. [CrossRef] [PubMed]

88. Vallejo-Diez, S.; Bernardo, D.; Moreno, M.L.; Muñoz-Suano, A.; Fernández-Salazar, L.; Calvo, C.; Sousa, C.; Garrote, J.A.; Cebolla, A.; Arranz, E. Detection of specific IgA antibodies against a novel deamidated 8-Mer gliadin peptide in blood plasma samples from celiac patients. *PLoS ONE* **2013**, *8*, e80982. [CrossRef] [PubMed]

89. Hischenhuber, C.; Crevel, R.; Jarry, B.; Mäki, M.; Moneret-Vautrin, D.A.; Romano, A.; Troncone, R.; Ward, R. Review article: Safe amounts of gluten for patients with wheat allergy or coeliac disease. *Aliment. Pharmacol. Ther.* **2006**, *23*, 559–575. [CrossRef] [PubMed]

90. Akobeng, A.K.; Thomas, A.G. Systematic review: Tolerable amount of gluten for people with coeliac disease. *Aliment. Pharmacol. Ther.* **2008**, *27*, 1044–1052. [CrossRef] [PubMed]

91. Shan, L.; Molberg, Ø.; Parrot, I.; Hausch, F.; Filiz, F.; Gray, G.M.; Sollid, L.M.; Khosla, C. Structural basis for gluten intolerance in celiac sprue. *Science* **2002**, *297*, 2275–2279. [CrossRef] [PubMed]

92. Morón, B.; Bethune, M.T.; Comino, I.; Manyani, H.; Ferragud, M.; López, M.C.; Cebolla, A.; Khosla, C.; Sousa, C. Toward the assessment of food toxicity for celiac patients: Characterization of monoclonal antibodies to a main immunogenic gluten peptide. *PLoS ONE* **2008**, *3*, e2294. [CrossRef] [PubMed]

93. Morón, B.; Cebolla, A.; Manyani, H.; Alvarez-Maqueda, M.; Megías, M.; del Thomas, M.C.; López, M.C.; Sousa, C. Sensitive detection of cereal fractions that are toxic to celiac disease patients by using monoclonal antibodies to a main immunogenic wheat peptide. *Am. J. Clin. Nutr.* **2008**, *87*, 405–414. [PubMed]

94. Comino, I.; Real, A.; De Moreno, M.L.; Montes, R.; Cebolla, A.; Sousa, C. Immunological determination of gliadin 33-mer equivalent peptides in beers as a specific and practical analytical method to assess safety for celiac patients. *J. Sci. Food Agric.* **2013**, *93*, 933–943. [CrossRef] [PubMed]

95. Halbmayr-Jech, E.; Hammer, E.; Fielder, R.; Coutts, J.; Rogers, A.; Cornish, M. Characterization of G12 sandwich ELISA, a next-generation immunoassay for gluten toxicity. *J. AOAC Int.* **2012**, *95*, 372–376. [CrossRef] [PubMed]

96. Real, A.; Comino, I.; Moreno Mde, L.; López-Casado, M.Á.; Lorite, P.; Torres, M.I.; Cebolla, Á.; Sousa, C. Identification and in vitro reactivity of celiac immunoactive peptides in an apparent gluten-free beer. *PLoS ONE* **2014**, *9*, e100917. [CrossRef] [PubMed]

97. De Moreno, M.L.; Muñoz-Suano, A.; López-Casado, M.Á.; Torres, M.I.; Sousa, C.; Cebolla, Á. Selective capture of most celiac immunogenic peptides from hydrolyzed gluten proteins. *Food Chem.* **2016**, *205*, 36–42. [CrossRef] [PubMed]

98. Comino, I.; Real, A.; Vivas, S.; Síglez, M.Á.; Caminero, A.; Nistal, E.; Casqueiro, J.; Rodríguez-Herrera, A.; Cebolla, A.; Sousa, C. Monitoring of gluten-free diet compliance in celiac patients by assessment of gliadin 33-mer equivalent epitopes in feces. *Am. J. Clin. Nutr.* **2012**, *95*, 670–677. [CrossRef] [PubMed]

99. Auricchio, S. An innovative approach to measure compliance to a gluten-free diet. *Am. J. Clin. Nutr.* **2012**, *95*, 537–538. [CrossRef] [PubMed]

100. Caminero, A.; Nistal, E.; Arias, L.; Vivas, S.; Comino, I.; Real, A.; Sousa, C.; de Morales, J.M.; Ferrero, M.A.; Rodríguez-Aparicio, L.B.; et al. A gluten metabolism study in healthy individuals shows the presence of faecal glutenasic activity. *Eur. J. Nutr.* **2012**, *51*, 293–299. [CrossRef] [PubMed]

101. Riestra, S. Enfermedades asociadas. In *Libro Blanco de la Enfermedad Celiaca*; Polanco, I., Ed.; España: Madrid, Spain, 2008; pp. 41–49.

102. Ludvigsson, J.F.; Green, P.H. Clinical management of coeliac disease. *J. Intern. Med.* **2011**, *269*, 560–571. [CrossRef] [PubMed]

103. Moreno, M.L.; Cebolla, Á.; Muñoz-Suano, A.; Carrillo-Carrion, C.; Comino, I.; Pizarro, Á.; León, F.; Rodríguez-Herrera, A.; Sousa, C. Detection of gluten immunogenic peptides in the urine of patients with coeliac disease reveals transgressions in the gluten-free diet and incomplete mucosal healing. *Gut* **2015**. [CrossRef] [PubMed]

104. Matoori, S.; Fuhrmann, G.; Leroux, J.C. Celiac disease: A challenging disease for pharmaceutical scientists. *Pharm. Res.* **2013**, *30*, 619–626. [CrossRef] [PubMed]

105. Tio, M.; Cox, M.R.; Eslick, G.D. Meta-analysis: Coeliac disease and the risk of all-cause mortality, any malignancy and lymphoid malignancy. *Aliment. Pharmacol. Ther.* **2012**, *35*, 540–551. [CrossRef] [PubMed]

106. Stoven, S.; Murray, J.A.; Marietta, E. Celiac disease: Advances in treatment via gluten modification. *Clin. Gastroenterol. Hepatol.* **2012**, *10*, 859–862. [CrossRef] [PubMed]
107. Soler, M.; Estevez, M.C.; de Moreno, M.L.; Cebolla, A.; Lechuga, L.M. Label-free SPR detection of gluten peptides in urine for non-invasive celiac disease follow-up. *Biosens. Bioelectron.* **2016**, *79*, 158–164. [CrossRef] [PubMed]

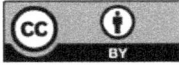

    [MDPI]

Article

Prevalence of Self-Reported Gluten Sensitivity and Adherence to a Gluten-Free Diet in Argentinian Adult Population

Francisco Cabrera-Chávez [1,†], Gimena V. A. Dezar [2,†], Anna P. Islas-Zamorano [1], Jesús G. Espinoza-Alderete [1], Marcela J. Vergara-Jiménez [1], Dalia Magaña-Ordorica [1] and Noé Ontiveros [1,3,*]

1   Nutrition Sciences Academic Unit, Universidad Autónoma de Sinaloa, Culiacán, Sinaloa 80019, Mexico; fcabrera@uas.edu.mx (F.C.-C.); islasap@hotmail.com (A.P.I.-Z.); jesus.93106@gmail.com (J.G.E.-A.); mjvergara@uas.edu.mx (M.J.V.-J.); dmagana@uas.edu.mx (D.M.-O.)

2   Facultad de Bioquímica y Ciencias Biológicas, Universidad Nacional del Litoral, Santa Fe 3000, Argentina; gdezar@unl.edu.ar

3   Regional Program for PhD in Biotechnology, FCQB, Universidad Autónoma de Sinaloa, Culiacán, Sinaloa 80019, Mexico

*   Correspondence: noeontiveros@gmail.com; Tel./Fax: +52-667-753-5454

†   These authors contributed equally to this work.

Received: 26 November 2016; Accepted: 16 January 2017; Published: 21 January 2017

Abstract: Background: Previous studies suggest that the prevalence of wheat/gluten sensitivity and adherence to a gluten-free diet (GFD) are high in Latin population despite a poor diagnosis of celiac disease. However, these prevalence rates still remain unknown in most Latin American countries. Methods: A cross-sectional survey study was conducted in Santa Fe, Argentina. Results: The estimated self-reported prevalence rates were (95% Confidence Interval [CI]): self-reported gluten sensitivity (SR-GS) 7.61% (6.2–9.2), SR-GS currently following a GFD 1.82% (1.2–2.7), celiac disease 0.58% (0.3–1.2), wheat allergy 0.33% (0.12–0.84), self-reported non-celiac gluten sensitivity (SR-NCGS) 6.28% (5.1–7.8), SR-NCGS currently following a GFD 0.91% (0.5–1.6), and adherence to a GFD 6.37% (5.1–7.9). SR-GS was more common in women (6.0%; $p < 0.001$) and associated with irritable bowel syndrome ($p < 0.001$). Among the GFD followers, 71.4% were doing it for reasons other than health-related benefits and 50.6% without medical/dietitian advice. In the non-SR-GS group, the main motivations for following a GFD were weight control and the perception that a GFD is healthier. Conclusion: In Argentina, gluten sensitivity is commonly reported and it seems that physicians/gastroenterologists are aware of celiac disease diagnosis. Trustable information about the benefits and potential consequences of following a GFD should be given to the general population.

Keywords: gluten; non-celiac gluten sensitivity; non-celiac wheat sensitivity; wheat allergy; celiac disease; prevalence

---

1. Introduction

The term "gluten-related disorders" encompasses all conditions related to gluten intake; it includes autoimmune, allergic, and non-autoimmune and non-allergic diseases [1,2]. Celiac disease is an autoimmune-like gluten-related disorder, which is triggered by gluten from wheat, rye and barley. This condition affects between 0.5% and 1% of the general population [3]. Wheat allergy is a condition that can be mediated or not by allergen-specific IgE antibodies and its prevalence in adult population is unknown in many countries [4]. A third gluten-related disorder is non-celiac gluten sensitivity (NCGS). These are cases where celiac disease and wheat allergy have been ruled-out, but symptomatic relief is reached after gluten withdrawal and a symptomatic relapse is confirmed upon reintroduction of gluten-containing food [5]. Because NCGS manifestations could be triggered by wheat components other than gluten, such as low-fermentable, poorly-absorbed, short-chain carbohydrates (FODMAPs) [6] and the wheat components amylase trypsin inhibitors [7], the abbreviation NCGS is evolving to non-celiac wheat sensitivity (NCWS) [8]. Experts have proposed diagnostic criteria for NCGS [9], but there is no a well-accepted gold standard for this purpose yet [8]. This and the lack of biological markers to support the diagnosis of NCGS make it difficult to estimate the population prevalence of this disorder. Alternatively, the self-reported gluten sensitivity (SR-GS) and/or self-reported NCGS (SR-NCGS) prevalence rates have been estimated. This prevalence rates varies among populations and fluctuates between 0.5% and 13% [10–13].

Following a gluten-free diet (GFD) is the only accepted treatment for gluten-related disorders. Patients following a GFD should be instructed by a trained physician/dietitian in order to avoid micronutrients deficiencies [14–16] and improve fiber intake [15]. Although the diet is considered a treatment, it seems that most people following a GFD are doing it for reasons other than health-related benefits and probably without medical/dietitian advice [11,12]. Studies addressing both the motivations for following a GFD without a physician-diagnosed gluten-related disorder and who instructs the diet in this group of people are scarce. The aim of the present study was to estimate the prevalence rates of SR-GS, SR-NCGS, and self-reported wheat allergy in adult population from Santa Fe, Argentina. The prevalence of adherence to a GFD as well as the motivations for adhering to the diet and who instructs the GFD were aspects also investigated.

2. Materials and Methods

2.1. Population Survey

We conducted a self-administered questionnaire-based cross-sectional study in Santa Fe, Argentina. All data were collected during the period from August to September 2016. The survey was conducted as previously described [11,12]. Briefly, respondents were approached in urban parks and outside shopping malls and supermarkets located in Santa Fe city. Inclusion criteria were: (1) Argentinian individuals; (2) ≥18 years old; and (3) subjects being able to read and answer the questionnaire by themselves. Assistance on specific terms was given when it was requested.

2.2. Questionnaire

A previously validated Spanish version of a self-administered questionnaire was utilized for the study purposes [11]. The questionnaire has two sections. The first section was designed for those who reported adverse reactions to oral wheat and/or gluten. The second section was designed for those who reported adverse reactions to foods other than wheat/gluten or reported no adverse reactions to foods [11,12]. The questionnaire was slightly modified to inquire about the motivations for following a GFD and who instructs the diet (Supplementary Materials Section S1).

2.3. Definitions

Adverse reactions to food were considered when the respondents reported that the food-induced symptoms occurred always or most of the time (recurrent) or sometimes (non-recurrent) [11,12]. Self-reported physician-diagnosed celiac disease or wheat allergy was considered when the respondents reported that a physician diagnosed them and were also following a GFD [11,12,17]. Additionally, self-reported wheat allergy was considered when the respondents reported recurrent adverse reactions convincing of food allergy and were also following a GFD, as previously described [11,12,18]. SR-GS was considered when the respondents met criteria for recurrent adverse reactions to oral wheat/gluten. Self-reported physician-diagnosed NCGS was considered when the respondents reported that a physician diagnosed them. SR-NCGS was considered when the respondents met the following: (1) respondents who did not meet criteria for self-reported physician-diagnosed celiac disease or wheat allergy; (2) respondents who did not meet criteria for self-reported wheat allergy; and (3) respondents who met criteria for recurrent adverse reactions to wheat/gluten (SR-GS) [12].

2.4. Statistical and Ethical Issues

Statistical analysis was carried out using PASW statistics version 18.0 (SPSS Inc., Chicago, IL, USA). Categorical variables were summarized by descriptive statistics, including total numbers, percentages, odds ratio, and 95% confidence interval (CI). Associations were analyzed by two-tailed Fisher's exact test. Continuous variables were summarized by mean and range with differences between groups calculated using the Student *t*-test. A *p* value < 0.05 was considered statistically significant. Prevalence rates were calculated using OpenEpi software version 3.03a [19]. Rates were reported as rate (95% CI) per 100 inhabitants. All respondents gave informed consent in writing to participate in the study. Ethics Review Board of the Universidad Nacional del Litoral approved the protocol. Ethical approval number Acta 09/16.

3. Results

3.1. Study Participants and Demographic Characteristics

A total of 1209 individuals completed the questionnaire in its entirety. The response rate was 53.3%. The mean age in years was 30 (range: 18–84) and the proportion of women was slightly higher than men (52.44%) ($p > 0.05$). The demographics and clinical characteristics of the studied population are given in Table 1. Non-food allergy and colitis were more common in men than in women ($p < 0.05$). Eating disorders were more common in women ($p < 0.05$). There were no significant differences by gender for the other self-reported physician-diagnosed conditions.

Table 1. Demographics and clinical characteristics of the studied population.

Variable *	%	*n*
Gender (male/female)	47.6/52.4	575/634
Non-food allergy	9.3	113
IBS **	5.5	66
Colitis	2.2	27
Lactose intolerance	1.9	23
Psychiatric disease	1.7	20
Food intolerance	1.3	16
Food allergy	1.2	15
Eating disorders	1.2	14
Diabetes mellitus	1.0	12
Gastrointestinal cancer	0.2	2
Hashimoto's thyroiditis	0.2	2

* Self-reported physician-diagnosed diseases were considered for analysis; ** Irritable Bowel Syndrome.

3.2. Estimated Prevalence Rates

Prevalence rates estimations are shown in Table 2. Adverse reactions to food, either recurrent or not, and SR-NCGS prevalence rates were significantly higher in women than in men ($p < 0.001$). The prevalence of SR-GS following a GFD was 1.82% ($n = 22$) (95% CI 1.2–2.7). Consequently, only 28.57% (22 out of 77) of the respondents following a GFD were doing it for health-related benefits. The characteristics of the respondents who reported current adherence to a GFD are shown in Figure 1. Previous studies estimated the prevalence rates of SR-NCGS based on GFD adherence and exclusion of celiac disease [20]. Under these criteria, the estimated prevalence rate of SR-NCGS in Argentinian population was 5.78% ($n = 70$) (95% CI 4.6–7.2). However, excluding the non-SR-GS respondents who reported current adherence to a GFD ($n = 55$) and those who met criteria for self-reported wheat allergy (($n = 4$); prevalence rate 0.33%; 95% CI 0.12–0.84), the prevalence rate of SR-NCGS currently following a GFD was 0.91% (*n* = 11) (95% CI 0.5–1.6). The prevalence of gluten avoiders (not following a GFD) was 16.13% (*n* = 195) (95% CI 14.2–18.3), but only 22.56% (*n* = 44) of them met criteria for SR-GS. The prevalence rates of adherence to a GFD or wheat/gluten avoidance were significantly higher among respondents <39 years old than those ≥39 years old (*p* < 0.01) (Figure 2). Stratified by gender, more women than men reported current adherence to a GFD (*p* > 0.05) or reported current avoidance of wheat/gluten-containing foods (*p* < 0.01).

Table 2. Self-reported prevalence rates estimations.

Assessment	(+) Cases *	Mean age in Years (Range)	Prevalence by Gender (95% CI)	*p* Value	General Prevalence (95% CI)
Adverse reactions to food	Total = 278 M ** = 79 F ** = 199	33.4 (18–84)	M 6.5 (5.2–8.0) F 16.5 (14.4–18.6)	<0.001	21.4 (19.3–23.7)
Adverse reactions to wheat/gluten	Total = 134 M = 31 F = 103	33.8 (18–74)	M 2.6 (1.8–3.7) F 8.5 (7.1–10.2)	<0.001	11.1 (9.4–12.9)
Recurrent adverse reactions to food	Total = 193 M = 50 F = 143	34.3 (18–79)	M 4.1 (3.2–5.4) F 11.8 (10.1–13.8)	<0.001	15.9 (14.0–18.1)
(a) Recurrent adverse reactions to wheat/gluten (SR-GS)	Total = 92 M = 19 F = 73	34.2 (18–74)	M 1.6 (1.0–2.4) F 6.0 (4.8–7.5)	<0.001	7.61 (6.2–9.2)
(b) Celiac disease ¶	Total = 7 M = 2 F = 5	26.7 (19–41)	M 0.2 (0.04–0.6) F 0.4 (0.2–1.0)	0.268	0.58 (0.3–1.2)
(c) Wheat allergy ¶	Total = 4 M = 1 F = 3	52.5 (37–59)	M 0.1 (0.01–0.5) F 0.2 (0.1–0.7)	0.350	0.33 (0.1–0.8)
(d) SR-NCGS	Total = 76 M = 15 F = 61	34.4 (18–74)	M 1.4 (0.9–2.2) F 5.5 (4.3–6.9)	<0.001	6.28 (5.1–7.8)
Adherence to GFD	Total = 77 M = 33 F = 44	33.8 (18–78)	M 2.7 (1.9–3.8) F 3.6 (2.7–4.8)	0.231	6.37 (5.1–7.9)

* Positive cases for the assessment; ** M: male; F: female; ¶ Two out of 9 celiac disease cases and 3 out of 7 wheat allergy cases did not report adherence to a GFD.

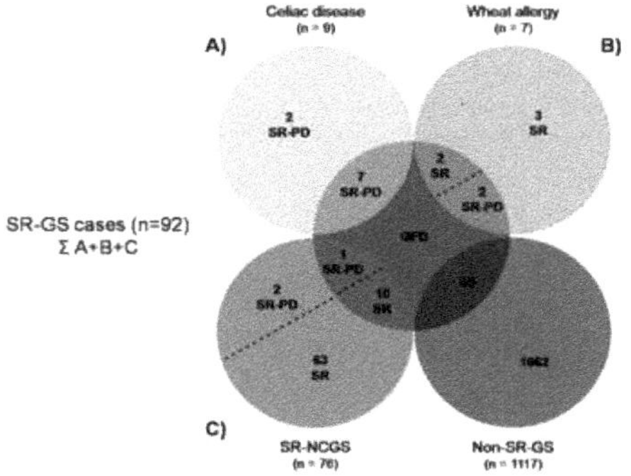

Figure 1. Characteristics of respondents following a GFD. SR: self-reported; SR-NCGS: self-reported non-celiac gluten sensitivity; Non-SR-GS: non self-reported gluten sensitivity; SR-PD: self-reported physician-diagnosed. (**A–C**) SR-celiac disease, SR-wheat allergy and SR-NCGS cases either following a GFD or not. Only those cases that reported adherence to a GFD were considered for prevalence rates estimations.

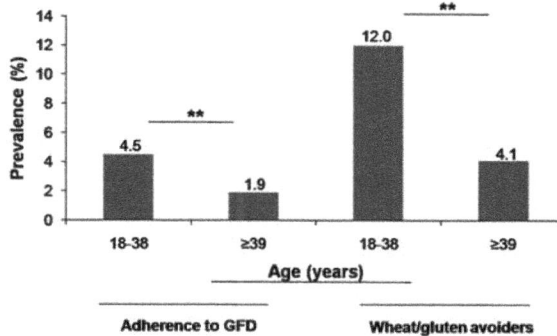

Figure 2. Prevalence of adherence to a GFD and avoidance of wheat/gluten-containing foods stratified by age (years). ** $p < 0.01$.

3.3. Characteristics of Subjects with SR-GS and Non-SR-GS

The characteristics of SR-GS and non-SR-GS respondents are shown in Table 3. Comparisons between these two groups showed significant differences for IBS ($p < 0.001$), eating disorders ($p < 0.05$) and lactose intolerance ($p < 0.01$). These self-reported physician-diagnosed diseases were more common in SR-GS than in non-SR-GS cases (Table 3). Statistical comparisons between SR-GS and those who reported recurrent adverse reactions to foods other than wheat/gluten were not significant for any of the self-reported physician-diagnosed diseases assessed ($p > 0.05$) (Supplementary Materials Table S1).

Table 3. Comparison between self-reported gluten sensitivity (SR-GS) and non-self-reported gluten sensitivity (non-SR-GS).

Variable *	SR-GS (n = 92) [¶]		Non-SR-GS (n = 1117) [¶]		Odds Ratio (95% CI)
	%	n	%	n	
Gender (male/female)	46.2/53.8	42/49	47.7/52.3	533/584	0.9 (0.6–1.4)
IBS	14.3	13	4.7	53	3.3 (1.7–6.4)
Food intolerance	3.3	3	1.2	13	2.9 (0.8–10.4)
Allergy	11.0	10	10.5	117	1.1 (0.5–2.1)
Psychiatric disease	0	0	1.8	20	-
Gastrointestinal cancer	1.1	1	0.1	1	12.4 (0.8–199.9)
Eating disorders	4.4	4	0.9	10	5.1 (1.6–16.6)
Autoimmune disease	2.2	2	1.1	12	2.1 (0.5–9.4)
Colitis	4.4	4	2.1	23	2.2 (0.7–6.5)
Lactose intolerance	6.6	6	1.5	17	4.6 (1.8–11.9)

* Self-reported physician-diagnosed diseases were considered for analysis; [¶] Age comparison between SR-GS (mean: 33.5; range: 18–74) and non-SR-GS (mean: 29.6; range: 18–84) was not significant ($p > 0.05$ by Student t-test).

3.4. Recurrent Symptoms Related to Wheat/Gluten Ingestion

Gastrointestinal symptoms were reported for 87 out of 92 SR-GS cases. The most commonly reported gastrointestinal symptoms were bloating ($n = 61$; 70.1%), abdominal discomfort ($n = 41$; 47.1%), and stomachache ($n = 40$; 46.0%) (Figure 3). Extraintestinal symptoms were reported for 45 SR-GS cases. The most common extraintestinal symptoms were tiredness ($n = 25$; 55.6%), lack of wellbeing ($n = 20$; 44.4%), and anxiety ($n = 13$; 28.9%) (Figure 3). These symptoms, either gastrointestinal or extraintestinal, were also the most common manifestations in SR-NCGS cases (Supplementary Materials Figure S1). Bloating and stomachache were the most common symptoms in those who reported adverse reactions to foods other than gluten (Supplementary Materials Figure S2). Comparisons between the SR-GS and self-reported recurrent adverse reactions to foods other than gluten groups showed significant differences for bloating and constipation ($p < 0.05$) (Supplementary Materials Table S2).

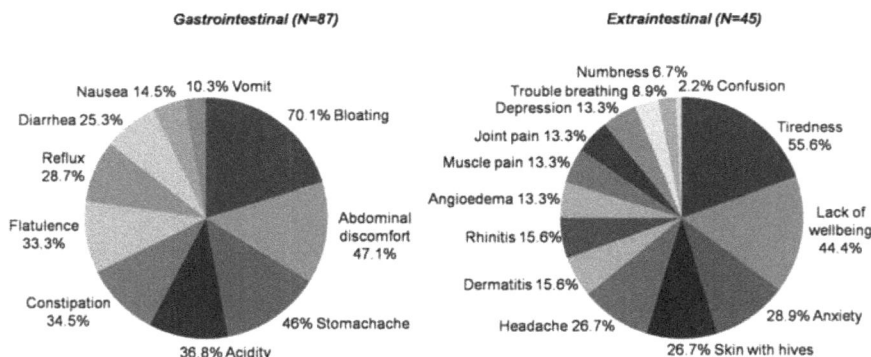

Figure 3. Recurrent self-reported symptoms in SR-GS cases.

3.5. Motivations for Following a GFD or for Avoiding Wheat/Gluten and who Instructs the GFD

In addition to the recurrent symptoms triggered by gluten intake, other motivations for following a GFD or for avoiding wheat/gluten from the diet were weight control and the perception that a GFD is healthier or avoiding wheat/gluten is healthy (Figure 4A,B). These motivations were also reported by most non-SR-GS cases that were following a GFD or were avoiding wheat/gluten from their diets (Figure 4C,D). Comparisons between the SR-GS and non-SR-GS groups currently following a GFD showed significant associations for weight control ($p < 0.05$) and the perception that a GFD is healthier ($p < 0.05$), these motivations were more commonly reported by the non-SR-GS group (Supplementary Materials Table S3). Regarding who instructs the GFD, 14 out of 22 (63.6%) SR-GS and 24 out of 55 (43.6%) non-SR-GS cases reported that they were seeing a physician/dietitian for gluten-free dietary advice ($p > 0.05$) (Figure 4A,C). Thus, among those who reported current adherence to a GFD ($n = 77$), 50.65% ($n = 39$) were doing it without medical/dietitian advice (Figure 4A,C).

Next, we stratified by gender the motivations for following a GFD and who instructs the diet. In the SR-GS group (15 women and seven men currently following a GFD), 50% ($n = 11$; seven women and four men) of the cases reported the symptoms triggered after wheat/gluten intake as the only reason for following a GFD (Supplementary Materials Table S4). Regarding who instructs the GFD, 45.45% ($n = 10$; seven women and three men) of the respondents from the SR-GS group reported that were seeing a physician/dietitian for gluten-free dietary advice (Supplementary Materials Table S4). In the non-SR-GS group (29 women and 26 men following a GFD), more women than men ($n = 18$; 62.07% vs. $n = 11$; 42.30%) reported weight control as the motivation for following a GFD ($p > 0.05$). A slightly higher proportion of men than women reported that a GFD was healthier ($n = 11$; 42.31% vs. $n = 11$; 37.93%) ($p > 0.05$). Regarding who instructs the GFD, more women than men ($n = 17$; 58.62% vs. $n = 7$; 26.92%) reported that were seeing a physician/dietitian for gluten-free dietary advice ($p < 0.05$). Consequently, more men than women ($n = 19$; 73.08% vs. $n = 12$; 41.38%) were following a GFD without medical/dietitian advice ($p < 0.05$).

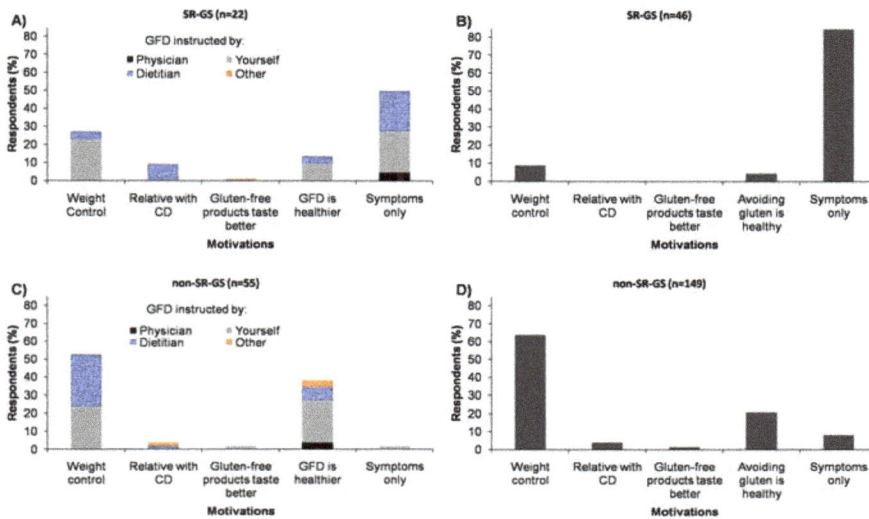

Figure 4. Motivations for following a GFD or avoiding wheat/gluten-containing foods and who instructs the GFD: (**A**) SR-GS individuals currently following a GFD; and (**B**) SR-GS individuals currently avoiding wheat/gluten-containing foods. In Figure 4A,B, in addition to the symptoms triggered by gluten intake, 11 and 6 individuals reported other motivations for following a GFD or avoiding wheat/gluten-containing foods, respectively; (**C**) Non-SR-GS individuals currently following a GFD; and (**D**) non-SR-GS individuals currently avoiding wheat/gluten-containing foods. In Figure 4C,D, 1 and 12 individuals reported non-recurrent adverse reactions to gluten intake as the motivation for following a GFD.

4. Discussion

This study has shown that recurrent adverse reactions to foods are commonly attributed to wheat/gluten intake. SR-GS was informed by 7.6% of the studied population. This prevalence estimation is consistent with previous survey studies carried out in Latin American countries and The Netherlands, which have estimated SR-GS prevalence rates between 5.3% and 7.8% [11–13]. Substantially higher SR-GS prevalence estimations (up to 13%) have been reported in the United Kingdom [17], but there are no enough data available to provide concise explanations about these discrepancies. According to others [13], media attention is a factor that might explain such differences. Findings consistent between the present and previously published survey studies include the following: SR-GS is predominant in women; the most common symptoms reported are bloating, abdominal discomfort, abdominal pain, tiredness, lack of wellbeing, and headache; SR-GS is significantly associated with IBS when compared to the general population [11–13,17]. Our results also corroborate that the percentage of self-reported physician-diagnosed IBS cases is slightly higher among those who met criteria for SR-GS than those who reported recurrent adverse reactions to foods other than wheat/gluten [11,12]. This further supports the notion that a single food (wheat) has a strong association with IBS. In fact, a recent study has shown that a high proportion of patients (up to 42.4%) with IBS met criteria for SR-NCGS [21].

The population prevalence of SR-NCGS should be estimated once self-reported celiac disease and wheat allergy have been ruled out in those who met criteria for SR-GS. Under these criteria, the prevalence of SR-NCGS in the studied population was 6.28%, which is similar to the SR-NCGS prevalence rates estimated in Mexican (4.5%) and Colombian populations (6.9%) utilizing the same instrument [11,12]. The self-reported physician-diagnosed prevalence of celiac disease in the Argentinian population was 0.58%, which is similar to that reported in the United Kingdom (0.8%) [17] and Australia (0.84%) [22]. Considering a general prevalence of celiac disease between 0.5% and 1% among populations [3] and two cases that reported a physician diagnosis of celiac disease but were not following a GFD, it can be inferred that a marked underdiagnosis of celiac disease is hardly probable in Santa Fe, Argentina. In previous studies carried out in other Latin American countries, no self-reported physician-diagnosed celiac disease cases were detected in Colombia and the self-reported physician-diagnosed prevalence of this condition in Mexican population was 0.08% (1/1238). More than fifteen years ago, studies carried out in Argentina could have estimated a self-reported physician-diagnosed prevalence rate of celiac disease of 0.05% (1/2000) [23]. However, almost ten years ago and different from Mexico and Colombia, Argentina's Ministry of Health implemented a nationwide program for the detection and control of celiac disease [24]. Furthermore, Argentinians have subsidies to help to manage the cost of the GFD once celiac disease diagnosis has been properly established [25]. These actions could increase awareness about celiac disease among healthcare professionals and the general population and, perhaps, motivate gluten sensitive people to see physicians/gastroenterologists to undergo proper assessment of celiac disease. Regarding wheat allergy, the prevalence of this disorder in the studied population was 0.33%. This prevalence rate is consistent with previous survey studies carried out in other Latin American countries [11,12] and elsewhere [4,26,27], which have reported prevalence rates between 0.24% and <1%.

Following a GFD without a known diagnosis of celiac disease has been proposed as a surrogate marker for SR-NCGS [20]. Under these criteria, the estimated SR-NCGS prevalence rate was 5.78% in the present study. Due to the inclusion of non-SR-GS cases that reported current adherence to a GFD, the main limitation of this approach is that overestimate the prevalence of SR-NCGS currently following a GFD. In fact, this prevalence rate was 0.91% in the studied population, which is closer to the NCGS prevalence rate expected in Italians (slightly higher than 1%) [28]. Furthermore, this prevalence rate is not far from that reported in U.S. population (0.548%) applying the criteria described above [20]. Although in the U.S. study the authors stated that in-person physical examinations were performed and health questionnaires were applied to the participants of the study, the characteristics of the participants who met criteria for SR-NCGS in relation to the symptoms triggered after wheat/gluten intake were not stated [20], and this could lead to misinterpretation of the results. Accordingly, we have indicated that SR-NCGS prevalence rates estimations should be interpreted with caution and special attention should be paid to study designs [11] and the given definitions of SR-GS and/or SR-NCGS.

According to previous studies, the self-reported prevalence rate of adherence to a GFD in adult population range between 1.67% and 5.9% [11,12,17,22,29]. In the present study, the self-reported prevalence rate was 6.37% being the highest self-reported prevalence rate of adherence to a GFD ever reported in population-based studies. Notably, many respondents who reported current adherence to a GFD (71.4%) or avoidance of wheat/gluten-containing foods (77.4%) were doing it for reasons other than health-related benefits. Consistent with previous studies [22,29,30], these reasons included weight control and the public perception that a GFD is healthier or avoiding wheat/gluten-containing foods is healthy. However, following a GFD in the absence of gluten-related disorders is unlikely to confer health benefits [31,32]. Furthermore, the diet could compromise some micronutrients intake [14–16], especially when adhering to the diet without dietary advice, and our results show that half of those who reported current adherence to a GFD (50.6%) were doing it without medical/dietitian advice.

Our results also show that a high proportion (70.6%) of the respondents who reported recurrent adverse reactions to wheat/gluten intake (SR-GS) were not following a GFD. Although our study did not address this issue, this lack of adherence to a GFD could be related to the severity of the symptoms triggered after wheat/gluten intake and/or the availability and cost of gluten-free products, as stated by others [13]. In fact, gluten-free products are more expensive than their wheat-based counterparts and have limited availability in Santa Fe, Argentina [33].

5. Conclusions

This is the third of a series of studies conducted to estimate the prevalence of self-reported gluten-related disorders and adherence to a GFD in Latin American countries. The present study shows that gluten sensitivity is common, predominant in women and strongly associated with IBS. The results also suggest that Argentinian physicians/gastroenterologists are aware of celiac disease diagnosis. However, most people who reported current adherence to a GFD were doing it for reasons other than health-related benefits. Furthermore, at least half of the gluten-free followers were doing it without medical/dietitian advice. Because the main motivations for following a GFD were weight control and the perception that a GFD is healthier, giving scientifically sound information to the general population about the health-related benefits of following a GFD in the absence of a proper diagnosis of gluten-related disorders seems to be urgent.

Supplementary Materials: The following are available online at http://www.mdpi.com/2072-6643/9/1/81/s1, S1: English and Spanish versions of the questionnaire; Table S1: Comparison between SR-GS and recurrent adverse reactions to foods other than wheat/gluten groups; Figure S1: Self-reported symptoms in the SR-NCGS group; Figure S2: Recurrent self-reported symptoms in the adverse reactions to foods other than gluten group; Table S3: Symptoms comparison between identified SR-GS and recurrent adverse reactions to foods other than wheat/gluten cases. Table S2: Motivations for following a GFD and avoiding wheat/gluten-containing foods; Table S4: Motivations for following a GFD and who instructs the GFD in the SR-GS group stratified by gender.

Acknowledgments: Authors are grateful to the nutrition sciences students from the Universidad Nacional del Litoral, especially to the epidemiology class (2016-2) of the Faculty of Biochemistry and Biological Sciences, for helping in data collection. We also wish to thanks to the Universidad Autónoma de Sinaloa for the financial support given to Anna P. Islas-Zamorano through the academic program "Verano Internacional de la Investigación Científica".

Author Contributions: F.C.-C. and G.V.A.D. conceived and designed the study and coordinated the survey; A.P.I.-Z. and J.G.E.-A. were responsible for substantial collection of the data and analyses and interpretation of the data; M.J.V.-J. and D.M.-O. designed the study, and analyzed and interpreted the data; N.O. conceived and designed the study, analyzed and interpreted the data, and drafted the manuscript with contributions from F.C.-C.; and A.P.I.-Z., F.C.-C. and N.O. Conceived and designed the questionnaire.

Conflicts of Interest: All authors declare no conflict of interest.

References

1. Catassi, C.; Bai, J.C.; Bonaz, B.; Bouma, G.; Calabrò, A.; Carroccio, A.; Castillejo, G.; Ciacci, C.; Cristofori, F.; Dolinsek, J. Non-celiac gluten sensitivity: The new frontier of gluten related disorders. *Nutrients* **2013**, *5*, 3839–3853. [CrossRef] [PubMed]
2. Sapone, A.; Bai, J.C.; Ciacci, C.; Dolinsek, J.; Green, P.H.; Hadjivassiliou, M.; Kaukinen, K.; Rostami, K.; Sanders, D.S.; Schumann, M. Spectrum of gluten-related disorders: Consensus on new nomenclature and classification. *BMC Med.* **2012**, *10*, 13. [CrossRef] [PubMed]
3. Gujral, N.F.; Hugh, J.; Thomson, A.B.R. Celiac disease: Prevalence, diagnosism pathogenesis and tratment. *World J. Gastroenterol.* **2012**, *18*, 6036–6059. [CrossRef] [PubMed]
4. Zuidmeer, L.; Goldhahn, K.; Rona, R.J.; Gislason, D.; Madsen, C.; Summers, C.; Sodergren, E.; Dahlstrom, J.; Lindner, T.; Sigurdardottir, S.T. The prevalence of plant food allergies: A systematic review. *J. Allergy Clin. Immunol.* **2008**, *121*, 1210–1218. [CrossRef] [PubMed]
5. Ontiveros, N.; Hardy, M.; Cabrera-Chavez, F. Assessing of celiac disease and nonceliac gluten sensitivity. *Gastroenterol. Res. Pract.* **2015**, *2015*, 723954. [CrossRef] [PubMed]
6. Biesiekierski, J.R.; Peters, S.L.; Newnham, E.D.; Rosella, O.; Muir, J.G.; Gibson, P.R. No effects of gluten in patients with self-reported non-celiac gluten sensitivity after dietary reduction of fermentable, poorly absorbed, short-chain carbohydrates. *Gastroenterology* **2013**, *145*, 320–328. [CrossRef] [PubMed]
7. Junker, Y.; Zeissig, S.; Kim, S.-J.; Barisani, D.; Wieser, H.; Leffler, D.A.; Zevallos, V.; Libermann, T.A.; Dillon, S.; Freitag, T.L. Wheat amylase trypsin inhibitors drive intestinal inflammation via activation of toll-like receptor 4. *J. Exp. Med.* **2012**, *209*, 2395–2408. [CrossRef] [PubMed]
8. Molina-Infante, J.; Carroccio, A. Suspected nonceliac gluten sensitivity confirmed in few patients after gluten challenge in double-blind, placebo-controlled trials. *Clin. Gastroenterol. Hepatol.* **2016**. [CrossRef] [PubMed]

9. Catassi, C.; Elli, L.; Bonaz, B.; Bouma, G.; Carroccio, A.; Castillejo, G.; Cellier, C.; Cristofori, F.; de Magistris, L.; Dolinsek, J. Diagnosis of non-celiac gluten sensitivity (NCGS): The salerno experts' criteria. *Nutrients* **2015**, *7*, 4966–4977. [CrossRef] [PubMed]

10. Molina-Infante, J.; Santolaria, S.; Sanders, D.; Fernández-Bañares, F. Systematic review: Noncoeliac gluten sensitivity. *Aliment. Pharmacol. Ther.* **2015**, *41*, 807–820. [CrossRef] [PubMed]

11. Ontiveros, N.; López-Gallardo, J.A.; Vergara-Jiménez, M.J.; Cabrera-Chávez, F. Self-reported prevalence of symptomatic adverse reactions to gluten and adherence to gluten-free diet in an adult Mexican population. *Nutrients* **2015**, *7*, 6000–6015. [CrossRef] [PubMed]

12. Cabrera-Chávez, F.; Granda-Restrepo, D.M.; Arámburo-Gálvez, J.G.; Franco-Aguilar, A.; Magaña-Ordorica, D.; Vergara-Jiménez, M.D.J.; Ontiveros, N. Self-reported prevalence of gluten-related disorders and adherence to gluten-free diet in Colombian adult population. *Gastroenterol. Res. Pract.* **2016**, *2016*. [CrossRef]

13. Van Gils, T.; Nijeboer, P.; IJssennagger, C.E.; Sanders, D.S.; Mulder, C.J.; Bouma, G. Prevalence and characterization of self-reported gluten sensitivity in The Netherlands. *Nutrients* **2016**, *8*, 714. [CrossRef] [PubMed]

14. Hallert, C.; Grant, C.; Grehn, S.; Grännö, C.; Hultén, S.; Midhagen, G.; Ström, M.; Svensson, H.; Valdimarsson, T. Evidence of poor vitamin status in coeliac patients on a gluten-free diet for 10 years. *Aliment. Pharmacol. Ther.* **2002**, *16*, 1333–1339. [CrossRef] [PubMed]

15. Wild, D.; Robins, G.; Burley, V.; Howdle, P. Evidence of high sugar intake, and low fibre and mineral intake, in the gluten-free diet. *Aliment. Pharmacol. Ther.* **2010**, *32*, 573–581. [CrossRef] [PubMed]

16. Dall'Asta, C.; Scarlato, A.P.; Galaverna, G.; Brighenti, F.; Pellegrini, N. Dietary exposure to fumonisins and evaluation of nutrient intake in a group of adult celiac patients on a gluten-free diet. *Mol. Nutr. Food Res.* **2012**, *56*, 632–640. [CrossRef] [PubMed]

17. Aziz, I.; Lewis, N.R.; Hadjivassiliou, M.; Winfield, S.N.; Rugg, N.; Kelsall, A.; Newrick, L.; Sanders, D.S. A UK study assessing the population prevalence of self-reported gluten sensitivity and referral characteristics to secondary care. *Eur. J. Gastroenterol. Hepatol.* **2014**, *26*, 33–39. [CrossRef] [PubMed]

18. Ontiveros, N.; Valdez-Meza, E.E.; Vergara-Jiménez, M.J.; Canizalez-Román, A.; Borzutzky, F.; Cabrera-Chávez, F. Parent-reported prevalence of food allergy in Mexican schoolchildren: A population-based study. *Allergol. Immunopathol.* **2016**, *44*. [CrossRef] [PubMed]

19. Dean, A.G.; Sullivan, K.M.; Soe, M.M. OpenEpi: Open Source Epidemiologic Statistics for Public Health, Version, Updated 2013/04/06. Available online: http://www.openepi.com (accessed on 24 November 2016).

20. DiGiacomo, D.V.; Tennyson, C.A.; Green, P.H.; Demmer, R.T. Prevalence of gluten-free diet adherence among individuals without celiac disease in the USA: Results from the continuous national health and nutrition examination survey 2009–2010. *Scand. J. Gastroenterol.* **2013**, *48*, 921–925. [CrossRef] [PubMed]

21. Aziz, I.; Branchi, F.; Pearson, K.; Priest, J.; Sanders, D.S. A study evaluating the bidirectional relationship between inflammatory bowel disease and self-reported non-celiac gluten sensitivity. *Inflamm. Bowel Dis.* **2015**, *21*, 847–853. [CrossRef] [PubMed]

22. Golley, S.; Corsini, N.; Topping, D.; Morell, M.; Mohr, P. Motivations for avoiding wheat consumption in Australia: Results from a population survey. *Public Health Nutr.* **2015**, *18*, 490–499. [CrossRef] [PubMed]

23. Gomez, J.C.; Selvaggio, G.S.; Viola, M.; Pizarro, B.; la Motta, G.; de Barrio, S.; Castelletto, R.; Echeverría, R.; Sugai, E.; Vazquez, H. Prevalence of celiac disease in Argentina: Screening of an adult population in the La Plata Area. *Am. J. Gastroenterol.* **2001**, *96*, 2700–2704. [CrossRef] [PubMed]

24. Ministerio de Salud. Crease el Programa Nacional Para la Detección y Control de Enfermedad Celiaca. Available online: http://www.msal.gob.ar/celiacos/pdf/resolucion-programa.pdf (accessed on 22 November 2016).

25. Ministerio de Salud. Resolución 1365/15: Actualiza el Monto a Cubrir por Obras Sociales y Prepagas a un Valor de $326.83 Mensuales. Available online: http://www.msal.gob.ar/celiacos/pdf/Resolución%201365.pdf (accessed on 22 November 2016).

26. Vierk, K.A.; Koehler, K.M.; Fein, S.B.; Street, D.A. Prevalence of self-reported food allergy in American adults and use of food labels. *J. Allergy Clin. Immunol.* **2007**, *119*, 1504–1510. [CrossRef] [PubMed]

27. Morita, E.; Chinuki, Y.; Takahashi, H.; Nabika, T.; Yamasaki, M.; Shiwaku, K. Prevalence of wheat allergy in Japanese adults. *Allergol. Int.* **2012**, *61*, 101–105. [CrossRef] [PubMed]

28. Volta, U.; Bardella, M.T.; Calabrò, A.; Troncone, R.; Corazza, G.R. An Italian prospective multicenter survey on patients suspected of having non-celiac gluten sensitivity. *BMC Med.* **2014**, *12*, 85. [CrossRef] [PubMed]

29. Kim, H.-S.; Patel, K.G.; Orosz, E.; Kothari, N.; Demyen, M.F.; Pyrsopoulos, N.; Ahlawat, S.K. Time trends in the prevalence of celiac disease and gluten-free diet in the US population: Results from the national health and nutrition examination surveys 2009–2014. *JAMA Intern. Med.* **2016**, *176*, 1716–1717. [CrossRef] [PubMed]
30. Pember, S.E.; Rush, S.E. Motivation for gluten-free diet adherence among adults with and without a clinically diagnosed gluten-related illness. *Calif. J. Health Promot.* **2016**, *14*, 68–73.
31. Wu, J.H.; Neal, B.; Trevena, H.; Crino, M.; Stuart-Smith, W.; Faulkner-Hogg, K.; Louie, J.C.Y.; Dunford, E. Are gluten-free foods healthier than non-gluten-free foods? An evaluation of supermarket products in Australia. *Br. J. Nutr.* **2015**, *114*, 448–454. [CrossRef] [PubMed]
32. Missbach, B.; Schwingshackl, L.; Billmann, A.; Mystek, A.; Hickelsberger, M.; Bauer, G.; König, J. Gluten-free food database: The nutritional quality and cost of packaged gluten-free foods. *PeerJ* **2015**, *3*. [CrossRef] [PubMed]
33. Cúneo, F.; Ortega, J. Disponibilidad, costo y valor nutricional de los alimentos libres de gluten en comercios de la ciudad de santa fe. *FABICIB* **2012**, *16*, 167–178. [CrossRef]

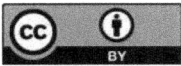

nutrients

MDPI

Article

Normal Bone Mineral Density Associates with Duodenal Mucosa Healing in Adult Patients with Celiac Disease on a Gluten-Free Diet

Tiziana Larussa, Evelina Suraci, Maria Imeneo, Raffaella Marasco and Francesco Luzza *

Department of Health Sciences, University of Catanzaro "Magna Graecia", Viale Europa, Germaneto,
Catanzaro 88100, Italy; tiziana.larussa@gmail.com (T.L.); e.suraci@libero.it (E.S.); graziaimeneo@hotmail.it (M.I.);
raffaellamarasco1@gmail.com (R.M.)
* Correspondence: luzza@unicz.it; Tel.: +39-0961-3697111; Fax: +39-0961-3697164

Received: 11 January 2017; Accepted: 23 January 2017; Published: 31 January 2017

Abstract: Impairment of bone mineral density (BMD) is frequent in celiac disease (CD) patients on a gluten-free diet (GFD). The normalization of intestinal mucosa is still difficult to predict. We aim to investigate the relationship between BMD and duodenal mucosa healing (DMH) in CD patients on a GFD. Sixty-four consecutive CD patients on a GFD were recruited. After a median period of a 6-year GFD (range 2–33 years), patients underwent repeat duodenal biopsy and dual-energy X-ray absorptiometry (DXA) scan. Twenty-four patients (38%) displayed normal and 40 (62%) low BMD, 47 (73%) DMH, and 17 (27%) duodenal mucosa lesions. All patients but one with normal BMD (23 of 24, 96%) showed DMH, while, among those with low BMD, 24 (60%) did and 16 (40%) did not. At multivariate analysis, being older (odds ratio (OR) 1.1, 95% confidence interval (CI) 1.03–1.18) and having diagnosis at an older age (OR 1.09, 95% CI 1.03–1.16) were associated with low BMD; in turn, having normal BMD was the only variable independently associated with DMH (OR 17.5, 95% CI 1.6–192). In older CD patients and with late onset disease, BMD recovery is not guaranteed, despite a GFD. A normal DXA scan identified CD patients with DMH; thus, it is a potential tool in planning endoscopic resampling.

Keywords: celiac disease; bone disorders; osteoporosis; histopathology; intestinal mucosa healing

1. Introduction

Celiac disease (CD) is a chronic autoimmune disorder occurring in genetically predisposed individuals, triggered by gluten and related prolamins contained in wheat, barley, and rye. The resulting malabsorption due to small intestinal injury leads to systemic damage, mostly related to nutritional deficiencies [1]. Serological screening tests are available to select individuals needing to undergo diagnostic endoscopic biopsy of the duodenal mucosa. They are immunoglobulin (Ig)A anti-tissue transglutaminase (tTG) and anti-endomysium antibodies-IgA (EMA), both showing a specificity close to 100% and a sensitivity greater than 90% [2]. Serology is also a useful tool in monitoring adherence and response to a gluten-free diet (GFD), although it may not be representative of a complete recovery of the intestinal mucosa [3].

Reduced bone mineral density (BMD) is found in more than 50% of newly diagnosed patients with CD, possibly due to impaired calcium and vitamin D absorption [4]. Besides micronutrient malabsorption, it is conceivable that chronic inflammation can predispose CD patients, whether on a GFD or not, to mineral metabolism derangement [5]. Indeed, a lack of calbindin and calcium-binding protein, the vitamin D-regulated protein implicated in calcium uptake from the intestinal lumen, has been described in the areas of damaged mucosa [6]. Hyperparathyroidism sustained by a chronic inflammatory state is another implicated factor, since high parathormone (PTH) values are frequent in

CD patients even in the presence of normal circulating vitamin D levels [7]. Release of proinflammatory cytokines such as interleukin (IL)-6, IL-1β, tumor necrosis factor (TNF)-α, and interferon (IFN)-γ has been implicated in bone remodeling during CD, as well as the receptor activator of nuclear factor kappaB (RANK)/RANK ligand (RANKL)/osteoprotegerin (OPG) axis, according to which the reabsorbing activity performed by RANKL is counteracted by the effects of its natural decoy receptor OPG [8]. A lower OPG/RANKL ratio was found in CD patients with recovery of intestinal mucosa and positively correlated with a reduced BMD [9]. A strict GFD restores mucosal damage and reverses the biochemical evidence of calcium malabsorption, resulting in normal BMD in these treated patients [10]. Nevertheless, a long-term impairment of bone mineralization can persist in some otherwise healthy CD patients adhering to a GFD and harboring negative serology [11]. In this regard, it is proper to recall that naturally gluten-free products are often low in B vitamins, calcium, vitamin D, iron, zinc, magnesium, and fiber, while enrichment of gluten-free products is not so common. Therefore, dietary advice other than gluten withdrawal seems to be necessary in CD patients in order to better choose the composition of foods and prevent complications due to malnutrition [12]. At the same time, incomplete mucosal recovery represents a challenge for clinicians, since it can occur in apparently asymptomatic CD patients despite adequate GFD and negative serology [13]. These findings suggest the importance of a follow-up biopsy after CD diagnosis and the need for parameters other than serology or dietary assessment to target the optimal timing of the endoscopic repeat procedure.

This study aimed at investigating the relationship between BMD assessment and mucosal duodenal status in adult CD patients on a GFD.

2. Materials and Methods

2.1. Patient Recruitment and Study Design

Between January 2012 and September 2015, 64 consecutive asymptomatic outpatients with CD (18 male and 46 female; median age 36 years, range 18–69) were selected for the study. Patients had to be adherent to a GFD for at least 2 years, harbored persistent (at least 18 months) negative CD-related serology, and reported no current gastrointestinal symptoms. Diagnosis of CD needed to be performed on the basis of clinical presentation, positive CD-related serology, and suggestive histological findings on duodenal biopsy [14]. All patients had atrophic disease at diagnosis and did not repeat biopsy before recruitment, neither a baseline BMD measurement was performed except for a subgroup of 25 patients. Exclusion criteria included pregnancy, breast-feeding, and a previous diagnosis of hematological diseases or hormonal and metabolic disorders which could account for low BMD. Data on height, weight, time since diagnosis, onset of symptoms, clinical presentation, age at menarche, cycle regularity, menopausal status, drug use, calcium intake, life style (such as levels of physical activity), smoking, history of fracture, and other relevant co-morbidities were collected. Each patient, in a time frame of 6 months from recruitment, was submitted to gastroscopy with duodenal resampling along with measurement of BMD and serological assay.

2.2. Dietary Assessment and Body Mass Index Calculation

Clinicians assessed dietary compliance by periodic interview during follow-up visits in order to demonstrate deliberate or inadvertent gluten intake. Adherence to a GFD was classified as good according to Leffler et al. in a standardized fashion by analysis of a 3-day food record [15]. The body mass index (BMI) was calculated as weight in kilograms divided by the square of height in meters (normal range 18–24.9 kg/m^2).

2.3. Serology and Laboratory Parameters

Blood samples were collected in the morning after a 12 h fast in order to measure serum levels of calcium, vitamin D, and PTH. Patients were tested for tTG and EMA antibodies (both IgA and IgG classes). Serum tTG antibodies were investigated by an enzyme-linked immunosorbent assay

(ELISA; A. Menarini diagnostics, Florence, Italy), a unit value of ≥ 5 being positive. Serum EMA was determined using an indirect immunofluorescence method with a monkey distal esophagus as a substrate; a dilution of 1:5 was considered positive (A. Menarini diagnostics).

2.4. Duodenal Mucosa Sampling and Histology

Patients underwent repeat duodenal biopsy after a period of at least 2 years since the beginning of the GFD (median 6 years, range 2–33). At least four biopsy specimens were collected from the distal duodenum during upper gastrointestinal endoscopy, fixed in 10% formalin and paraffin-embedded. Intraepithelial lymphocytes have been identified using CD3 immunostaining, and a value of ≤ 25 lymphocytes/100 epithelial cells was considered normal. Histological changes were classified according to Marsh criteria (Stage 0: normal mucosa; Stage 1: increased number of intraepithelial lymphocytes; Stage 2: crypts proliferation; Stages 3a-3b-3c: respectively mild, moderate, and severe villous atrophy) [16]. Marsh Stage 0 at repeat biopsy was considered duodenal mucosa healing (DMH). All evaluations were carried out in a blinded fashion by the same pathologist without prior knowledge of patient history.

2.5. Measurement of Bone Mineral Density

At the time of duodenal resampling, BMD in the lumbar spine and femoral neck was measured by means of dual-energy X-ray absorptiometry (DXA) according to standard procedures. Values were expressed as standard deviation scores, which compare individual BMD determinations to those of young adults (T-score). Based on the World Health Organization criteria, patients with a T-score (in the lumbar spine or femoral neck or both) between -2.5 and -1 were considered osteopenic, while a T-score < -2.5 identified osteoporosis [17].

2.6. Ethical Considerations

The study was carried out according to the Declaration of Helsinki. The patients received oral and written information about the study. All participators were informed that participation was voluntarily and that they could withdraw at any time without consequences. The study protocol was approved by the local research Ethical Committee, and written informed consent was obtained from all the participants.

2.7. Statistics

At univariate analysis, BMD and duodenal mucosa status were analyzed in relation to all the considered variables by means of an unpaired Student's *t*-test, a chi-square test, or a Fisher's exact test, as required. A difference was considered significant if the *p*-value was less than 0.05. The odds ratio (OR) of having low BMD and DMH, given the presence of a particular variable, was used as a measure of association and adjusted for the effect of confounding variables by multivariate logistic regression analysis (SPSS Statistic 16.0; IBM, Armonk, NY, USA).

3. Results

3.1. Clinical Findings and Serology

Table 1 shows the demographic and clinical characteristics of the participants. No patient had a history of bone fractures or of any endocrine, kidney, or liver disorder accountable for bone derangement. Patients did not receive supplementation with vitamins, calcium, or iron, nor had they taken medications capable of acting on bone metabolism, such as steroids. The three patients on menopausal status did not assume hormone replacement therapy for their condition. Intestinal resections or small bowel diseases causing malabsorption were absent. All patients showed a good adherence to a GFD. No special diet regimen was found (such as vegetarian or vegan diet), nor were excess or deficiency levels of physical activity worth noting. Serum calcium, vitamin D, and parathyroid hormone levels were normal, and both anti-tTG and EMA were negative in all patients.

Table 1. Characteristics of the 64 patients with celiac disease on a gluten-free diet.

Variables	Values
Sex	18 (28) males; 46 (72) females
Age, years	36.1 ± 10.7 (range 18–69)
Age at diagnosis, years	28 ± 14.3 (range 2–64)
Duration of GFD, years	8.3 ± 6.6 (range 2–33)
BMI (Kg/m²)	21.9 ± 1.8 (range 19.1–25.6)
Clinical presentation	
Malabsorption	36 (56)
Diarrhea	16 (25)
Dyspepsia	7 (11)
Extraintestinal symptoms	2 (3)
Screen-detected	3 (5)
Smoke	19 (29)
Menopausal status	3 (7)
History of fracture	0 (0)

BMI = body mass index; GFD = gluten-free diet; SD = standard deviation. Values are numbers (%) or means ± SD as indicated.

3.2. BMD and Histology

Forty (62%) of the 64 CD patients displayed low BMD, with 2 (5%) accounting for osteoporosis and 38 (95%) for osteopenia. BMD was normal in the remaining 24 patients (38%). With the exception of age at evaluation and diagnosis, and duration of the GFD, characteristics of patients did not differ between subjects with normal and low BMD at univariate analysis (Table 2). However, only being older and having CD diagnosis at an older age remained independently associated with low BMD at multivariate analysis (Table 2). DMH was found in 47 (73%) patients, while 17 (27%) showed duodenal mucosa lesions ($n = 9$, Marsh Stage 1; $n = 2$, Marsh Stage 2; and $n = 6$, Marsh Stage 3). All patients but one with normal BMD ($n = 23$, 96%) showed DMH. Among patients with low BMD, 24 (60%) showed DMH, while 16 (40%) did not (Table 3). Characteristics of the 64 CD patients on a GFD according to duodenal mucosa status are summarized in Table 3. Even though age, age at diagnosis, and BMI closely approached statistical significance, at multivariate analysis, a normal BMD was the only variable independently associated with DMH (OR 17.5, 95% CI 1.6–192).

Table 2. Characteristics of the 64 patients with celiac disease on a gluten-free diet according to bone mineral density as assessed by dual energy X ray absorptiometry.

Variables	Normal BMD $n = 24$	Low BMD $n = 40$	p	OR (95% CI) Adjusted [a]	p
Sex					
Male	7 (29)	11 (28)	0.83	1.56 (0.41–5.86)	0.51
Female	17 (71)	29 (72)			
Age, years	30.1 ± 10.6	39.6 ± 9.5	0.0002	1.1 (1.03–1.18)	0.004
Age at diagnosis *, years	20.1 ± 14.9	37.7 ± 11.9	0.0002	-	-
BMI (Kg/m²)	22.3 ± 1.7	21.7 ± 1.8	0.08	0.8 (0.6–1.17)	0.31
Smoke	7 (29)	12 (30)	0.97	0.86 (0.23–3.15)	0.82
Clinical presentation [b]					
Malabsorption	12 (50)	24 (60)	0.34		
Diarrhea	7 (29)	9 (23)	0.48		
Dyspepsia	3 (13)	4 (10)	0.71	0.83 (0.18–3.66)	0.81
Extraintestinal symptoms	0 (0)	2 (4)	0.27		
Screen-detected	2 (8)	1 (3)	0.26		
Duration of GFD [c], years	10.1 ± 7.6	7.2 ± 5.7	0.04	0.65 (0.19–2.18)	0.48

CI = confidence interval; MVA = multivariate analysis; OR = odds ratio; SD = standard deviation; BMD = bone mineral density; BMI = body mass index; GFD = gluten-free diet. Values are numbers (%) or means ± SD as indicated. Means were compared with the use of a Student's *t*-test and proportions with the use of a chi-square test or Fisher's exact test. OR with 95% CI in brackets is given. * Due to collinearity with age, this variable entered a separate MVA with all other variables than age and leads to OR 1.09, 95% CI 1.03–1.16, $p = 0.003$, while the other variables did not reach the statistical significance ($p > 0.05$). [a] All variables except age at diagnosis (due to collinearity with age) entered MVA. Male gender, smoking, conventional clinical presentation, and patients with GFD ≤ 7 as references in MVA. [b] Clinical presentation entered MVA analysis as categorical variable, assuming malabsorption and diarrhea as conventional presentation and screen-detected, extraintestinal symptoms and dyspepsia as unusual presentation. [c] Duration of GFD entered MVA as categorical variable, subgrouping subjects with GFD ≤ 7 ($n = 36$) and those with GFD ≥ 8 ($n = 28$).

Table 3. Characteristics of the 64 patients with celiac disease on a gluten-free diet according to duodenal mucosa healing as assessed by Marsh classification.

Variables	Mucosal Healing n = 47	Mucosal Lesions n = 17	p	OR (95% CI) Adjusted [a]	p
Bone mineral density					
Normal	23	1	0.001	17.5 (1.6–192)	0.019
Low	24	16			
Sex					
Male	12	6	0.53	0.5 (0.11–2.52)	0.43
Female	35	11			
Age, years	35.1 ± 10.5	39.8 ± 11.3	0.06	1.1 (0.9–1.34)	0.34
Age at diagnosis, years	26.4 ± 14	32.5 ± 14.7	0.07	0.9 (0.76–1.08)	0.26
BMI (Kg/m^2)	22.1 ± 1.8	21.4 ± 1.7	0.08	0.9 (0.64–1.48)	0.91
Smoke	13	6	0.55	2.7 (0.56–13.5)	0.20
Clinical presentation [b]					
Malabsorption	28 (60)	8 (47)	0.4		
Diarrhea	10 (21)	6 (35)	0.32		
Dyspepsia	6 (13)	1 (6)	0.66	1.3 (0.23–7.6)	0.75
Extraintestinal symptoms	0 (0)	2 (12)	0.06		
Screen-detected	3 (6)	0 (0)	0.55		
Duration of GFD [c], years	8.7 ± 6.4	7.3 ± 7.6	0.23	0.17 (0.01–1.65)	0.12

CI = confidence interval; MVA = multivariate analysis; OR = odds ratio; SD = standard deviation; BMI = body mass index; GFD = gluten-free diet. Values are numbers (%) or means ± SD as indicated. Means were compared with the use of a Student's *t*-test and proportions with the use of a chi-square test or Fisher's exact test. OR with 95% CI in brackets is given. [a] All variables entered MVA. Male gender, smoking, conventional clinical presentation, and patients with GFD ≤ 7 as references in MVA. [b] Clinical presentation entered MVA analysis as categorical variable, assuming malabsorption and diarrhea as conventional presentation and screen-detected, extraintestinal symptoms and dyspepsia as unusual presentation. [c] Duration of GFD entered MVA as categorical variable, subgrouping subjects with GFD ≤ 7 (*n* = 36) and those with GFD ≥ 8 (*n* = 28).

4. Discussion

In spite of long-term strict adherence to a GFD and persistent negative CD-related serology, a high prevalence of low BMD (62%) has been shown in CD patients of this study. These findings suggest that risk factors other than villous atrophy are possibly involved in bone injury, such as diagnosis of CD in adult life, irregular adherence to a GFD, lactose intolerance, and nutritional deficiency related to naturally gluten-free foods or to the composition of gluten-free products.

At the same time, a significant proportion of patients (27%) displayed duodenal mucosa lesions, and they all had a low BMD. It has been already observed that DMH after a GFD is not achieved in a considerable proportion of CD patients, notwithstanding prolonged and strict adherence to the diet [3]. Pekki et al. found, both at diagnosis and after one year GFD, a relationship between an impaired T-score and duodenal mucosa lesions as verified by follow-up biopsies [18]. Therefore, even in the presence of a negative serology and lack of intestinal symptoms, a low BMD could be taken into account when considering a persistent duodenal mucosa lesion. As an additional value, this study focuses on the fact that a normal BMD predicts DMH, since all but one patient who displayed a normal BMD showed DMH (96%) and independently associated with DMH (OR 17.5).

Compared to patients with abnormal DXA findings, patients with both normal BMD and DMH were younger, had an earlier diagnosis, and a longer period of GFD. Nevertheless, adjustment of variables with each other no longer confirmed that age, age at diagnosis, and duration of the GFD were independently associated with duodenal mucosa status at multivariate analysis—only a normal BMD has this association. It is remarkable that, in the same series, negative CD-related serology was associated in only 73% of patients who showed DMH. Even though the presence of non-atrophic lesions of the intestinal mucosa (i.e., Marsh Stages 1 and 2) cannot be considered sufficient to establish the diagnosis of CD, they should be regarded as a lack of histological recovery after a long-term strict adherence to a GFD [19,20]. Accordingly, we established that DMH corresponds to Marsh Stage 0.

An impaired bone mineralization is a frequent finding during CD, at both diagnosis and after a GFD, widely ranging from 38% to 72% and 9% to 47%, respectively [21]. In the subgroup of 25 patients who performed DXA at the time of CD diagnosis, 22 (88%) had an impaired bone mineralization (data not shown), and this may explain the high proportion of low BMD (62%) still found after a GFD in all the study patients.

In untreated CD patients, calcium malabsorption is due mechanically to intestinal mucosal damage and functionally to the presence of intraluminal unabsorbed fatty acids which bind calcium in the intestinal lumen and may reduce dietary vitamin D absorption [22]. In our series, it was confirmed that no patient displayed abnormal levels of circulating calcium, vitamin D, and PTH [23]. Even though serum calcium levels may not adequately reflect calcium absorption, we did not search for bone resorption markers since they are rarely used in clinical practice, while being an accurate method of bone health assessment [24]. Moreover, chronic release of proinflammatory cytokines and other factors of bone remodeling, such as estrogens, androgens, insuline-like growth factor-1, and PTH contribute to low BMD in CD patients and they are still under investigation [25]. All the above conditions are reversed by a GFD, which repairs mucosal damage. Nevertheless, diet is found to improve but often not to normalize BMD, suggesting that further strategies are needed to manage bone derangement in CD patients [26]. Current data did not support evidence for additional benefits derived from dietary supplementation (e.g., with calcium and vitamin D) in adult CD patients. However, in some special situations, such as osteoporosis detected in celiac postmenopausal women, it could be useful to begin treatment with hormone replacement therapy or bisphosphonates. In addition, education on the importance of lifestyle changes, such as regular exercise, smoking cessation, and excessive alcohol intake, should be provided [27].

Many risk factors for derangement of bone mineralization and its relationship with the duodenal mucosa status have been here assessed in a homogeneous group of CD patients on a GFD. Indeed, age at evaluation and diagnosis, and the duration of the GFD, were significantly different between patients with low and normal BMD, while no other differences in acknowledged risk factors were found between the two groups, nor the clinical presentation of CD. This means that older patients, diagnosed at a later age and with a shorter GFD period, are at higher risk of bone derangement. Studies on pediatric CD population support these findings, as BMD normalization is achieved in young CD patients initiating a GFD early [28]. Furthermore, adjustment of variables with each other indicates only age and age at diagnosis as independent risk factors associated with BMD. Consequently, the duration of the GFD needed to normalize BMD remains unclear [29]. Given that CD is a risk factor for bone health impairment and that GFD alone is not enough to restore BMD, efforts should be focused to identify predicting factors for bone demineralization in CD patients.

The novel finding of this study is that DXA may have a place in the follow-up of CD patients, particularly to help selecting patients who need a control biopsy and those who did not. Indeed, the association between normal BMD and DMH excludes patients with a normal DXA from endoscopic biopsy resampling, shifting the attention on CD patients who display an abnormal DXA and, possibly, harbor duodenal mucosa lesions.

Data on the correlation between bone derangement and Marsh Stage in newly diagnosed CD patients have been produced, and this supports the role of malabsorption in determining low BMD in untreated individuals [30]. However, little is known about the mucosal intestinal recovery and the causes of its delay. To date, the time for scheduling repeat biopsies is still debated and no agreement exists on the best time to plan biopsy follow-up [31]. If a normal BMD will be confirmed to associate with DMH in CD patients on a GFD, the use of DXA could be proposed as an adjunctive tool in the management of CD patients during the follow-up.

5. Conclusions

This study confirms that BMD derangement and incomplete DMH are frequent findings in adult CD patients on a GFD. Furthermore, the novel finding that a normal BMD associates with DMH suggests that DXA may be a useful tool in the management of adult CD patients and the timely planning of endoscopic biopsy resampling.

Acknowledgments: The authors would like to thank Ashour Michael for revision of the English language.

Author Contributions: E.S., M.I., and R.M. collected the data and contributed with critical revision of the manuscript. T.L. and F.L. contributed equally to the design of the study. T.L. analyzed the data and wrote the article. F.L. revised the manuscript for important intellectual content and interpretation of the data. All authors approved the final version of the manuscript.

Conflicts of Interest: The authors declare no conflict of interest.

References

1. Di Sabatino, A.; Corazza, G.R. Coeliac Disease. *Lancet* **2009**, *373*, 1480–1493. [CrossRef]
2. Feighery, C.; Conlon, N.; Jackson, J. Adult population screening for coeliac disease: Comparison of tissue-transglutaminase antibody and anti-endomysial antibody tests. *Eur. J. Gastroenterol. Hepatol.* **2006**, *18*, 1173–1175. [CrossRef] [PubMed]
3. Lanzini, A.; Lanzarotto, F.; Villanacci, V.; Mora, A.; Bertolazzi, S.; Turini, D.; Carella, G.; Malagoli, A.; Ferrante, G.; Cesana, B.M.; et al. Complete recovery of intestinal mucosa occurs very rarely in adult celiac patients despite adherence to gluten free diet. *Aliment. Pharmacol. Ther.* **2009**, *29*, 1299–1308. [CrossRef] [PubMed]
4. Zanchetta, M.B.; Longobardi, V.; Bai, J.C. Bone and Celiac Disease. *Curr. Osteoporos. Rep.* **2016**, *14*, 43–48. [CrossRef]
5. Bianchi, M.L.; Bardella, M.T. Bone in celiac disease. *Osteoporos. Int.* **2008**, *19*, 1705–1716. [CrossRef] [PubMed]
6. Staun, M.; Jarnum, S. Measurement of the 10,000-molecular weight calcium-binding protein in small-intestinal biopsy specimens from patients with malabsorption syndromes. *Scand. J. Gastroenterol.* **1988**, *23*, 827–832. [CrossRef] [PubMed]
7. Lemieux, B.; Boivin, M.; Brossard, J.H.; Lepage, R.; Picard, D.; Rousseau, L.; D'Amour, P. Normal parathyroid function with decreased bone mineral density in treated celiac disease. *Can. J. Gastroenterol.* **2001**, *15*, 302–307. [CrossRef] [PubMed]
8. Tilg, H.; Moschen, A.R.; Kaser, A.; Pines, A.; Dotan, I. Gut, inflammation and osteoporosis: Basic and clinical concepts. *Gut* **2008**, *57*, 684–694. [CrossRef] [PubMed]
9. Fiore, C.E.; Pennisi, P.; Ferro, G.; Ximenes, B.; Privitelli, L.; Mangiafico, R.A.; Santoro, F.; Parisi, N.; Lombardo, T. Altered osteoprotegerin/RANKL ratio and low bone mineral density in celiac patients on long-term treatment with gluten-free diet. *Horm. Metab. Res.* **2006**, *38*, 417–422. [CrossRef] [PubMed]
10. Sategna-Guidetti, C.; Grosso, S.B.; Grosso, S.; Mengozzi, G.; Aimo, G.; Zaccaria, T.; Di Stefano, M.; Isaia, G.C. The effects of 1-year gluten withdrawal on bone mass, bone metabolism and nutritional status in newly-diagnosed adult coeliac disease patients. *Aliment. Pharmacol. Ther.* **2000**, *14*, 35–43. [CrossRef] [PubMed]
11. Grace-Farfaglia, P. Bones of contention: Bone mineral density recovery in celiac disease—A systematic review. *Nutrients* **2015**, *7*, 3347–3369. [CrossRef] [PubMed]
12. Bardella, M.T.; Fredella, C.; Prampolini, L.; Molteni, N.; Giunta, A.M.; Bianchi, P.A. Body composition and dietary intakes in adult celiac disease patients consuming a strict gluten-free diet. *Am. J. Clin. Nutr.* **2000**, *72*, 937–939. [PubMed]
13. Kaukinen, K.; Peräaho, M.; Lindfors, K.; Partanen, J.; Woolley, N.; Pikkarainen, P.; Karvonen, A.L.; Laasanen, T.; Sievänen, H.; Mäki, M.; et al. Persistent small bowel mucosal villous atrophy without symptoms in coeliac disease. *Aliment. Pharmacol. Ther.* **2007**, *25*, 1237–1245. [CrossRef] [PubMed]
14. National Institute of Health Consensus Development Conference Statement on Celiac Disease, June 28–38, 2004. *Gastroenterology* **2005**, *128*, S1–S9.
15. Leffler, D.A.; Edwards George, J.B.; Dennis, M.; Cook, F.; Schuppan, D.; Kelly, C.P. A prospective comparative study of five measures of gluten-free diet adherence in adults with coeliac disease. *Aliment. Pharmacol. Ther.* **2007**, *26*, 1227–1235. [CrossRef] [PubMed]
16. Oberhuber, G. Histopathology of celiac disease. *Biomed. Pharmacother.* **2000**, *54*, 368–372. [CrossRef]

17. Kanis, J.A.; Melton, L.J., 3rd; Christiansen, C.; Johnston, C.C.; Khaltaev, N. The diagnosis of osteoporosis. *J. Bone Miner. Res.* **1994**, *9*, 1137–1141. [CrossRef] [PubMed]

18. Pekki, H.; Kurppa, K.; Mäki, M.; Huhtala, H.; Sievnen, H.; Laurila, K.; Collin, P.; Kaukinen, K. Predictors and Significance of Incomplete Mucosal Recovery in Celiac Disease After 1 Year on a Gluten-Free Diet. *Am. J. Gastroenterol.* **2015**, *110*, 1078–1085. [CrossRef] [PubMed]

19. Lebwohl, B.; Murray, J.A.; Rubio-Tapia, A.; Green, P.H.; Ludvigsson, J.F. Predictors of persistent villous atrophy in coeliac disease: A population-based study. *Aliment. Pharmacol. Ther.* **2014**, *39*, 488–495. [CrossRef] [PubMed]

20. Tuire, I.; Marja-Leena, L.; Teea, S.; Katri, H.; Jukka, P.; Paivi, S.; Heini, H.; Markku, M.; Pekka, C.; Katri, K. Persistent duodenal intraepithelial lymphocytosis despite a long-term strict gluten-free diet in celiac disease. *Am. J. Gastroenterol.* **2012**, *107*, 1563–1569. [CrossRef] [PubMed]

21. Larussa, T.; Suraci, E.; Nazionale, I.; Abenavoli, L.; Imeneo, M.; Luzza, F. Bone mineralization in celiac disease. *Gastroenterol. Res. Pract.* **2012**, *2012*. [CrossRef] [PubMed]

22. Pazianas, M.; Butcher, G.P.; Subhani, J.M.; Finch, P.J.; Ang, L.; Collins, C.; Heaney, R.P.; Zaidi, M.; Maxwell, J.D. Calcium absorption and bone mineral density in celiacs after long term treatment with gluten-free diet and adequate calcium intake. *Osteoporos. Int.* **2005**, *16*, 56–63. [CrossRef] [PubMed]

23. Molteni, N.; Bardella, M.T.; Vezzoli, G.; Pozzoli, E.; Bianchi, P. Intestinal calcium absorption as shown by stable strontium test in celiac disease before and after gluten-free diet. *Am. J. Gastroenterol.* **1995**, *90*, 2025–2028. [PubMed]

24. Di Stefano, M.; Mengoli, C.; Bergonzi, M.; Corazza, G.R. Bone mass and mineral metabolism alterations in adult celiac disease: Pathophysiology and clinical approach. *Nutrients* **2013**, *5*, 4786–4799. [CrossRef] [PubMed]

25. Larussa, T.; Suraci, E.; Nazionale, I.; Leone, I.; Montalcini, T.; Abenavoli, L.; Imeneo, M.; Pujia, A.; Luzza, F. No evidence of circulating autoantibodies against osteoprotegerin in patients with celiac disease. *World J. Gastroenterol.* **2012**, *18*, 1622–1627. [CrossRef] [PubMed]

26. Di Stefano, M.; Veneto, G.; Corrao, G.; Corazza, G.R. Role of lifestyle factors in the pathogenesis of osteopenia in adult coeliac disease: A multivariate analysis. *Eur. J. Gastroenterol. Hepatol.* **2000**, *12*, 1195–1199. [CrossRef] [PubMed]

27. Capriles, V.D.; Martini, L.A.; Arêas, J.A. Metabolic osteopathy in celiac disease: Importance of a gluten-free diet. *Nutr. Rev.* **2009**, *67*, 599–606. [CrossRef] [PubMed]

28. Mora, S.; Barera, G.; Beccio, S.; Proverbio, M.C.; Weber, G.; Bianchi, C.; Chiumello, G. Bone density and bone metabolism are normal after long-term gluten-free diet in young celiac patients. *Am. J. Gastroenterol.* **1999**, *94*, 398–403. [CrossRef] [PubMed]

29. Usta, M.; Urganci, N. Does gluten-free diet protect children with celiac disease from low bone density? *Iran. J. Pediatr.* **2014**, *24*, 429–434. [PubMed]

30. García-Manzanares, A.; Tenias, J.M.; Lucendo, A.J. Bone mineral density directly correlates with duodenal Marsh stage in newly diagnosed adult celiac patients. *Scand. J. Gastroenterol.* **2012**, *47*, 927–936. [CrossRef] [PubMed]

31. Galli, G.; Esposito, G.; Lahner, E.; Pilozzi, E.; Corleto, V.D.; Di Giulio, E.; Aloe Spiriti, M.A.; Annibale, B. Histological recovery and gluten-free diet adherence: A prospective 1-year follow-up study of adult patients with coeliac disease. *Aliment. Pharmacol. Ther.* **2014**, *40*, 639–647. [CrossRef] [PubMed]

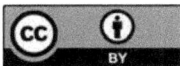

nutrients

MDPI

Article

Contact Dermatitis Due to Nickel Allergy in Patients Suffering from Non-Celiac Wheat Sensitivity

Alberto D'Alcamo [1], Pasquale Mansueto [1], Maurizio Soresi [1], Rosario Iacobucci [1], Francesco La Blasca [1], Girolamo Geraci [2], Francesca Cavataio [3], Francesca Fayer [1], Andrea Arini [4], Laura Di Stefano [1], Giuseppe Iacono [5], Liana Bosco [6] and Antonio Carroccio [1,*]

[1]   Dipartimento di Biologia e Medicina Interna e Specialistica (DiBiMIS), Internal Medicine Unit, University Hospital, Palermo 90100, Italy; adalcamo@hotmail.it (A.D.); pasquale.mansueto@unipa.it (P.M.); maurizio.soresi@unipa.it (M.S.); iacobuccirosario@gmail.com (R.I.); francescolablasca@gmail.com (F.L.B.); francesca.fayer@libero.it (F.F.); lauradist@virgilio.it (L.D.S.)
[2]   Surgery Department, University Hospital, Palermo 90100, Italy; girolamo.geraci@unipa.it
[3]   Pediatric Unit, "Giovanni Paolo II" Hospital, Sciacca (ASP Agrigento) 90100, Italy; francesca_cv@inwind.it
[4]   DiBiMIS, Gastroenterology Unit, University Hospital, Palermo 90100, Italy; a.arini@libero.it
[5]   Pediatric Gastroenterology Unit, "ARNAS Di Cristina" Hospital, Palermo 90100, Italy; stoai@inwind.it
[6]   Dipartimento di Scienze e Tecnologie Biologiche Chimiche e Farmaceutiche (Ste.Bi.CeF), University of Palermo, Palermo 90100, Italy; liana.bosco@unipa.it
*   Correspondence: acarroccio@hotmail.com; Tel.: +39-0925-962-492; Fax: +39-0925-84757

Received: 17 December 2016; Accepted: 23 January 2017; Published: 2 February 2017

Abstract: Background: Non-celiac wheat sensitivity (NCWS) is a new clinical entity in the world of gluten-related diseases. Nickel, the most frequent cause of contact allergy, can be found in wheat and results in systemic nickel allergy syndrome and mimics irritable bowel syndrome (IBS). Objective: To evaluate the frequency of contact dermatitis due to nickel allergy in NCWS patients diagnosed by a double-blind placebo-controlled (DBPC) challenge, and to identify the characteristics of NCWS patients with nickel allergy. Methods: We performed a prospective study of 60 patients (54 females, 6 males; mean age 34.1 ± 8.1 years) diagnosed with NCWS from December 2014 to November 2016; 80 age- and sex-matched subjects with functional gastrointestinal symptoms served as controls. Patients reporting contact dermatitis related to nickel-containing objects underwent nickel patch test (Clinicaltrials.gov registration number: NCT02750735). Results: Six out of sixty patients (10%) with NCWS suffered from contact dermatitis and nickel allergy and this frequency was statistically higher ($p = 0.04$) than observed in the control group (5%). The main clinical characteristic of NCWS patients with nickel allergy was a higher frequency of cutaneous symptoms after wheat ingestion compared to NCWS patients who did not suffer from nickel allergy ($p < 0.0001$). Conclusions: Contact dermatitis and nickel allergy are more frequent in NCWS patients than in subjects with functional gastrointestinal disorders; furthermore, these patients had a very high frequency of cutaneous manifestations after wheat ingestion. Nickel allergy should be evaluated in NCWS patients who have cutaneous manifestations after wheat ingestion.

Keywords: non-celiac wheat sensitivity; nickel allergy; cutaneous symptoms; irritable bowel syndrome

1. Introduction

In recent years a new clinical entity has emerged which includes patients who consider themselves to be suffering from problems caused by wheat and/or gluten ingestion, even though they do not have celiac disease (CD) or wheat allergy. This clinical condition has been named non-celiac gluten sensitivity (NCGS) [1–3], although in a recent article we suggested the term "non-celiac wheat sensitivity" (NCWS) [4], because to date it is not known what component of wheat actually causes the symptoms.

Other areas of doubt in NCWS regard its pathogenesis; while some papers have reported intestinal immunologic activation [5–9], others have linked NCWS to the dietary short–chain carbohydrate load (fermentable oligo-di-monosaccharides and polyols: FODMAPs) [10,11]. We recently demonstrated that a high percentage of patients with NCWS develop autoimmune disorders and are antinuclear antibody (ANA) positive, supporting an immunologic involvement in NCWS [12]. Furthermore, some papers have also reported a high frequency (22% to 35%) of coexistent atopic diseases in NCWS patients [13,14], and we suggested that a percentage of NCWS patients could actually suffer from non-immunoglobulin E (IgE)-mediated wheat allergy [15]. Nickel is the fourth most used metal and the most frequent cause of contact allergy in the industrialized world. As a natural element of the earth's crust, small amounts are found in water, soil, and foods, including wheat. Nickel allergy not only affects the skin but can also result in systemic manifestations. Systemic nickel allergy syndrome (SNAS) can have signs and symptoms that are cutaneous (urticaria/angioedema, flares, itching), and/or gastrointestinal (meteorism, colic, diarrhea) [16]. It has been reported that 15% of NCWS patients suffered from allergy to nickel [13], but that study did not further characterize this subgroup of patients, and the NCWS diagnosis was not reached by means of a double-blind placebo-controlled (DBPC) challenge as recommended [3]. The present study was designed to: (A) evaluate the frequency of contact dermatitis due to nickel allergy in NCWS patients diagnosed by a DBPC challenge; and (B) identify the clinical, serological, and histological characteristics of NCWS patients who were positive for nickel allergy compared to NCWS patients without nickel allergy.

2. Materials and Methods

2.1. Study Design and Population

We prospectively included adult patients with functional gastroenterological symptoms according to the Rome III criteria [17], and a definitive diagnosis of NCWS. The patients were recruited between December 2014 and November 2016 at three centres: (1) Department of Internal Medicine at the University Hospital in Palermo; (2) Department of Internal Medicine of the Hospital of Sciacca; (3) the Gastroenterology Units of the "ARNAS Di Cristina" Hospital in Palermo. These patients were randomly selected, by a computer generated method, among those who were cured by elimination diet with the exclusion of wheat and tested positive to the DBPC diagnostic wheat challenge. Sixty NCWS patients (54 females, 6 males; mean age 34.1 ± 8.1 years) were included in the study. Fifty-five patients had reported gastrointestinal symptoms that could be related to wheat ingestion; five others had showed fibromyalgia-like symptoms and/or anaemia, without gastrointestinal symptoms. The characteristics of the NCWS patients suffering from nickel allergy were compared to those of the NCWS patients who did not suffer from nickel allergy. A control group of 80 patients with functional gastroenterological symptoms was selected to compare the frequency of nickel allergy in NCWS and non-NCWS patients. These controls were randomly chosen by a computer-generated method from subjects diagnosed during the same period, age-matched (±2 years) and sex-matched (±5%) to the NCWS patients. The controls had undergone the same elimination diet as the NCWS patients and had not shown any clinical improvement.

2.2. Diagnostic Criteria

NCWS diagnosis. All subjects met the recently proposed criteria [1]: negative serum anti-tissue transglutaminase and anti-endomysium (EmA) IgA and IgG antibodies; absence of intestinal villous atrophy; IgE-mediated immunoallergy tests negative for wheat (skin prick tests and/or serum–specific IgE detection). Additional criteria for our patients were: resolution of the gastrointestinal symptoms on a standard elimination diet, without wheat, cow's milk, egg, tomato, chocolate, or other food(s) causing self-reported symptoms; as well as symptom reappearance on a DBPC wheat challenge, performed as described previously [9]. As in previous studies, a DBPC cow's milk protein challenge and other "open" food challenges were also performed (see Supplementary Materials for details about the elimination diet and the DBPC challenge method). Exclusion criteria were: age <18 years; positive EmA in the culture medium of the duodenal biopsies, even if the villi–to–crypts ratio in the duodenal mucosa was normal; self-exclusion of wheat from the diet and refusal to reintroduce it before entering the study; other organic cutaneous and/or gastrointestinal diseases; and concomitant treatment with steroids and/or antihistamines.

Contact dermatitis diagnosis. Allergic contact dermatitis was diagnosed by an independent physician who blindly reviewed the skin in all the subjects included in the study. The diagnosis was posed in patients with local eczematous lesions on the skin in close contact with nickel-containing objects. Suspected systemic nickel allergy syndrome (SNAS) was defined as a reaction characterized not only by diffused eczematous lesions (systemic contact dermatitis), but also by extracutaneous signs and symptoms, mainly gastrointestinal, after ingestion of nickel–rich foods (i.e., tomato, cocoa, beans, mushrooms, vegetables, wheat flour, etc.) [16]. In all cases, the diagnosis was confirmed by means of the epicutaneous patch test which provoked delayed lesions.

Associated autoimmune disease diagnosis. A structured and previously validated questionnaire [12] was used to diagnose autoimmune diseases.

Atopic disease diagnosis. As in previous studies, the following diseases were diagnosed according to standard criteria: rhinitis, conjunctivitis, bronchial asthma, and atopic dermatitis.

2.3. Laboratory Methods

Serology for CD, duodenal histology studies, and Human Leucocyte Antigens (HLA)-DQ typing were performed on all patients to exclude a CD diagnosis, as described previously (Supplementary Materials, [13,14]).

Nickel allergy. All of the NCWS patients reporting contact dermatitis related to nickel-containing objects were patch tested. Patch tests were performed in our laboratory, with the Italian Society of Allergological, Occupational and Environmental Dermatology (SIDAPA) standard series (Lofarma S.p.A., Milano, Italy), using a commercial method (Curatest® F, Lohmann & Rauscher; Neuwied, Germany); allergens were applied on the upper back and removed after 72 h. The sites were examined on removal and 24 h or 48 h after removal according to the recommended International Contact Dermatitis Research Group guidelines. Reactions were graded as: negative; macular erythema; weak reaction (non-vesicular erythema, infiltration or papules); strong reaction (edema or vesicles); extreme reaction (spreading, bullous and ulcerative lesions); or irritant. The treating physician determined the relevance of each positive result on the basis of the patient's history and known exposure. Weak, strong, and extreme reactions at the final reading were considered positive reactions.

Duodenal histology. Duodenal histology was classified according to Corazza and Villanacci [18].

Serum anti-nuclear antibodies (ANA). ANA were identified by Human epithelial type 2 (HEp-2) cells, using an indirect immunofluorescence technique; a titer of 1:40 or higher was considered positive and the sera were titered at progressive dilutions until they became negative.

2.4. Statistical Analysis

Data were expressed as mean ± Standard deviation (SD) when the distribution was Gaussian and differences were calculated using the Student t test. Otherwise, data were expressed as median and range and analyzed using the Mann-Whitney U test. Fisher's exact or the χ^2 tests were used where appropriate. $p < 0.05$ was considered significant. All analyses were performed using the SPSS software package (version 16.0, released 2007, SPSS Inc., Chicago, IL, USA). The study protocol conformed to the ethical guidelines of the Declaration of Helsinki, and was approved by our institution's human research committee (University Hospital of Palermo, identification code 4/2015), and registered at clinicaltrials.gov (registration number: NCT02750735).

3. Results

Table 1 shows the clinical characteristics of the patients, compared to the control group composed of patients with functional gastroenterological disorders who did not improve on the elimination wheat-free diet. In general, in NCWS patients there was a significantly higher percentage of self-reported wheat intolerance and coexisting atopic diseases than in IBS controls.

Table 1. Clinical characteristics of the NCWS patients compared to the control group composed of patients suffering from IBS who did not improve on elimination diet.

	NCWS Patients (*n* = 60)	IBS Controls (*n* = 80)	*p* Value
Sex	54 F, 6 M	72 F, 8 M	Not Applicable, matching factor
Age	34.1 ± 8.1 years	35.4 ± 9.0 years	Not Applicable, matching factor
Self-reported wheat intolerance	33 cases (55%)	20 cases (25%)	0.05
Family history of celiac disease	6 cases (10%)	2 cases (2.5%)	0.07
Coexistent atopic diseases	25 cases (42%)	7 cases (8.7%)	0.0001

Note: Family history of CD indicates a CD diagnosis in a first-degree relative. NCWS, non-celiac wheat sensitivity; IBS, irritable bowel syndrome; F, Female; M, Male; CD, celiac disease.

3.1. Frequency of Contact Dermatitis Due to Nickel Allergy

Six (10%) of the 60 NCWS patients reported contact dermatitis related to nickel-containing objects and all tested positive on nickel patch. In the control group contact dermatitis related to nickel-containing objects was observed in 4 out of 80 patients (5%), and nickel patch was positive in all. This different frequency was statistically significant ($p = 0.04$).

3.2. Clinical Characteristics of the NCWS Patients with Nickel Allergy

Table 2 summarizes the clinical characteristics of the NCWS patients with associated contact dermatitis and nickel allergy compared to NCWS patients who did not suffer from contact dermatitis and nickel allergy. Patients with NCWS and nickel allergy had a higher frequency of cutaneous symptoms, considered as a whole, after wheat ingestion, than NCWS patients who did not have associated nickel allergy (100% vs. 7%; $p < 0.0001$). In particular, cutaneous erythema after wheat ingestion was present in all NCWS patients suffering from nickel allergy, whereas widespread itching and urticaria were observed in 50% and 33% of them respectively. In the NCWS patients without nickel allergy, all of the above cutaneous symptoms were present in less than 10% of the cases. No other clinical characteristics were different in the two groups, including the frequency and kind of gastrointestinal symptoms, the associated atopic and autoimmune diseases, and multiple food hypersensitivity, which showed a trend to a higher frequency in NCWS patients with nickel allergy (83% vs. 46% in NCWS without nickel allergy; $p = 0.07$).

Table 2. Clinical characteristics of the NCWS patients with contact dermatitis due to nickel allergy (*n* = 6) compared to NCWS patients who did not suffer from contact dermatitis (*n* = 54).

	NCWS without Contact Dermatitis *n* = 54 (90%)	NCWS with Contact Dermatitis and Nickel Allergy *n* = 6 (10%)	*p* Value
Male Sex	5 (9.3%)	1 (16.6%)	not significant
Age (years) (x ± SD)	35.0 ± 8.1	33.8 ± 9.2	not significant
Symptom Duration (months; median and range)	70 (6–240)	66 (3–216)	not significant
Coexistent Atopic Diseases	20 (37%)	5 (83%)	0.07 ns
Coexistent Autoimmune Diseases	15 (28%)	2 (33%)	not significant
Abdominal Bloating	48 (89%)	6 (100%)	not significant
Abdominal Pain	45 (83%)	6 (100%)	not significant
Diarrhea	32 (59%)	4 (66%)	not significant
Constipation	11 (20%)	1 (17%)	not significant
Vomit	5 (9%)	1 (17%)	not significant

Table 2. Cont.

	NCWS without Contact Dermatitis n = 54 (90%)	NCWS with Contact Dermatitis and Nickel Allergy n = 6 (10%)	p Value
GERD-Like Symptoms	26 (48%)	3 (50%)	not significant
Extra-intestinal Symptoms	37 (68%)	5 (83%)	not significant
Cutaneous Symptoms after Wheat Ingestion	4 (7%)	6 (100%)	0.0001
Diffuse Itching	3 (5%)	3 (50%)	0.002
Cutaneous Erythema	4 (7%)	6 (100%)	0.0001
Urticaria	3 (5%)	2 (33%)	not significant
Multiple Food Hypersensitivity	25 (46%)	5 (83%)	not significant
Serum ANA Positivity	18 (33%)	2 (33%)	not significant
HLA DQ2 or DQ8 Positive	27 (50%)	3 (50%)	not significant
Increased Number of IEL in Duodenal Mucosa (Grade A Histology)	29 (54%)	3 (50%)	not significant

SD: standard deviation; ns: not significant; GERD: gastro-esophageal reflux disease; HLA: Human Leucocyte Antigens; IEL: intra-epithelial lymphocytes; ANA, anti-nuclear antibodies.

4. Discussion

NCWS is a relatively new clinical entity in the world of "gluten-related disease" [1,19,20], although its pathogenesis remains uncertain [20,21]. A role for FODMAP malabsorption as a determinant of the abdominal symptoms in NCWS patients has been advocated [10,11], and wheat is actually one of the foods richest in FODMAPs, but FODMAP intolerance cannot explain both the extra-intestinal symptoms and the increasing evidence of immunologic involvement in many NCWS patients [5,7–9,22,23].

The present study focused attention on the frequency of contact dermatitis and nickel allergy in NCWS and the clinical characteristics of the subjects who had this association. We found a 10% frequency of contact dermatitis and nickel allergy in NCWS, which is statistically higher than observed in the control group composed of IBS patients who did not suffer from NCWS (whose symptoms were not improved on the elimination diet, with the exclusion of wheat). This finding is consistent with our previous observation that one third of NCWS patients with an IBS-like clinical manifestation had associated atopic diseases [14], and the high prevalence of atopic diseases (42%) observed in the patients involved in the present study. Furthermore, an Italian multicentre study of about 500 patients found that more than 20% of suspected NCWS patients had an allergy to one or more inhalants (26% to mites), food, or metals [13].

Regarding the clinical characteristics of the patients with NCWS associated with nickel allergy, we found that they had a significantly higher frequency of cutaneous manifestations after wheat ingestion than NCWS patients who did not suffer from contact dermatitis and nickel allergy. In particular, cutaneous erythema was present in all of the patients. In contrast, cutaneous manifestations were present in only 7% of the NCWS patients not suffering from nickel allergy. On this basis it could be suggested that the patients with NCWS who have cutaneous symptoms after wheat ingestion should be investigated for suspected nickel allergy.

Some limits of our study must be mentioned. Our study design did not permit evaluation of the frequency of nickel allergy in NCWS as we performed the nickel patch only with the patients who reported contact dermatitis. Other NCWS patients could have suffered from nickel allergy without contact dermatitis signs. We studied patients who were referred to tertiary centres with experience in CD and NCWS, so this created a selection bias. Consequently, our results cannot be extended to the broad population of self-treated or diagnosed NCWS patients. The sample size of NCWS patients was relatively small and it must be remembered that the general prevalence of nickel allergy in western countries is high and similar to the prevalence reported in NCWS patients in our study [24].

Furthermore, we have not performed any study to evaluate the hypothesis that nickel allergy could contribute to the pathogenesis of NCWS. It has been demonstrated that some immunologic pathways involved in the nickel-induced mucositis and dermatitis, i.e., the inflammatory response via the activation of TLR4 and the infiltration of lymphocytes that secrete Interleukin (IL)-17 and Interferon-gamma (IFN)-γ [25,26], have also been supposed or demonstrated in NCWS [5,7–9,27].

The strength of our data are the patient selection based on a NCWS diagnosis made by using the DBPC challenge method, and the study design specifically constructed to reveal the presence of nickel allergy.

5. Conclusions

In conclusion, our study suggests that contact dermatitis due to nickel allergy is more frequent in NCWS patients than in subjects with functional gastrointestinal disorders. Furthermore, as these patients had a very high frequency of cutaneous manifestations after wheat ingestion, we suggest that NCWS patients who have cutaneous symptoms should be investigated for suspected nickel allergy.

Supplementary Materials: The following are available online at http://www.mdpi.com/2072-6643/9/2/103/s1.

Acknowledgments: We wish to thank Frank Adamo for revising the English text. Funding/Support: The study was supported by the Italian Foundation for Celiac Disease (FC) Grant for Project 013/2014.

Author Contributions: Antonio Carroccio had full access to all of the data in the study and takes responsibility for the integrity of the data and accuracy of the data analysis. Study concept and design: Antonio Carroccio, Pasquale Mansueto and Alberto D'Alcamo. Acquisition of data: Antonio Carroccio, Alberto D'Alcamo, Giuseppe Iacono, Francesca Cavataio, Laura Di Stefano, Rosario Iacobucci, Francesco La Blasca, Francesca Fayer, Liana Bosco and Pasquale Mansueto. Endoscopy study: Andrea Arini, Girolamo Geraci and Francesca Cavataio. Analysis and interpretation of data: Antonio Carroccio, Alberto D'Alcamo, Maurizio Soresi, Giuseppe Iacono and Pasquale Mansueto. Drafting of the manuscript: Antonio Carroccio and Pasquale Mansueto. Critical revision of the manuscript for important intellectual content: All authors. Statistical analysis: Maurizio Soresi.

Conflicts of Interest: The authors declare no conflict of interest.

Abbreviations

ANA: anti-nuclear antibodies; anti-tTG: anti-tissue transglutaminase; CD: celiac disease; DBPC: double-blind placebo-controlled; EmA: anti-endomysium antibodies; FODMAPs: fermentable oligo-di-monosaccharides and polyols; IBS: irritable bowel syndrome; NCGS: non-celiac gluten sensitivity; NCWS: non-celiac wheat sensitivity; SD: standard deviation; SNAS: systemic nickel allergy syndrome.

References

1. Sapone, A.; Bai, J.C.; Ciacci, C.; Dolinsek, J.; Green, P.H.; Hadjivassiliou, M.; Kaukinen, K.; Rostami, K.; Sanders, D.S.; Schumann, M.; et al. Spectrum of gluten related disorders: Consensus on new nomenclature and classification. *BMC Med.* **2012**, *10*, 13. [CrossRef] [PubMed]

2. Catassi, C.; Bai, J.C.; Bonaz, B.; Bouma, G.; Calabrò, A.; Carroccio, A.; Castillejo, G.; Ciacci, C.; Cristofori, F.; Dolinsek, J.; et al. Non-celiac gluten sensitivity: The new frontier of gluten related disorders. *Nutrients* **2013**, *5*, 3839–3853. [CrossRef] [PubMed]

3. Catassi, C.; Elli, L.; Bonaz, B.; Bouma, G.; Carroccio, A.; Castillejo, G.; Cellier, C.; Cristofori, F.; de Magistris, L.; Dolinsek, J.; et al. Diagnosis of Non-Celiac gluten sensitivity (NCGS): The Salerno Experts' Criteria. *Nutrients* **2015**, *7*, 4966–4977. [CrossRef] [PubMed]

4. Carroccio, A.; Rini, G.; Mansueto, P. Non-celiac wheat sensitivity is a more appropriate label than non-celiac gluten sensitivity. *Gastroenterology* **2014**, *146*, 320–321. [CrossRef] [PubMed]

5. Sapone, A.; Lammers, K.M.; Mazzarella, G.; Mikhailenko, I.; Cartenì, M.; Casolaro, V.; Fasano, A. Differential mucosal IL-17 expression in two gliadin-induced disorders: Gluten sensitivity and the autoimmune enteropathy celiac disease. *Int. Arch. Allergy Immunol.* **2010**, *152*, 75–80. [CrossRef] [PubMed]

6. Sapone, A.; Lammers, K.M.; Casolaro, V.; Cammarota, M.; Giuliano, M.T.; De Rosa, M.; Stefanile, R.; Mazzarella, G.; Tolone, C.; Russo, M.I.; et al. Divergence of gut permeability and mucosal immune gene expression in two gluten-associated conditions: Celiac disease and gluten sensitivity. *BMC Med.* **2011**, *9*, 23. [CrossRef] [PubMed]

7. Brottveit, M.; Beitnes, A.C.; Tollefsen, S.; Bratlie, J.E.; Jahnsen, F.L.; Johansen, F.E.; Sollid, L.M.; Lundin, K.E. Mucosal cytokine response after short-term gluten challenge in celiac disease and non-celiac gluten sensitivity. *Am. J. Gastroenterol.* **2013**, *108*, 842–850. [CrossRef] [PubMed]

8. Vazquez-Roque, M.I.; Camilleri, M.; Smyrk, T.; Murray, J.A.; Marietta, E.; O'Neill, J.; Carlson, P.; Lamsam, J.; Janzow, D.; Eckert, D.; et al. A controlled trial of gluten-free diet in patients with irritable bowel

syndrome-diarrhea: Effects on bowel frequency and intestinal function. *Gastroenterology* **2013**, *144*, 903–911. [CrossRef] [PubMed]

9. Di Liberto, D.; Mansueto, P.; D'Alcamo, A.; Pizzo, M.L.; Presti, E.L.; Geraci, G.; Fayer, F.; Guggino, G.; Iacono, G.; Dieli, F.; et al. Predominance of type 1 innate lymphoid cells in the rectal mucosa of patients with non-celiac wheat sensitivity: Reversal after a wheat-free diet. *Clin. Transl. Gastroenterol.* **2016**, *7*, e178. [CrossRef] [PubMed]

10. Biesiekierski, J.R.; Peters, S.L.; Newnham, E.D.; Rosella, O.; Muir, J.G.; Gibson, P.R. No effects of gluten in patients with self-reported non-celiac gluten sensitivity after dietary reduction of fermentable, poorly absorbed, short-chain carbohydrates. *Gastroenterology* **2013**, *145*, 320–328. [CrossRef] [PubMed]

11. De Giorgio, R.; Volta, U.; Gibson, P. Sensitivity to wheat, gluten and FODMAPs in IBS: Facts or fiction? *Gut* **2016**, *65*, 169–178. [CrossRef] [PubMed]

12. Carroccio, A.; D'Alcamo, A.; Cavataio, F.; Soresi, M.; Seidita, A.; Sciumè, C.; Geraci, G.; Iacono, G.; Mansueto, P. High proportions of people with Non-Celiac Wheat Sensitivity have autoimmune disease or anti-nuclear antibodies. *Gastroenterology* **2015**, *149*, 596–603. [CrossRef] [PubMed]

13. Volta, U.; Bardella, M.T.; Calabrò, A.; Troncone, R.; Corazza, G.R. An Italian prospective multicenter survey on patients suspected of having non-celiac gluten sensitivity. *BMC Med.* **2014**, *12*, 85. [CrossRef] [PubMed]

14. Carroccio, A.; Mansueto, P.; Iacono, G.; Soresi, M.; D'alcamo, A.; Cavataio, F.; Brusca, I.; Florena, A.M.; Ambrosiano, G.; Seidita, A.; et al. Non-celiac wheat sensitivity diagnosed by double-blind placebo-controlled challenge: Exploring a new clinical entity. *Am. J. Gastroenterol.* **2012**, *107*, 1898–1906. [CrossRef] [PubMed]

15. Carroccio, A.; Mansueto, P.; D'alcamo, A.; Iacono, G. Non-celiac wheat sensitivity as an allergic condition: Personal experience and narrative review. *Am. J. Gastroenterol.* **2013**, *108*, 1845–1851. [CrossRef] [PubMed]

16. Fabbro, S.K.; Zirwas, M.J. Systemic contact dermatitis to foods: Nickel, BOP, and more. *Curr. Allergy Asthma Rep.* **2014**, *14*, 463. [CrossRef] [PubMed]

17. Rome Foundation. Rome III Diagnostic Criteria. Available online: http://www.romecriteria.org/criteria (accessed on 26 September 2016).

18. Corazza, G.R.; Villanacci, V. Celiac disease. *J. Clin. Pathol.* **2005**, *58*, 573–574. [CrossRef] [PubMed]

19. Fasano, A.; Sapone, A.; Zevallos, V.; Schuppan, D. Non celiac gluten-sensitivity. *Gastroenterology* **2015**, *148*, 1195–1204. [CrossRef] [PubMed]

20. Aziz, I.; Hadjivassiliou, M.; Sanders, D.S. The spectrum of nonceliac gluten-sensitivity. *Nat. Rev. Gastroenterol. Hepatol.* **2015**, *12*, 516–526. [CrossRef] [PubMed]

21. Volta, U.; Caio, G.; Tovoli, F.; De Giorgio, R. Non-celiac gluten sensitivity: Questions still to be answered despite increasing awareness. *Cell. Mol. Immunol.* **2013**, *10*, 383–392. [CrossRef] [PubMed]

22. Hollon, J.; Puppa, E.L.; Greenwald, B.; Goldberg, E.; Guerrerio, A.; Fasano, A. Effect of gliadin on permeability of intestinal biopsy explants from celiac disease patients and patients with non-celiac gluten sensitivity. *Nutrients* **2015**, *7*, 1565–1576. [CrossRef] [PubMed]

23. Caio, G.; Volta, U.; Tovoli, F.; De Giorgio, R. Effect of gluten free diet on immune response to gliadin in patients with non-celiac gluten sensitivity. *BMC Gastroenterol.* **2014**, *14*, 26–32. [CrossRef] [PubMed]

24. Ricciardi, L.; Arena, A.; Arena, E.; Zambito, M.; Ingrassia, A.; Valenti, G.; Loschiavo, G.; D'Angelo, A.; Saitta, S. Systemic nickel allergy syndrome: Epidemiological data from four Italian allergy units. *Int. J. Immunopathol. Pharmacol.* **2014**, *27*, 131–136. [CrossRef] [PubMed]

25. Di Tola, M.; Marino, M.; Amodeo, R.; Tabacco, F.; Casale, R.; Portaro, L.; Borghini, R.; Cristaudo, A.; Manna, F.; Rossi, A.; et al. Immunological characterization of the allergic contact mucositis related to the ingestion of nickel-rich foods. *Immunobiology* **2014**, *219*, 522–530. [CrossRef] [PubMed]

26. Dyring-Andersen, B.; Skov, L.; Løvendorf, M.B.; Bzorek, M.; Søndergaard, K.; Lauritsen, J.P.; Dabelsteen, S.; Geisler, C.; Bonefeld, C.M. CD4(+) T cells producing interleukin (IL)-17, IL-22 and interferon-γ are major effector T cells in nickel allergy. *Contact Dermat.* **2013**, *68*, 339–347. [CrossRef] [PubMed]

27. Junker, Y.; Zeissig, S.; Kim, S.; Barisani, D.; Wieser, H.; Leffler, D.A.; Zevallos, V.; Libermann, T.A.; Dillon, S.; Freitag, T.L.; et al. Wheat amylase trypsin inhibitors drive intestinal inflammation via activation of toll-like receptor 4. *J. Exp. Med.* **2012**, *209*, 2395–2408. [CrossRef] [PubMed]

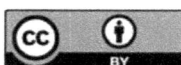

nutrients

MDPI

Article

Gluten Contamination in Naturally or Labeled Gluten-Free Products Marketed in Italy

Anil K. Verma [1,*], Simona Gatti [1,2], Tiziana Galeazzi [1], Chiara Monachesi [1], Lucia Padella [1], Giada Del Baldo [2], Roberta Annibali [2], Elena Lionetti [1,2] and Carlo Catassi [1,2]

[1] Celiac Disease Research Laboratory, Department of Pediatrics, Università Politecnica delle Marche, 60123 Ancona, Italy; simona.gatti@hotmail.it (S.G.); t.galeazzi@univpm.it (T.G.); chiara.monachesi28@gmail.com (C.M.); luciapadella@libero.it (L.P.); mariaelenalionetti@gmail.com (E.L.); c.catassi@univpm.it (C.C.)

[2] Department of Pediatrics, Università Politecnica delle Marche, 60123 Ancona, Italy; giadadelbaldo@gmail.com (G.D.B.); robertannibali@hotmail.it (R.A.)

*   Correspondence: anilkrvermaa@gmail.com or a.k.verma@pm.univpm.it; Tel.: +39-071-596-28-34; Fax: +39-071-36281

Received: 14 December 2016; Accepted: 3 February 2017; Published: 7 February 2017

Abstract: Background: A strict and lifelong gluten-free diet is the only treatment of celiac disease. Gluten contamination has been frequently reported in nominally gluten-free products. The aim of this study was to test the level of gluten contamination in gluten-free products currently available in the Italian market. Method: A total of 200 commercially available gluten-free products (including both naturally and certified gluten-free products) were randomly collected from different Italian supermarkets. The gluten content was determined by the R5 ELISA Kit approved by EU regulations. Results: Gluten level was lower than 10 part per million (ppm) in 173 products (86.5%), between 10 and 20 ppm in 9 (4.5%), and higher than 20 ppm in 18 (9%), respectively. In contaminated foodstuff (gluten > 20 ppm) the amount of gluten was almost exclusively in the range of a very low gluten content. Contaminated products most commonly belonged to oats-, buckwheat-, and lentils-based items. Certified and higher cost gluten-free products were less commonly contaminated by gluten. Conclusion: Gluten contamination in either naturally or labeled gluten-free products marketed in Italy is nowadays uncommon and usually mild on a quantitative basis. A program of systematic sampling of gluten-free food is needed to promptly disclose at-risk products.

Keywords: celiac disease; gluten-free products; naturally gluten-free; R5 ELISA; oats; buckwheat; lentils

1. Introduction

Celiac disease (CD) is an autoimmune condition characterized by permanent intolerance to dietary gluten, a protein complex found in wheat, rye and barley, occurring in genetically predisposed individuals [1]. The hallmarks of active CD are the presence of serum autoantibodies (e.g., IgA antitransglutaminase and antiendomysial antibodies) and a small intestinal enteropathy characterized, in typical cases, by villous atrophy, crypt hypertrophy and increased number of intraepithelial lymphocytes (IELs). Treatment of CD is based on the lifelong exclusion of gluten-containing food from the diet. The gluten-free diet (GFD) determines the gradual disappearance of symptoms and serum autoantibodies, and the normalization of the intestinal histological architecture [2].

Unfortunately, CD patients are highly sensitive to the toxic effect of gluten. It has been shown that the protracted ingestion of traces of gluten (10–50 mg on a daily basis) may damage the integrity of the small intestinal mucosa, an increased number of IELs being the first marker of mucosal deterioration [3]. By combining these toxicity data with the observed food intake, it has been calculated that gluten-free products with less than 20 mg/kg (or parts per millio*n* = ppm) of gluten contamination are safe over a wide range of daily consumption [4]. The 20 ppm threshold for gluten-free food has been endorsed by the Codex Alimentarius [5] and other agencies, e.g., the US Food and Drug Administration (FDA) and the European Food Safety Authority (EFSA) [6].

Despite the availability of a wide range of natural (by origin) and industrially-prepared gluten-free food, complete avoidance of gluten from the diet is difficult to maintain. Gluten is indeed a "pervasive" nutrient that may contaminate otherwise gluten-free items along the production chain, from the field to the milling, stockage and manufacture steps [7]. Furthermore wheat flour or purified gluten are largely added by the food industry to naturally gluten-free food, due to its technological properties, particularly the high visco-elasticity. Protracted intake of items contaminated with gluten traces may cause persistent intestinal damage and symptoms in treated CD patients [8].

The scarcity of published data on the possible gluten contamination of nominally gluten-free products is a matter of concern. This is the reason why we decided to undertake the current study, by measuring gluten in a large sample of gluten-free products that are currently on the market in Italy, using the only method (R5 ELISA) approved by the EU regulation. We present here the final results of these analyses on 200 commercially available gluten-free products.

2. Materials and Methods

2.1. Collection of Food Products

A sampling plan was developed to analyze gluten-free products, including substitutes of wheat-based food, and other starch-rich food, e.g., legumes, that are extensively used in day-to-day meal preparation by individuals following a gluten-free diet. Selected products included different brands of (a) gluten-free flour, pasta, snacks, cookies, muesli, breakfast cereals, bread, and pizza; (b) rice, oats, buckwheat, quinoa, amaranth, mixed cereals, lentils, and chickpeas. Between April and October 2016, a total of 200 commercially available food products of common use were purchased in randomly chosen supermarkets in Ancona, Italy.

Food products were carefully identified and categorized into two broad categories, i.e., naturally (by origin) gluten-free products (Group 1) and labeled "gluten-free" products (Group 2). Group 1 was further divided into 1a, reporting no information of gluten content (defined herein as "products with unknown gluten content"), and 1b, reporting "may contain traces of gluten" on the label. Group 2, i.e., certified gluten-free products, were categorized as 2a, including products fulfilling the EU regulation for gluten-free products (UE 828/2014) plus the quality certification released by the Italian Celiac Society (identified by the "Crossed Ear" symbol on the package) or 2b, including gluten-free products fulfilling the EU regulation for gluten-free products only (Figure 1).

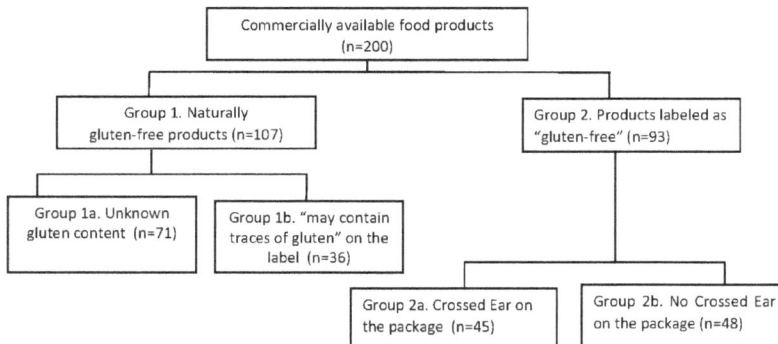

Figure 1. Types of food products analyzed in this study.

2.2. Determination of Gluten Content

All food products were subjected to gluten content determination by the Ridascreen Gliadin sandwich R5 enzyme-linked immunosorbent assay R-7001 (R-Biopharm, Darmstadt, Germany) at the Celiac Disease Research Laboratory of the Department of Pediatrics, Università Politecnica delle Marche, Ancona, Italy. During each run of ELISA, manufacturer's guidelines were strictly followed. Briefly, the steps of the ELISA procedure were as follows.

2.2.1. Extraction and Preparation of Samples

All samples were given a unique laboratory code and their details (including brand, cost, ingredient, food type, etc.) were recorded on an Excel sheet. Five grams of each sample were homogenized and crushed in a laboratory blender (solid food products). Each time after the crushing of a particular sample, parts of the blender were removed and washed with alkaline-enzyme detergent and rinse with 70% ethanol and dried before processing of another sample. Homogenized samples were stored in sterile tubes. Ridascreen R-7006 cocktail solution, containing detergents and reducing agent, was used for the extraction of samples. One-quarter gram of processed solid samples and 0.25 mL of liquid samples were measured in separate pre-labeled falcon tubes. In tannin and polyphenol containing products additionally 0.25 g of skimmed milk powder was added. After this preparation, 2.5 mL of cocktail solution was added in each tube under a chemical hood and tubes were vortexed and kept in water bath at 50 °C for 40 min. After the incubation, tubes were allowed to maintain room temperature and 7.5 mL of freshly prepared 80% ethanol was mixed in each tube and kept on a shaker for 1 h. Samples were then transferred into 1.5 mL of Eppendorf tubes and centrifuged at least 2500 g for 10 min, supernatant was separated and collected into another 1.5 mL Eppendorf tube and stored at room temperature. To avoid any possible cross contamination, samples were crushed in different rooms and at different time intervals.

2.2.2. Gluten Quantification

Extracted food samples were diluted at 1:12.5 in provided sample dilution, standard and samples were added in duplicate into pre-defined ELISA wells and enzyme conjugate was added to each well followed by wash of ELISA plate by washing buffer and kept for incubation for 30 min at room temperature. Substrate and chromogen were added and the reaction was stopped by provided stop solution and reading was obtained at the absorbance of 450 nm. Samples that showed an absorption value above the highest standard value were further diluted to get the absorption value within the range. The lower limit of the quantification was 2.5 ppm (mg/kg) of gliadin, corresponding to 5 ppm (mg/kg) of gluten. Results were calculated by the suggested method and then entered in the Excel sheet.

Food products containing gluten level lower than 20 ppm were considered as gluten-free while products with gluten level between 20 and 100 ppm were classified as products with low gluten contamination and products with more than 100 ppm of gluten were considered significantly contaminated. All products with a gluten level higher than 20 ppm were re-extracted and analyzed second time.

2.3. Quality Control

Each time absorption value of ELISA standards was assured with the quality assurance certificate provided with the ELISA kit. The result of each run was discussed with research group members and random results were sent to the principal company for expert comments and suggestion. At different time intervals, all the group members gathered and discussed the procedure and further action.

2.4. Cost Analysis: Correlation between the Cost of the Product and Gluten Contamination

If at least 5 products with similar ingredients from different brands were available, the mean price was calculated. Then, for each product the price index (PI) was calculated as the product price divided by the mean price of the category. The PI was then categorized in 3 groups (price categories): PI < 0.75 (products with a low price), PI: 0.75–1.25 (products with an average price), PI > 1.25 (products with a high price).

2.5. Statistics

Data are presented as proportions, means and S.D., medians and range, as appropriate. The Kruskal-Wallis one-way analysis of variance was used to determine if there was statistically significant difference of gluten contamination between the four groups of products (1a, 1b, 2a, and 2b), and, if significant, post hoc test was used for multiple comparisons. Comparison between proportions of contaminated (>20 ppm) and not contaminated (<20 ppm) samples within each group was calculated by the Fisher's test. Spearman's test was used to correlate quantitative variables (prices and gluten levels). Results were found significant when $p < 0.05$. The statistical analysis was performed using the Software Program Stata System (SPSS) v17.0 (Chicago, IL, USA).

3. Results

Detection of Gluten Contamination

Overall, 200 food products were analyzed: 107 in Group 1 (group 1a, $n = 71$; group 1b, $n = 36$) and 93 in Group B (group 2a, $n = 45$; group 2b, $n = 48$). Overall 173 (86.5%) products were detected with gluten level lower than 10 ppm, nine (4.5%) products contained between 10 and 20 ppm of gluten, and 18 (9%) products were detected with gluten level above the maximum tolerable of 20 ppm (15 products containing less and three products more than 100 ppm of gluten) (Table 1).

The proportion of contaminated products (gluten > 20 ppm) according to the staple ingredient and to the food category is reported in Tables 2 and 3, respectively. In products belonging to group 1, 16 items (8%) were contaminated with more than 20 ppm of gluten, 12 (6%) from sub-group 1a (gluten content unknown) and four (2%) products from sub-group 1b ("may contain gluten") products. In group 2 (products labeled as gluten free), only two (1%) products were found to have gluten level higher than 20 ppm. These products belonged to subgroup 2b, whereas no "Crossed-Ear" product was found to contain gluten at 20 or more ppm (Figure 2). Overall, we found a significant different proportion of contamination between the four groups of products (Kruskal-Wallis, $p < 0.01$). By multiple comparison, a significant higher proportion of contaminated products was found in group 1a as compared to group 2a (16% vs. 0, $p < 0.01$) (Table 2). No significant difference was found in the proportion of contaminated products between groups 1a and 1b and between groups 2a and 2b, respectively (Table 2, Figure 3). By comparing the staple ingredients, we found a significant higher proportion of contaminated products in oats, buckwheat and lentils as compared to chickpeas, corn, mixed seeds, quinoa, and chocolate. By comparing the food categories, the lunch/dinner products were significantly more contaminated as compared to snacks.

Overall 53 products belonging to six different food categories (lentils, chickpeas, beans, oats, buckwheat and quinoa) were considered for the cost analysis. The PI was not significantly correlated to the content of gluten ($r = -0.009$; $p = 0.51$). However, a significantly different distribution of price categories was found according to the level of gluten contamination. As shown in Figure 4, a higher proportion of low price foods were found in products with levels of gluten > 20 ppm ($p < 0.01$).

Table 1. Level of gluten contamination in the 200 examined products.

Gluten Content (ppm)	Number of Products	Median (Range) (ppm)	Mean ± SD (ppm)
<10	173	<5 (<0.5–9.3)	n.a.
10–20	9	13.9 (10.4–17.1)	14.1 ± 2.2
>20	18	31.7 (20.4–126.2)	49.2 ± 35.9

n.a. = not applicable (due to the (<5) values).

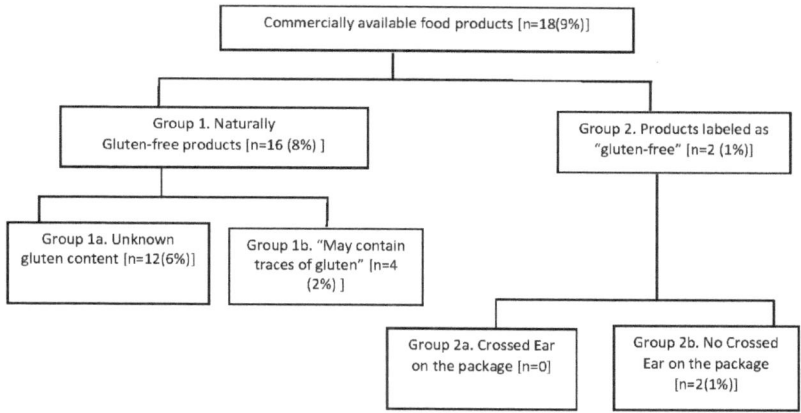

Figure 2. Number of food products containing gluten >20 ppm in different groups.

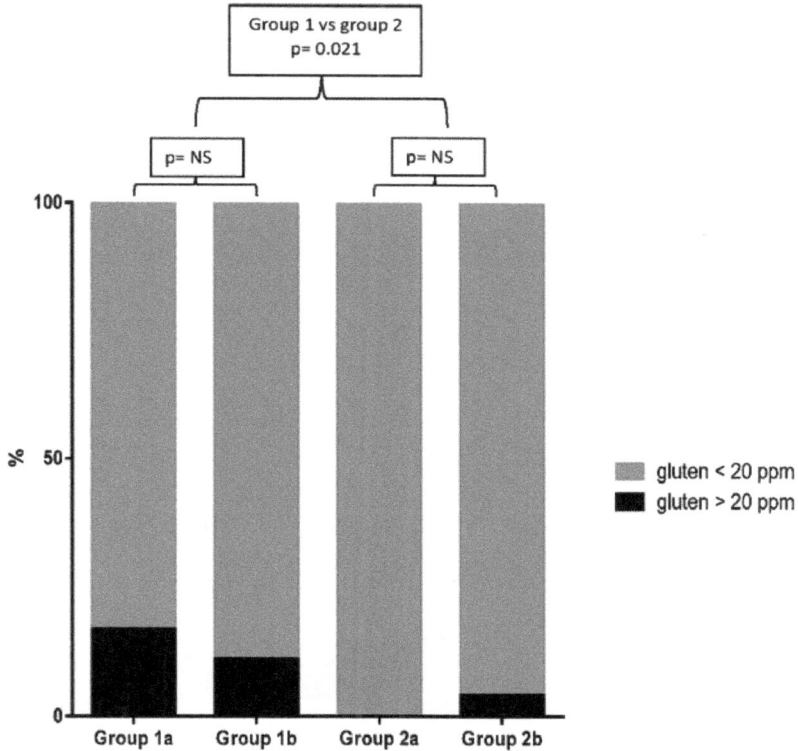

Figure 3. Percentage of contaminated products in each food group.

Table 2. Proportion of items containing >20 ppm of gluten by staple ingredient (contaminated/tested products).

Item	Overall *	Group 1 Naturally Gluten Free Products		Group 2 Products Labeled as "Gluten Free"		*p*	*p*
		Group 1a	Group 1b	Group 2a	Group 2b	Kruskal-Wallis	Multiple Comparisons
Amaranth	0/2	0/1	0/1	-	-	1.000	
Buckwheat	5/12	3/5	1/3	0/1	1/3	0.695	
Chickpeas	0/6	0/4	0/2	-	-	1.000	
Chocolate	0/9	0/1	0/3	-	0/5	1.000	
Coconut	1/3	1/2	-	-	0/1	0.480	
Corn	0/40	0/8	0/5	0/23	0/4	1.000	
Dry fruit	0/2	0/2	-	-	-	-	
Fruit Candy	0/4	0/1	-	-	0/3	1.000	
Fruit Jam	0/4	0/2	-	-	0/2	1.000	
Kidney Bean	0/7	0/5	0/2	-	-	1.000	
Lentil	4/17	2/6	2/11	-	-	0.495	
Mixed Cereal	1/25	0/2	0/2	0/10	1/11	0.736	
Mixed Seeds	0/12	0/8	0/1	0/1	0/2	1.000	
Oats	4/5	4/5	-	-	-	-	
Others	1/14	0/4	1/3	-	0/7	0.160	
Peanuts	1/4	1/4	-	-	-	-	
Quinoa	0/10	0/5	0/1	0/1	0/3	1.000	
Rice	1/24	1/6	0/2	0/9	0/7	0.392	
Total	18/200	12/71	4/36	0/45	2/48	0.010	1a vs. 2a *p* = 0.012

* Kruskal-Wallis *p* < 0.001; Multiple comparisons: *p* < 0.001: mixed seeds vs. oats, quinoa vs. oats, chocolate vs. oats, corn vs. oats; *p* = 0.001: chickpeas vs. oats; *p* = 0.002: corn vs. buckwheat.

Table 3. Proportion of items containing >20 ppm of gluten by food category (contaminated/tested products).

Food Category	Overall *	Group 1 Naturally Gluten Free Products		Group 2 Products Labeled as "Gluten Free"		*p*	*p*
		Group 1a	Group 1b	Group 2a	Group 2b	Kruskal-Wallis	Multiple Comparisons
Breakfast	0/11	0/4	0/1	0/4	0/2	1.000	
Lunch/dinner	15/88	10/45	4/25	0/12	1/6	0.348	
Snacks	2/95	2/22	0/10	0/28	0/35	0.082	
Bread	0/3	-	-	0/1	0/2	1.000	
Pizza	1/3	-	-	-	1/3	-	
Total	18/200	12/71	4/36	0/45	2/48	0.010	1a vs. 2a *p* = 0.012

* Kruskal-Wallis *p* = 0.004; Multiple comparisons: Lunch/dinner versus snacks: *p* = 0.006.

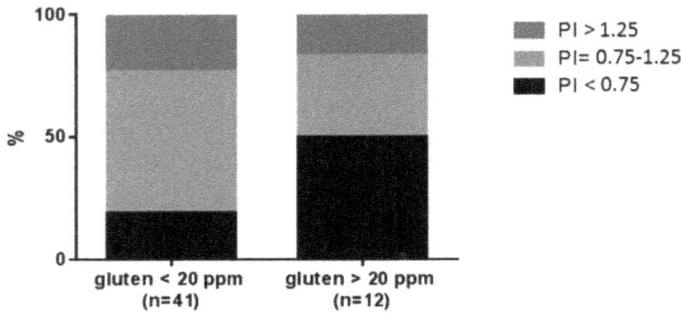

Figure 4. Distribution of price indexes (PIs) according to the level of gluten contamination.

4. Discussion

Our large survey shows that gluten contamination is low in gluten-free food marketed in Italy, both in terms of the percentage of contaminated products (9%), and the amount of gluten in contaminated products (almost exclusively in the range of the low gluten content 20–100 ppm). However, naturally (by origin) gluten-free products are at significantly higher risk of contamination as compared to products certified as gluten-free; indeed, we found that 16% of naturally gluten-free products with unknown gluten content are contaminated with respect to none of the certified gluten-free products with the crossed-ear symbol. Of note, among the certified gluten-free products without crossed-ear symbol we found that two out of 48 (4%) were contaminated with respect to none of the products with crossed-ear symbol; although this difference is not significant, it may suggest that the more stringent controls performed on "Crossed Ear" gluten-free products guarantee less risk of gluten contamination.

Our findings are more encouraging than previous studies in some American countries, e.g., contamination was found in 20.5% of gluten-free products marketed in the USA [7] and 21.5% in Brazil [9] respectively, and are in line with previous data from Canada [10] and Europe [4]. Compared to the past, the picture has clearly improved, most likely due to the worldwide implementation of the 20 ppm maximum threshold of gluten contamination established by the Codex Alimentarius in the year 2008 [5]. Based on these data and the dietary habits of the Italian population, the safety threshold of 10–50 mg of daily gluten would hardly be exceeded even by CD patients consuming very large quantities of gluten-free items (provided that no other contaminated food is eaten at the same time).

Quantification of gluten in food is difficult, for several reasons. Firstly gluten is not a single protein but a mix of different protein components (microheterogeneity) generally classified as gliadins, glutenins, globulins and albumins [11]. Measuring all these different fractions is clearly unpractical. Gliadins are the major component on a quantitative basis, and it is generally assumed that the ratio between gliadins (the fraction that is measured with the R5 test) and overall gluten is 1:2 (50%) [12,13]. Other analytical problems include the difficulty in (a) specifically quantifying all the different celiac-toxic peptides contained in gluten; (b) extracting gluten from the different food matrixes; and (c) measuring hydrolysed gluten peptides (e.g., in fermented food such as beer). Several tools have been developed for gluten quantification in food, such as the R5, the G12 and the α-20 antibody-based ELISA kits [14,15]. In the present study we used the R5 method, an ELISA test based on specially designed monoclonal antibodies raised against a pentapeptide from rye. It detects prolamins of wheat (gliadins), rye (secalins) and barley (hordeins), i.e., all the cereals that are toxic for celiac patients, in both raw (flours) and processed food products [16]. It is the only method certified by the Association of Officials Analytical Chemists (AOAC), and is considered as the method of choice for gluten detection in food, according to the Codex Alimentarius Commission and other International Agencies [5,6]. Most recent studies on gluten contamination have been performed using the same R5 test, a finding that allows comparisons among the results of different surveys [4,7,9,10,17].

As reported in previous studies [4,7,9,10,17], we found that products at significant higher risk of contamination of gluten are oats (four out of five examined items), buckwheat (5/12) and lentils-based (4/17) products. Several studies have shown that medium-high amounts of gluten-uncontaminated oats can be safely ingested by patients with CD [18,19]. Official recommendations acknowledge the safety of products containing purified oats, and several national associations for CD allow inclusion of oats in the diet of people with CD [19]. Unfortunately, the commercial oat supply is often contaminated with wheat. In Canada 88% of 133 oat samples were contaminated above 20 ppm [10]. There are possibilities for cross-contamination in the field, in the transport of the grain, in the storage of the grain, and in the milling and packaging facilities [7,10]. This is a deplorable situation since oats is rich in soluble dietary fiber, vitamins and minerals, and may unquestionably improve the nutritional value and increase the palatability of the GFD, while expanding food choices and ultimately improving the life quality of people with CD. Buckwheat is a gluten-free pseudocereal that belongs to the Polygonaceae family. Buckwheat grain is a highly nutritional food component that has been shown to provide a wide range of beneficial effects. Health benefits attributed to Buckwheat include plasma cholesterol level reduction, neuroprotection, anticancer, anti-inflammatory, antidiabetic effects, and improvement of hypertension. In addition, buckwheat has been reported to possess prebiotic and antioxidant activities [20]. The possible gluten contamination of buckwheat has been correlated with the high content of fiber [21]. The frequent gluten contamination of lentils was somewhat unexpected, since this food is a legume and not a cereal, and its production chain is far different from wheat. Lentils are an edible pulse that is part of the human diet since the Neolitic age, being one of the first crops domesticated in the Near East. Lentils are a rich source of numerous nutrients, including protein, starch, folate, thiamin, pantothenic acid, vitamin B6, phosphorus, iron and zinc [22]. The origin of gluten contamination of lentils remains unclear. Many patients or caregivers check lentils seed by seed, and have reported that rare wheat seeds can be found mixed with lentils, most likely due to contamination occurring in the field. The practice of inspecting and washing lentils before cooking should be recommended when the package does not report any gluten-free labeling.

It is important to underscore that oats, buckwheat and lentils are nutritious dietary components that may increase the variety of carbohydrate- and fiber-rich food in the gluten-free diet. For this reason, we hope that the food industry will pay more attention in ensuring and certifying a gluten-free food chain for these important ingredients.

Finally, in the present study we also aimed to evaluate if the gluten contamination is, to some extent, related to the cost of the product. It is worth noting that we found that a higher proportion of low price foods were contaminated with respect to higher price foods ($p < 0.01$), suggesting that the lower the price the lower the quality of control on the gluten contamination.

Despite the GFD, many treated CD patients frequently show incomplete resolution of the histological intestinal damage at the follow-up intestinal biopsy, suggesting ongoing gluten ingestion [8]. Since our data and other surveys [4] found that gluten contamination of wheat substitutes does not represent a big issue in recent years, this persistent enteropathy is probably related to different sources of contamination, such as voluntary dietary transgressions, particularly in adolescents, or contaminated meals consumed outside home. Consumption of food prepared away from home plays an increasingly large role in the diet. In the US in 1970, 25.9 percent of all food spending was on food away from home; by 2012, that share rose to its highest level of 43.1 percent (data of the US Department of Agriculture, 2016; www.ers.usda.gov). In restaurants, pizzerias and cafeterias the chance of getting gluten-contamined GF food is higher than home, due to inadequate personnel training, careless use of tools/workbench and so forth. An active policy of training and education on the requirements for the GFD should be addressed to employees at food services.

5. Conclusions

Gluten contamination in either naturally or commercial gluten-free products marketed in Italy is nowadays uncommon and usually mild on a quantitative basis. Crossed Ear and higher cost gluten-free products are in general safer than other products. Caution is however needed to interpret these findings, due to the intrinsic limitations of the analytical method for determining gluten traces in food matrixes. A program of systematic sampling of gluten-free food is needed to promptly disclose at-risk products, to ensure the safety of available products and ultimately improve the long-term wellbeing of individuals affected with CD or other gluten-related disorders.

Author Contributions: Anil K. Verma designed and performed the laboratory tests; Anil K. Verma, Simona Gatti, Giada Del Baldo; Tiziana Galeazzi and Roberta Annibali, acquired the data; Anil K. Verma and Carlo Catassi wrote and drafted the manuscript; Simona Gatti and Tiziana Galeazzi conceived and designed the experiments; Simona Gatti, Tiziana Galeazzi, Chiara Monachesi, Lucia Padella, Elena Lionetti and Carlo Catassi gave technical and material support; Tiziana Galeazzi supervised the laboratory experiments; Simona Gatti, Tiziana Galeazzi, Elena Lionetti and Carlo Catassi critically revised the manuscript; Elena Lionetti and Carlo Catassi analyzed and interpreted the data. Carlo Catassi designed the overall study concept and gave administrative and financial support and supervised the study. All authors revised and approved the final version.

Conflicts of Interest: Carlo Catassi has received consultancy funds from Schär. Other authors declare no conflict of interest.

References

1. Fasano, A.; Catassi, C. Current approaches to diagnosis and treatment of celiac disease: An evolving spectrum. *Gastroenterology* **2001**, *120*, 636–651. [CrossRef] [PubMed]
2. Lionetti, E.; Castellaneta, S.; Francavilla, R.; Pulvirenti, A.; Tonutti, E.; Amarri, S.; Barbato, M.; Barbera, C.; Barera, G.; Bellantoni, A.; et al. Introduction of gluten, HLA status, and the risk of celiac disease in children. *N. Engl. J. Med.* **2014**, *371*, 1295–1303. [CrossRef] [PubMed]
3. Catassi, C.; Fabiani, E.; Iacono, G.; D'Agate, C.; Francavilla, R.; Biagi, F.; Volta, U.; Accomando, S.; Picarelli, A.; De Vitis, I.; et al. A prospective, double-blind, placebo-controlled trial to establish a safe gluten threshold for patients with celiac disease. *Am. J. Clin. Nutr.* **2007**, *85*, 160–166. [PubMed]
4. Gibert, A.; Kruizinga, A.G.; Neuhold, S.; Houben, G.F.; Canela, M.A.; Fasano, A.; Catassi, C. Might gluten traces in wheat substitutes pose a risk in patients with celiac disease? A population-based probabilistic approach to risk estimation. *Am. J. Clin. Nutr.* **2013**, *97*, 109–116. [CrossRef] [PubMed]
5. Codex Alimentarius Commission. *Foods for Special Dietary Use for Persons Intolerant to Gluten Codex STAN 118-1979*; Codex Alimentarius Commission: Rome, Italy, 2008.
6. European Commission, COMMISSION REGULATION No 41/2009 of 20 January 2009 Concerning the Composition and Labelling of Foodstuffs Suitable for People Intolerant to Gluten. 2009. Available online: http://eur-lex.europa.eu/LexUriServ/LexUriServ.do?uri=OJ:L:2009:016:0003:0005:EN:PDF (accessed on 14 December 2015).
7. Lee, H.J.; Anderson, Z.; Ryu, D. Gluten contamination in foods labeled as "gluten free" in the United States. *J. Food Prot.* **2014**, *77*, 1830–1833. [CrossRef] [PubMed]
8. Lanzini, A.; Lanzarotto, F.; Villanacci, V.; Mora, A.; Bertolazzi, S.; Turini, D.; Carella, G.; Malagoli, A.; Ferrante, G.; Cesana, B.M.; et al. Complete recovery of intestinal mucosa occurs very rarely in adult coeliac patients despite adherence to gluten-free diet. *Aliment. Pharmacol. Ther.* **2009**, *15*, 1299–1308. [CrossRef] [PubMed]
9. Farage, P.; de Medeiros Nóbrega, Y.K.; Pratesi, R.; Gandolfi, L.; Assunção, P.; Zandonadi, R.P. Gluten contamination in gluten-free bakery products: A risk for coeliac disease patients. *Public Health Nutr.* **2016**, *15*, 1–4. [CrossRef] [PubMed]
10. Koerner, T.B.; Cléroux, C.; Poirier, C.; Cantin, I.; Alimkulov, A.; Elamparo, H. Gluten contamination in the Canadian commercial oat supply. *Food Addit. Contam. Part A Chem. Anal. Control Expo. Risk Assess.* **2011**, *28*, 705–710. [CrossRef] [PubMed]
11. Zilić, S.; Barać, M.; Pešić, M.; Dodig, D.; Ignjatović-Micić, D. Characterization of proteins from grain of different bread and durum wheat genotypes. *Int. J. Mol. Sci.* **2011**, *12*, 5878–5894.
12. Wieser, H.; Antes, S.; Seilmeier, W. Quantitative determination of gluten protein types in Wheat flour by reversed-phase high-performance liquid chromatography. *Cereal Chem.* **1998**, *75*, 644–650. [CrossRef]
13. Haas-Lauterbach, S.; Immer, U.; Richter, M.; Koehler, P. Gluten fragment detection with a competitive ELISA. *J. AOAC Int.* **2012**, *5*, 377–381. [CrossRef]
14. Halbmayr-Jech, E.; Hammer, E.; Fielder, R.; Coutts, J.; Rogers, A.; Cornish, M. Characterization of G12 sandwich ELISA, a next-generation immunoassay for gluten toxicity. *J. AOAC Int.* **2012**, *95*, 372–376. [CrossRef] [PubMed]
15. Mujico, J.R.; Dekking, L.; Kooy-Winkelaar, Y.; Verheijen, R.; van Wichen, P.; Streppel, L.; Sajic, N.; Drijfhout, J.W.; Koning, F. Validation of a new enzyme-linked immunosorbent assay to detect the triggering proteins and peptides for celiac disease: interlaboratory study. *J. AOAC Int.* **2012**, *95*, 206–215. [CrossRef] [PubMed]
16. Valdés, I.; García, E.; Llorente, M.; Méndez, E. Innovative approach to low-level gluten determination in foods using a novel sandwich enzyme-linked immunosorbent assay protocol. *Eur. J. Gastroenterol. Hepatol.* **2003**, *15*, 465–474. [CrossRef] [PubMed]
17. Koerner, T.B.; Cleroux, C.; Poirier, C.; Cantin, I.; La Vieille, S.; Hayward, S.; Dubois, S. Gluten contamination of naturally gluten-free flours and starches used by Canadians with celiac disease. *Food Addit. Contam. Part A Chem. Anal. Control Expo. Risk Assess.* **2013**, *30*, 2017–2021. [CrossRef] [PubMed]
18. La Vieille, S.; Pulido, O.M.; Abbott, M.; Koerner, T.B.; Godefroy, S. Celiac Disease and Gluten-Free Oats: A Canadian Position Based on a Literature Review. *Can. J. Gastroenterol. Hepatol.* **2016**, *2016*, 1870305. [CrossRef] [PubMed]

19. Gatti, S.; Caporelli, N.; Galeazzi, T.; Francavilla, R.; Barbato, M.; Roggero, P.; Malamisura, B.; Iacono, G.; Budelli, A.; Gesuita, R.; et al. Oats in the Diet of Children with Celiac Disease: Preliminary Results of a Double-Blind, Randomized, Placebo-Controlled Multicenter Italian Study. *Nutrients* **2013**, *5*, 4653–4664. [CrossRef] [PubMed]
20. Giménez-Bastida, J.A.; Zieliński, H. Buckwheat as a Functional Food and Its Effects on Health. *J. Agric. Food Chem.* **2015**, *63*, 7896–7913. [CrossRef] [PubMed]
21. La Vieille, S.L.; Dubois, S.; Hayward, S.; Koerner, T.B. Estimated Levels of Gluten Incidentally Present in a Canadian Gluten-Free Diet. *Nutrients* **2014**, *6*, 881–896. [CrossRef] [PubMed]
22. Mudryj, A.N.; Yu, N.; Aukema, H.M. Nutritional and health benefits of pulses. *Appl. Physiol. Nutr. Metab.* **2014**, *39*, 1197–1204. [CrossRef] [PubMed]

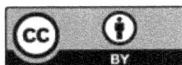

![nutrients](nutrients logo) MDPI

Review

Evolutionary Developments in Interpreting the Gluten-Induced Mucosal Celiac Lesion: An Archimedian Heuristic

Michael N. Marsh [1],* and Calvin J. Heal [2]

[1] Luton and Dunstable Hospitals University NHS Trust, and Wolfson College, University of Oxford, Linton Road, Oxford OX2 6UD, UK

[2] Centre for Biostatistics, Faculty of Biology, Academic Health Science Centre, University of Manchester, Manchester M13 9PL, UK; calvin.heal@manchester.ac.uk

* Correspondence: mikemarshmd@uwclub.net; Tel.: +44-1608-8100-29

Received: 19 December 2016; Accepted: 22 February 2017; Published: 28 February 2017

Abstract: The evolving history of the small intestinal biopsy and its interpretation—and misinterpretations—are described in this paper. Certain interpretative errors in the technical approaches to histological assessment are highlighted—even though we may never be rid of them. For example, mucosal "flattening" does not reduce individual villi to their cores, as still seems to be widely believed. Neither is the mucosa undergoing an atrophic process—since it can recover structurally. Rather, the intestinal mucosa manifests a vast hypertrophic response resulting in the formation of large plateaus formed from partially reduced villi and their amalgamation with the now increased height and width of the inter-villous ridges: this is associated with considerable increases in crypt volumes. Sections through mosaic plateaus gives an erroneous impression of the presence of stunted, flat-topped villi which continues to encourage both the continued use of irrelevant "atrophy" terminologies and a marked failure to perceive what random sections through mosaic plateaus actually look like. While reviewing the extensive 40+ year literature on mucosal analysis, we extracted data on intraepithelial lymphocytes (IEL) counts from 607 biopsies, and applied receiver-operating characteristic (ROC)-curve analysis. From that perspective, it appears that counting IEL/100 enterocyte nuclei in routine haematoxylin and eosin (H&E) sections provides the most useful discriminator of celiac mucosae at histological level, with an effective cut-off of 27 IEL, and offering a very high sensitivity with few false negatives. ROC-curve analysis also revealed the somewhat lesser accuracies of either $CD3^+$ or $\gamma\delta^+$ IEL counts. Current official guidelines seem to be somewhat inadequate in clearly defining the spectrum of gluten-induced mucosal pathologies and how they could be optimally interpreted, as well as in promoting the ideal manner for physicians and pathologists to interact in interpreting intestinal mucosae submitted for analysis. Future trends should incorporate 3-D printing and computerised modelling in order to exemplify the subtle micro-anatomical features associated with the crypt-villus interzone. The latter needs precise delineation with use of mRNA in-section assays for brush border enzymes such as alkaline phosphate and esterase. Other additional approaches are needed to facilitate recognition and interpretation of the features of this important inter-zone, such as wells, basins and hypertrophic alterations in the size of inter-villous ridges. The 3-D computerised models could considerably expand our understandings of the microvasculature and its changes—in relation both to crypt hypertrophy, in addition to the partial attrition and subsequent regrowth of villi from the inter-villous ridges during the flattening and recovery processes, respectively.

Keywords: computerised image-analysis; celiac mucosa; Marsh classification; ROC-curve analysis; IEL; lymphocyte immuno-subtypes; mesenteric immune system; invalid Marsh III a,b,c sub-classification

1. Introduction

It may be true that a "Copernican revolution" has seen earlier concepts of celiac disease—perceived as a unitary, gluten-induced disease of the gastro-intestinal tract—changed to one exhibiting multisystem involvements, as well as a growing spectrum now known as gluten-related disorders. These include true gluten sensitivity, gluten allergy, and the more recent "wheat gluten intolerance syndrome". Nevertheless, aspects of the changes wrought throughout the intestinal tract still remain a central issue for celiac disease diagnosis, as well as for those having a primary interest in the mechanisms bringing about those changes and their structural correlates.

Clinically, our current understandings of 'celiac disease' derive from the late 19th century, but as two conditions. Paediatricians used celiac disease following Samuel Gee [1] while adult physicians used 'idiopathic steatorrhea'. The advent of peroral biopsy techniques led to the realisation (1960–1970) that each constituted a single, lifelong condition [2,3]. These biopsy techniques closely followed Wood's instrument [4] for retrieving gastric mucosa from patients with achlorhydria. Although Margot Shiner in London pioneered one approach (1956), William H. Crosby's revolutionary capsule (1958), engineered by Heinz Kugler, enjoyed worldwide usage.

Here, already, we have seen many notable evolutionary advances—Dicke, Wood, Shiner, Crosby—and then Rubin. We therefore suggest that if this collection of papers has its referential foundations in Greek philosophical science, then we should also include Archimedes. That is because many "heureka" moments have been characterised, not as notional views concerning a more generalised pathogenesis, but as sequential moments of inspirational "breakthrough". These have served in exemplifying—and uniquely advancing—our understandings of each mucosal stage in celiac disease pathogenesis.

It is upon these specific, time-based advances that the evolutionary structuring in our interpretation of mucosal immune-pathology has progressively evolved, and on which this essay is based. At the same time, we note that this review will not deal with the complex issues surrounding enteropathy-associated T-cell lymphoma (EATL): that requires its own detailed account.

2. Early (Mis-) Interpretations of Intestinal Biopsies

Science never progresses by step-wise, logically perfect steps. Humankind always prefers comfort of the known against the threatening unknown. Paulley's operative specimens [5], although rejected in ignorance, were as good as later capsule biopsies. Likewise, Dicke's new findings about gluten protein in pathogenesis were robustly rejected because of Haas's "curative" banana diet; his assertions were later vindicated [6,7].

Shiner's tube gained scant interest, although in those early days when fresh intestinal tissue abnormalities were unknown and awaiting informed interpretation, her classification succeeded. This was (unfortunately) based on her view that mucosal flattening is an '*atrophic*' process, probably guided by Wood's description of true gastric atrophy in pernicious anaemia. Viewed histologically, however, each lesion resembles the other. A closer reading of Wood's studies would have further indicated that a gross misinterpretation was at stake here. The celiac lesion is not atrophic since on gluten restriction, villous regrowth occurs, as was first shown by Charlotte Anderson, thus becoming another diagnostic yardstick [8]. This misinterpretation persists after more than fifty decades.

Furthermore, more careful correlations between dissecting microscopy and histology would not have extended 'atrophy' nomenclature into 'partial', 'subtotal', and 'total villous atrophy'. These were histological misinterpretations of mosaic surface plateaus, resulting in reports of 'branched', or 'stunted', flat-topped 'villi' [9]. These were not villi, being far too short (<150 μm, compared with normal 350–600 μm). Again, this second misinterpretation persists today.

Two further novel approaches to mucosal structure came at this time. The first used wax reconstructions leading to the recognition of "basins" and "wells" [10]. Here several individual crypt tubes fed upwards into circular basins, which themselves coalesced into the larger wells ~200 μm in diameter and depth, accommodating up to 20 individual crypt openings. It is regrettable that more extensive use of wax models was not deployed in furthering knowledge.

The second approach employed autolysed specimens, thereby exposing the more robust sub-epithelial structures covered by basement membrane [11] including the delicate inter-villous ridges, as also revealed later [12] by scanning EM (see their Figures 1,2,9 and 10). During flattening, theseridges grow higher and thicker, engulfing shortened villi into the characteristic mosaic plateaus [13], whose surfaces lie ~150–200 μm *above* the crypt openings, and confirming histochemical studies [14], in particular of Padykula, who demonstrated the presence of normal (villous) enterocyte enzymes lining their vertical walls (Figure 1). That information is unknown today, and thus contributes little to histological analysis, or its understandings.

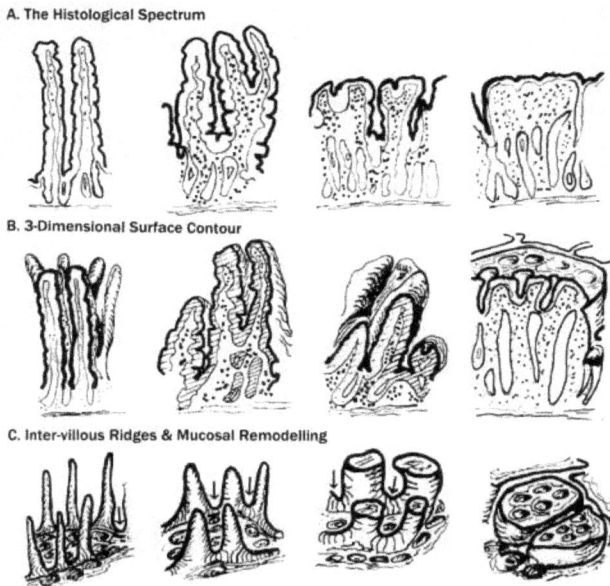

Figure 1. This overview represents intestinal mucosa through its remodelling process from "normal" to typically "flat" celiac appearances [15]. This is not merely an "atrophic" process, but one involving considerable hypertrophic remodelling of the entire mucosal profile. (**A**) The upper series of diagrams, crosswise, illustrate progression as commonly observed in histological section (Marsh Stages 0-III); (**B**) The second line of diagrams depicts the three-dimensional background to flattening, showing the rapid pliancy of villi in their reversion to leaves, ridges, convolutions and finally mosaic plateaus; (**C**) The third line of sketches illustrate *de-epithelialised* mucosae, emphasising the inter-villous ridges (arrowed). Normally, ridges are thin, delicate structures, but as remodelling proceeds, they undergo progressive increments in height and thickness, seemingly filling up the gaps between the now extensively reduced and deformed villi. This fusion results in mosaic plateaus which extend upwards by ~200 μm above the crypt-villus junctional zone (itself complicated by 'circumvillar basins' and crypt 'wells'). At this evolutionary (plateau) stage, it should be appreciated that if a random section passed through consecutive wells, the histologic appearances could well be misinterpreted as "blunted villi", as often happens in practice. Alternatively, if the sectioning ran between the wells, an entirely flat mucosa would be seen, illustrating one major difficulty inherent in histologic interpretation, especially of the mosaic "terrain". (Reprinted from Gastroenterology, 151(5), Marsh, Michael N. and Rostami, Kamran, What is a Normal Mucosa? pp. 784–788: Copyright 2016, with permission from Elsevier [15]).

3. The Immunological Functions of Intestinal Mucosa

Growing disinterest in the idea that celiac enterocytes lack a gluten-digesting "peptidase" (another failure here in recognising the non-specificity of brush border protein digestion) was supplanted by an immune-based pathogenesis. This was buttressed by definitions of the mesenteric immune system by Gowans and Knight who revealed the recirculatory properties of lymphocytes, particularly transference of thoracic duct 'blasts' to lamina propria in becoming plasma cells [16]. The latter sustain the local IgA system [17], including its mucosal product—secretory IgA. The functional capacity of this system [18], both throughout the small intestine and the colonic mucosa, was demonstrated [19] elegantly in mice orally primed with the antigen ferritin, an observation ultimately prompting our work in Manchester on rectal gluten challenge [20] and employing logistic regression analysis by Professor Ensari [21].

It is important to know that luminal antigen primes naïve lymphocytes in Peyer's Patches and other primary lymphoid tissues within the intestine to emigrate and recirculate to other mucosal surfaces [22]. This is an important defence against enteric infections, and of protective relevance [23] to lactating humans and animals. Activated recirculating lymphocytes, detected in blood following specific enteric infection in humans, interact with the special $\beta 7$–MAdCAM-1 receptor exhibited by lamina propria post-capillary venules [24]. More interesting has been the recent demonstration of blood-borne CD4$^+$ gluten-induced T lymphocytes responsive to DQ2-peptide complexes following an oral gluten loading [25,26], again exemplary of the recirculatory potential of mesenteric immune cells reacting to an environmental (dietary) antigen. This has the potential for precise celiac disease diagnosis, and is consistent with the increased numbers of anti-gluten IgA-secreting plasma cells within the mucosa, albeit based on the suspect use [27] of comparative high power fields.

The growing impetus towards diagnostic 'measurement' of intestinal biopsies was now based [28] on counts of intra-epithelial lymphocytes (IEL) per 100 villous epithelial cell nuclei. This technique is still the cornerstone of histological diagnosis today, despite its inherent flaw in relating one variable to another variable. "Normal" ranges or diagnostic "cut-off" levels for IEL [28–36] (Table 1) range between 20 and 40 IEL, indicating uncertainties over the actual interface. When collated, their fragility becomes strikingly apparent—due to small groups, ill-defined "controls", interest in other enteropathies (HIV infection), or distribution of IEL at villous tips. Overall, our notions of "the normal range" are distinctly precarious, while the marked overlap between diseasecontrols and celiac patients has never been clarified with additional statistical analyses.

Table 1. Summary of papers on intraepithelial lymphocytes (IEL) counts.

Paper	Methods	Number of Biopsies	Upper Range	Comments
Ferguson and Murray, 1971 [28]	H&E staining IEL/100 enterocytes 7 μm sections	40	40	Used controls, celiac and autoimmune conditions. Incorrect about normally distributed IEL. Highest IEL count recorded, of 155
Batman et al., 1989 [29]	H&E staining 5 μm sections	8	33	Study of HIV enteropathy
Hayat et al., 2002 [30]	H&E staining 4 μm sections	20	25	Counts made on uninterrupted length of epithelium >500 epithelial cells: Controls defined only by a "normal" sugar permeability
Mahadeva et al., 2002 [31]	H&E staining 3 μm sections	??	22	Major interest in normal villi with IEL infiltrate Really difficult to infer group numbers here
Kakar et al., 2003 [32]	H&E staining	12	39	Interest in normal villi with IEL infiltrates

Table 1. *Cont.*

Paper	Methods	Number of Biopsies	Upper Range	Comments
Veress et al., 2004 [33]	H&E staining CD3+ counts	64	20 5–9	3 μm H&E sections: If IEL to EC ratio >5:1, do CD3 count
Biagi et al., 2004 [34]	H&E staining	17	45	Major interest in villous tip counts
Nasseri-Moghaddam et al., 2008 [35]	H&E staining CD45+ counts	46	46 47	Establishing normal criteria by histology and immuno-cytology
Siriweera et al., 2015 [36]	H&E staining	75	8	Retrospective study on 38 control specimens and 37 celiacs. Inexplicably small upper ranges for both groups

4. Re-Evaluating Intraepithelial Lymphocyte (IEL) Counts Derived from the Existing Literature

In order to highlight this impasse, we have reworked and extended previously published data culled from a vast literature (from single case reports to smaller group studies over a 40-year period, as reviewed in this paper) in order to address this issue. In total, data relating to 607 biopsies (386 celiacs) were available for re-evaluation thus providing an important, yet hitherto unknown, extension to the existing literature.

(a) It is crucial that the considerable overlap between counts of IEL obtained either histologically, or estimated through their immunophenotypes (Figure 2), is acknowledged. From this, two important conclusions follow: (i) that immuno-subtyping IEL does not offer much in the way of improving diagnostic accuracy—again because of massive overlapping; and (ii) that a "normal" IEL count [15] does not exist.

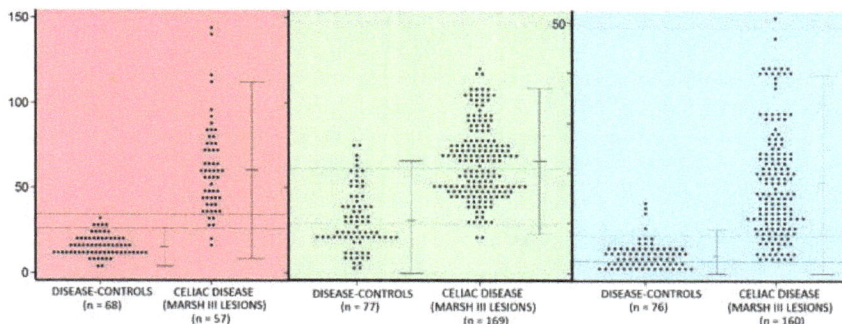

Figure 2. A cumulative assembly of sporadically published reports provided 607 biopsies (386 celiacs), illustrating the numerical distributions of IEL in hematoxylin and eosin (H&E) sections (red), CD3+ (green), and $\gamma\delta^+$ (blue) immuno-subtypes,with their accompanying disease-control groups.(**a**) For IEL (H and E) the mean (±95% Confidence Limits) was 15 (4–26) for controls and 60 (9–111) for celiacs; (**b**) The results for CD3+ cells were 31 (0–66) for disease controls, and 66 (23–109) for celiacs; (**c**) For $\gamma\delta^+$ cells, the mean was 23 (0–39) in the celiac group compared with 4 (0–9) for the controls. Marked overlaps between disease controls and celiac patients (indicated by the paired horizontal lines) occurred with all IEL counts: 43 for histological (H&E) counts, 110 for CD3+ counts, and 69 for $\gamma\delta^+$ cells, respectively.

Each set of counts was not normally distributed. But the 'normalised' means after log-transformation differed from the numerical means by only ~5 lymphocytes, indicating that for most practical purposes, IEL counts do not require this treatment.

(b) If these data from each type of measurement (histologically, or by CD3⁺ and γδ⁺ immunophenotyping) are graphically depicted, using a cumulative, biopsy-on-biopsy approach, they all exhibit a continuous, rather than a bi-modal, dose-response (Figure 3). In other words, both control and celiac IEL follow a continuous form of response to gluten ingestion, depending on intrinsic and extrinsic factors: they do not behave as separate clonal populations.

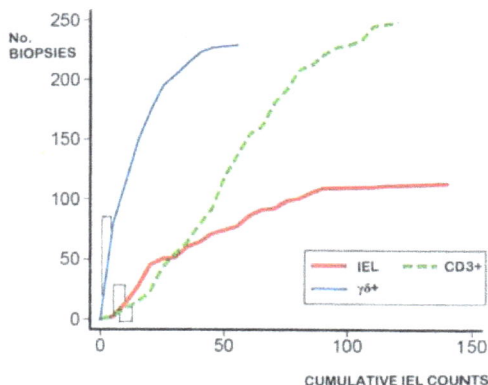

Figure 3. Cumulative IEL counts biopsy-on-biopsy, for histologically counted IEL (red), and immunostained CD3⁺ (green), and γδ⁺ (blue) cells. The cumulative overlap between disease control and celiac biopsies is indicated by paired, vertical lines for each of the three data strands.

Each graph is reminiscent of a dose-response, consistent with the view that changes in the IEL population, by whichever technique identified, represent graded responses to environmental antigenic challenge. Thus, they do not reveal bimodal behaviour in demonstrating differences between IEL in 'control' mucosae, compared with 'celiac' mucosae. This explains why there is an overlap and hence no specific, diagnostic cut-off for any of the lymphocyte populations illustrated.

(c) A notional cut-off with optimal sensitivities and specificities requires calculation (Figure 4). From the data given here (Table 2), ROC-curve analysis suggests an optimal cut-off level of 27 IEL per 100 enterocytes in H&E sections, a level incurring three false-negatives and five false-positives. The results for CD3⁺ and γδ⁺ cells were, within this analysis, apparently less accurate, as shown comparatively in Table 2.

If there is any comfort in these results, then counting IEL in histological sections is a very useful method for differentiating control from celiac biopsies (Table 2). The difficulty arises more with mis-diagnosed (false-positive) disease controls, because other diagnostic parameters may not be available to explain a raised IEL count.

This is diagnostically important on grounds that while repeat biopsies are often performed on celiac patients during gluten restriction, they are rarely done with disease controls. Therefore, we must be ever watchful that so-called "normal ranges" may not be a secure as some papers might suggest. This issue is critically well illustrated by one of Ferguson and Murray's (1971) patients with "abdominal pains". Her initial biopsy was "flat", yielding one of the highest recorded IEL counts of 155. One year later, however, on repeat biopsy, the IEL count was then 26. The actual diagnosis and the causal reason(s) for this marked difference were never explained [28].

Conversely, if a celiac (nowadays) is histologically misdiagnosed (false-negative below arbitrary cut-off), other parameters (family history; DQ 2/8 haplotyping; EMA and AGA antibodies, etc.) strengthen the physician's arm.

Table 2. Summary of ROC-curve Analyses.

Lymphocyte Subtype	H&E Stained	CD3$^+$	$\gamma\delta^+$
AUC	0.985	0.891	0.943
OPTIMALCUT-OFF	27	40	6
FALSE-POSITIVE	5	21	10
FALSE-NEGATIVE	3	11	15

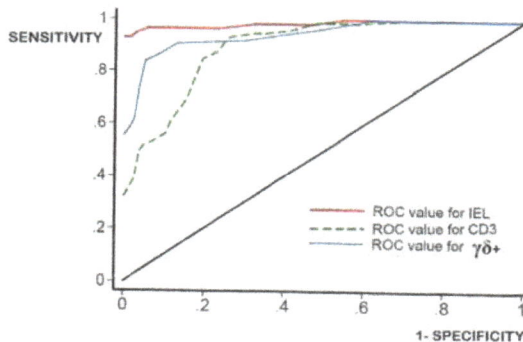

Figure 4. Receiver-operating characteristic (ROC)-curve analysis shows that IEL (H&E) counts per 100 enterocytes (red) are the most accurate procedure, compared with either CD3$^+$(green-), or $\gamma\delta^+$ (blue-) immunostained IEL. This analysis produced a cut-off of 27 IEL, with three false-negatives and six false positives. Intra-observer IEL count differences would be required to establish the degree of variation around any cut-off proposed. That important variation is often forgotten (especially if the counting has only been done by one histopathologist) and therefore rarely factored into any 'norms' offered. See Table 2 for further data analysis relevant to each of the three modes of IEL identified. Note, however, that the use of ROC-curve analysis considerably reduces the overlap between control and celiac biopsies (compare raw numerical distributions, Figure 2).

5. Objective (Computerised) Measurements of Intestinal Mucosa

One approach by Whitehead [37] used a point-counting grid producing ratios and 'absolute' values: however, the observer decides on which bit of mucosa the ends of the grid-lines fall, needing some degree of concentration. In Manchester, we used a test square of muscularis mucosae of 100 μm length (10^4 μm^2) providing an invariant reference over which we 'rebuilt' the mucosa in terms of villous, crypt and lamina propria volumes (as μm^3 per 10^4 μm^2 of muscularis): 'absolute' cell counts within each space were determined independently [38], based on Weibel's approach.

This method is similar to currently employed techniques using an external scanner which takes millions of observations from an external, independent vantage point, thus creating, say, the three-dimensional structure of a jet engine or hydraulic pump, or the interior of a stately home. It is regrettable that the field of mucosal morphology has, so far, not taken advantage of such powerful computerised programmes in order to reconstruct the 3-D micro-world of the mucosa and its internal structures, especially the microvasculature. Such application to specimens undergoing regrowth during a gluten-free diet would add enormously to our understanding of the regenerative processes involved. Pseudo-colouring could also be employed to highlight structures or areas of specific interest. Our cumulative results (Figure 5) probably represent the largest assembly of data unaffected by relative measurements. When set out in this way, the data afford a panoramic view of the major structural changes taking place across the mucosa as it progressively undergoes its hypertrophic response in remodelling its surface contour.

Some weak criticisms were raised that since the muscularis itself is caught up in the 'mucosal celiac process', it is invalid. But that is nonsense. Two objections arise—first, if it were thickened, which is irrelevant since we are only interested in area, and second, if it were "stretched". We excluded the latter [39] by demonstrating identical inter-crypt distances in horizontally sectioned control and celiac biopsies.

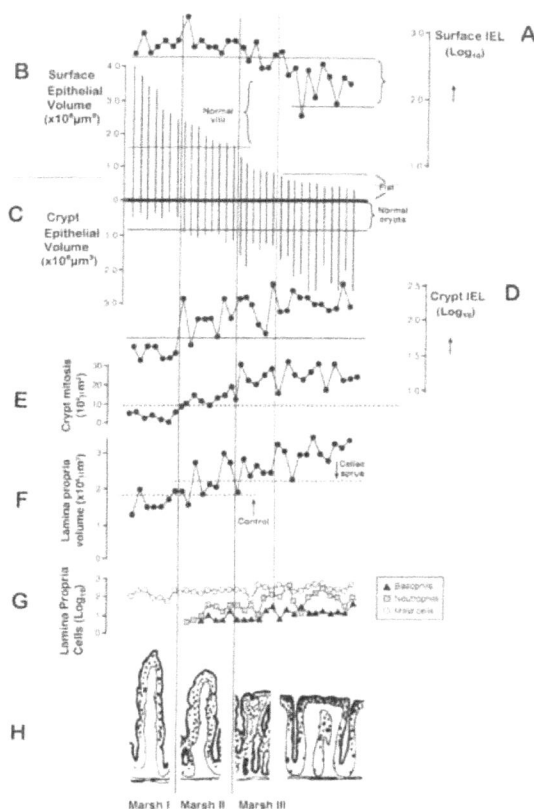

Figure 5. This represents mucosal metamorphosis from "normal" to "flat", based on computerised image analysis relevant to an invariant square (10^4 μm^2) of muscularis mucosae. Here, a comprehensive overview provides a clear picture of the progressive morphometric/immunopathologic alterations observed and hardly possible by viewing a vast collection of micrographs illustrating the same changes. (**A**) This line shows the progressive reduction in absolute surface epithelial IEL populations ($\log_{10}$ transformed). With Marsh Stage III lesions, the IEL count falls *within the normal range*; (**B**) Here, volumes of surface epithelium ($\times 10^6$ μm^3) are shown as vertical lines, in order of flattening; (**C**) This line reveals the progressive increase in crypt epithelial volumes, which are doubled (Marsh Stage II lesions), and quadrupled (Marsh Stage III); (**D**) Changes in crypt IEL populations ($\log_{10}$) are rarely demonstrated or measured. Here we show that their number begins to change at the Marsh II Stage, progressively increasing thereafter; (**E**) Parallel with the crypt IEL rises, there is a brisk increase in crypt cell mitotic activity, which is well established at Marsh Stage II; (**F**) The lamina propria begins to increase in volume ($\times 10^6$ μm^3) at Stage II, indicative of marked inflammatory changes initiated within, and involving its structures; (**G**) As the lamina swells, an influx of inflammatory cells occurs (all as $\log_{10}$ counts), including basophils, mucosal mast cells, and a notably brisk rise in neutrophils; (**H**) All data are related to specific stages (Marsh I, II and III). The Marsh II lesion (despite being considered either "non-specific" or difficult to identify) enjoys a strikingly prominent role, since marked changes are already operative at this pivotal point in the sequence, indicating that the entire mucosa seems to be "active" once this stage is reached. These composite relationships have never been demonstrated in other histological studies of celiac mucosae.

6. Classification of Mucosal Remodelling: A Major Hypertrophic Process

In overcoming these technical problems especially in circumventing inappropriate "atrophy" terminology, a novel classification [40] based on recognisable, immunopathologically phased stages (Marsh 0–III) during mucosal remodelling was proposed. Incidentally, the paper was also the first major systematic review of celiac disease, intended to divert its scientific basis away from 1950s-era thinking towards the molecular era of the 21st century. Thus, in addition to the mucosal Stage Classification, it considered possible HLA polymorphisms, relevant gliadin epitopes, and suggested a radical overhaul of lymphoma classification and treatment.

The development [40] of this classification was gradual and hesitant, depending on several contributory elements [41]: it was not an Archimedian"heuristic" of intense inspiration.

First came the realisation from many sporadic case reports [42–48] that the celiac mucosa evolves (a) over time, (b) at different rates, (c) with differing functional (clinical) outcomes, thereby (d) providing the obvious realisation that a flat mucosa is not a "given", as was assumed from the beginning when biopsies were first observed. Histologically, the biopsies obtained in these sporadic cases were often regarded as "normal"—although some subtle changes may have been present, once the structural progression had been clarified [49].

Second, time/dose response studies on treated patients [50] showed a progression of villous infiltration, modest crypt hypertrophy, followed by flattening and finally massive increases in crypt depth. The Marsh Stage II lesion (villous infiltration with a doubling of crypt size) was seemingly identical to that described by Mowat and Ferguson [51] as a mucosal T-cell dependent phenomenon.

Third, came the realisation that many family relatives of known celiac patients exhibit lymphocyte-infiltrated villi with or without modest crypt hypertrophy. This observation came as we repeated the original intestinal 'permeability' study [52] by Tim Peters's group in London (dealing then only with celiac patients with a flat lesion). In the repeat study [53], only celiac relatives who did *not* have gross lesional pathology were included. The realisation, for the first time, that identifiable minor changes occurred widely was, indeed, a "heureka" moment. It was very evident that lymphocytic infiltration of normal-looking villi was a frequently unrecognised but critical abnormality (except perhaps in some of the individual case reports mentioned above). But these further observations confirmed the reality of the classification, operative now for 25 years, which incorporates the major phases in the immunohistological progression to a flat lesion (Figure 5).

Based on that classification, we are now in a position to evaluate the structural remodelling of the mucosa.

6.1. The Surface Epithelium

We use Figure 5 for guidance. The top line, A, in this diagram represents the IEL population, expressed logarithmically (with absolute counts) and its progressive reduction towards the control range with mucosal flattening. In comparison, the progressive reductions in villous surface volumes are expressed as vertical lines along the second horizontal strand (B). The mean volume for an infiltrated mucosa is 2.6 (1.5–3.6) $\times$ 10^6 μm^3, compared with 0.4 (0.2–0.6) $\times$ 10^6 μm^3 for flat lesions: that is, a five-sixths volume reduction.

But these data can be interrogated further, in respect of IEL populations, because we also measured [54] individual cell volumes. These allowed us to calculate the number of enterocytes within each specified volume of epithelium, from which absolute ratios of IEL per 100 enterocytes could be determined, as follows.

Average cell volumes were 780 μm^3 (~800) for control enterocytes compared with 600 μm^3 for flat mucosae, although we do not know why Stage III enterocytes suffer 25% volume reductions. From those measurements, the absolute population of enterocytes in surface epithelium is ~3000 compared with 600 enterocytes for flat specimens. Flattening thus incurs a ~80% loss of surface enterocytes. Therefore, using data (line A, Figure 5), celiac disease specimens contain 190 (150–240) IEL, representing a less marked reduction of ~50% compared with enterocyte losses (Table 3). That is why, relatively, a flat mucosa *appears* to be infiltrated by lymphocytes: in fact, that is clearly not the case.

Table 3. Numerical values for intestinal mucosa (computerisedimage analysis).

	Disease Controls	**Celiac Disease**
Surface Epithelium		
Volume ($\times 10^6$ μm^3)	2.3 (1.5–3.6)	0.4 (0.2–0.6)
Cell Height (μm)	37 (30–43)	33 (27–33)
Cell Width (μm)	5.1 (4.1–6.2)	4.7 (3.8–5.8)
Cell Volume (μm^3)	800 (500–1250)	600 (390–920)
No. Enterocytes/Volume	3000 (1935–4435)	600 (320–1100)
No. IEL/Volume	350 (275–450)	190 (150–240)
IEL/100 enterocytes		
('Absolute' by Image Analysis)	12 (10–16)	32 (27–37)
(Ferguson, per 100 cells)	24 (11–53)	61 (31–122)
Enterocytes per Lymphocyte	8 (7–11)	3 (2–4)
CRYPTS		
Volume ($\times 10^6$ μm^3)	0.5–0.6	1.7
IEL ('Absolute'/volume)	30 (12–48)	173 (121–225)
LAMINA PROPRIA		
Volume (10^6 μm^3)	1.4 (1.12–1.6)	3.1 (2.8–3.5)
Cells/Volume		
('Absolute')		
Mast Cells	14 (10–20)	38 (22–54)
Eosinophils	18 (16–20)	62 (50–74)
Basophils		0.7 (0.48–1.12)
Neutrophils		45 (25–65)

Second, use of 'absolute' data permits determining ratios of IEL per 100 enterocytes (Figure 3). For diseasecontrols the values were 12 (10–16), and 32 (27–37) for flat lesions. However, when the same specimens were counted according to Ferguson (using 1 μm toluidine blue-stained Epon sections viewed under oil immersion optics), the values were *doubled* over the absolute counts: 24 (11–53) for disease controls, and 61 (31–122) for celiacs.

This difference is greatly significant, and rests on the failure of the Ferguson technique to identify every epithelial cell thought to have been counted. The deficit results from the fact that only enterocyte nuclei are counted [55] and not individual epithelial cells, which cannot be sequentially identified during counting. The difference between nuclei counted (rather than individual enterocytes) is of the order of a 50% reduction, resulting in the spuriously doubled IEL count. The inherent problems are illustrated (Figure 6). The basic problem is the attempted matching of one moving variable against another: a no-win situation.

The alternative (right-hand panel) is closer to reality, comprising an idealised epithelium scaled to data obtained by transmission/scanning EM studies. The lines in the upper (plan) diagram reflect random sectioning planes through this epithelium. It should be carefully noted that, on average, only ~50% nuclear profile discs appear in any section, as represented imaginatively in A,B,C below. Thus, the high numbers of "lost" enterocyte nuclei now becomes apparent. However, since IEL counts are made relative to the simultaneously changing world of enterocyte (nuclei) populations, values are spuriously increased twofold. The basic flaw is discussed elsewhere (reference [56]: and see Figure 5).

From that (Ferguson) position, nevertheless, it is usually asserted that IEL are increased within flat mucosae, but that needs qualifying. The computerised data reveal an absolute six-fold reduction in enterocytes for flat mucosae, whereas the IEL population is only reduced two-fold. Therefore, *relatively*, the IEL density obviously remains high, as inferred correctly [15] by Guix and Whitehead. Further proof is afforded by other calculations made possible by our approach, since a single IEL is associated with 9 (7–11) enterocytes in control mucosae, but only 3 (2–4) enterocytes in flat celiac mucosae, emphasising the markedly increased "concentration" of IELs in flat biopsies, largely exaggerated by the precipitous loss (80%) of surface enterocytes. On those grounds, how would we answer the critical question 'Is the flat mucosa actually infiltrated at Marsh Stage III, and by what extent'?

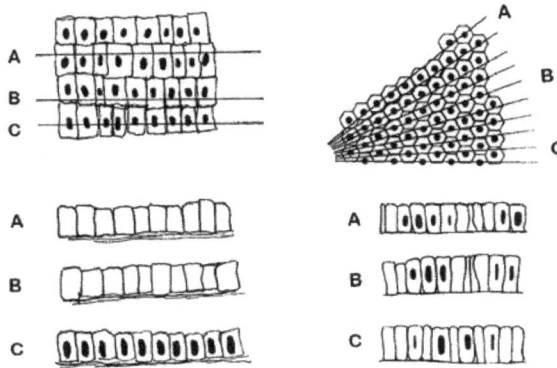

Figure 6. The **left-hand panel** indicates that enterocytes do not lie in an orthogonally arranged grid pattern on the basement membrane (plan view, upper diagram). Therefore, "counts" of enterocytes (or more importantly their nuclei) cannot be accomplished with the ease often assumed in the Methods sections of many publications. This model obviously predicts the possibility of observing large tracts of enterocytes without nuclei (as in the imagined sections at (**A**,**B**)), an event never encountered in histopathological practice. Only occasionally would a palisade that included a run of every adjacent enterocyte, and their contained nuclei, be observable (**C**). Therefore, this model is wrong. The alternative (**right-hand panel**) is closer to reality, comprising an idealised epithelium, scaled to data obtained by transmission/scanning EM studies. The lines in the upper (plan) diagram reflect random sectioning planes through this epithelium. But, it should be carefully noted that, on average, only ~50% nuclear profile discs appear in any section, as represented imaginatively in A,B,C below. Thus, the high numbers of "lost" enterocyte nuclei now becomes apparent. However, since IEL counts are made relative to the simultaneously changing world of enterocyte (nuclei) populations, values are spuriously increased twofold. The basic flaw is discussed elsewhere (reference [55]: and see Figure 5).

It has also been shown [56] that IEL in flat mucosae are considerably larger than those in control mucosal specimens but it is unlikely that these are gluten-induced 'blasts,' as they would presumably be of similar calibre in the early infiltrated Stage I and II lesions. The lymphocytes in these early lesions, however, are small and non-mitotic. It is possible that, resulting from widespread shedding of the surface epithelium, some attempt at repairing a depleted IEL population from within the epithelium is operational. In support of that idea, we have to take into account [57,58] the raised mitotic activity of IEL in flat (Marsh III) mucosae. But that is another problem remaining to be resolved, as well as the immunophenotype of lymphocytes involved. We are totally ignorant of those details.

6.2. The Crypts

In comparison with the great interest in surface epithelium, the crypts have always played the "Cinderella" role, as the forgotten companion. In earlier studies [59] from Trier's lab in Boston, the use of mucosal explants revealed the rapidly accelerated flow of cells upwards towards the surface, complementing previous washout studies which likewise suggested a massive loss of enterocytes in untreated patients. That was followed by Nicholas Wright's elegant investigations which showed [60] that (i) the growth fraction in the crypts is enlarged; (ii) the actual duration of crypt cell mitosis is shortened (from the normal rate of 1 h to approximately 40 min); and (iii) the inter-mitotic interval is reduced, so that successive mitoses are speeded up. These observations revealed the degree to which the hypertrophic crypt response is geared up for the assumed losses of surface enterocytes.

In Figure 5C, it is evident that the crypts are small and non-infiltrated in mucosae where villi are subject to infiltration. But things change markedly as flattening proceeds (Marsh Stage II) with a doubling of crypt volumes and increased lymphocytic infiltration (Figure 5D) accompanied by the first evidence of increased crypt cell mitotic activity (Figure 5E). These changes are highly reminiscent of the enlarged crypts together with normal, infiltrated villi [61] in mild graft-versus-host reactions where recipient and donor tissue were of identical genetic histocompatibility backgrounds: a phenomenon termed the 'innocent bystander effect' [62] in the intestine by Elson.

It is thus evident that the mucosal (Marsh) Stage II development reveals important outcomes, since additional mechanisms are now clearly in place which progress lesion pathology towards its final state. It is questionable whether the progressive hypertrophy of the crypts to almost four-fold (once flattening has been achieved) is still a continuing T-cell-mediated effect, or whether loss of surface cells still has to be accommodated by a massively increased crypt cell production rate, and migratory profile. Neither do we know why the initial infiltration of crypts is delayed, why the later increased lymphocyte infiltration does not impair their vast hypertrophic crypt responses even though mucosal surface contours are reduced, or why crypt IEL are significantly enlarged over control mucosae [63], although of similar size distribution to surface IEL.

6.3. The Lamina Propria

Further evidence for this proposal is seen in the lamina propria (Figure 5F) which has begun to swell at Stage (Marsh) II, accompanied by a brisk influx of neutrophils, always indicative of mucosal inflammation and a rise in basophils and mucosal mast cells (Figure 5G), many seemingly degranulated [64]. That reflects the two-fold swelling of lamina propria partly due to local vasodilatation of the microvasculature whose vessels are swollen, with enlarged endothelial nuclei, thickened basal laminae, and cells such as eosinophils and basophils emigrating across their walls into the surrounding tissues [65]: fibrinogen staining provides a rough indicator of the extravasated vascular fluids.

Current celiac research seems to have lost sight of the influence of mucosal mast cells, their T-cell dependency [66–68] and contributory roles in the evolutionary genesis of the celiac lesion, especially within the subepithelial zone, and contributors to the local T-cell-mediated hypersensitivity reaction to gluten. Computerised morphometry showed that mucosal mast cell populations are increased 2.5 times, eosinophils 4.5 times, and basophils 20-fold over control values, and all gluten dependent. The influx of eosinophils and basophils through the microvasculature suggests a bone marrow origin. Mucosal mast cells were never seen in the vascular compartment, so are presumably differentiated locally, or from incoming precursors not distinguishable histologically.

7. Interpreting the Marsh Classification

The changes noted in this diagram (Figure 5) as the mucosa progresses from villous infiltration to flattening is illustrated (Figure 5H) by appropriate diagrams (Marsh Stages I through III). It is to this classification of the mucosal changes that we now pass.

7.1. So-Called "Non-Specificity" of the Marsh I and II Lesions

Many have dismissed early Marsh I and II lesion as 'non-specific' [69,70]. On the other hand, there are those who have understood that Marsh I/II lesions should be investigated prospectively [31], thus to exclude true glutensensitivity: as these authors summarise—*'a raised IEL count with normal villous architecture is of sufficient clinical importance to be highlighted in routine duodenal biopsy reports'.*

To clarify this position for histopathologists, a series of differential diagnoses has been set out by the Bucharest Consensus [71], under the terminological umbrella of "microscopic enteritis". It is to be hoped that these widelyagreed guidelines will be recognised and employed. And within a family setting and DQ 2/8 haplotypes, the possibility of celiac disease remains a high probability. Individuals with these mucosal changes should be closely followed up, or even treated [72], particularly if they have disabling symptoms associated with malabsorption of important nutrients. Despite a lesser mucosal involvement there is often considerable abdominal symptomatology and pain, osteoporosis and iron deficiency anemia, features surely necessitating a gluten-free diet—even only if a defined, agreed, short-term trial to monitor clinical response and reversal of malabsorptive defects is undertaken. Given the growing literature, it is now *unacceptable to refuse a diet on the grounds that the mucosa is not* flat. By now, it should be widely recognised that there is neither a specific, nor certainly a uniquely related diagnostic mucosal change.

7.2. Irrelevance of the Marsh III Sub-Classification

The division [73] of the Marsh III lesion into three subdivisions (a, b, c), as a "guide to histopathologists" has been widely, but surprisingly uncritically, employed. This proposed analytical system is a failure because of the following flaws:

(a) *Absence of appropriate criteria*: these subdivisions were never precisely defined morphologically as verification of the proposed subdivisions. It is interesting to envisage how (and why) so many histologists thought they were identifying real structures. Even the micrographs illustrated in a later publication [74] written by histopathologists, for the help of other histologists, failed to correspond to the originals, again demonstrative of the subjective nature of the whole scheme.

Oberhuber's approach has now been further degraded by additional studies:

(b) *morphological*—which highlight the misinterpretations of sectioned mosaic plateaus as supposedly representing 'blunted', 'degenerate' 'villi' [75];

(c) *immunohistochemical*—demonstrating that varied sub-immunophenotype IEL are equally represented in each subdivision, when their density should have increased with the worsening histological picture alleged to represent each successive stage: a, b, c [76];

(d) *mathematical*—the regression equations employed by Charlesworth and colleagues failed to identify the a,b,c subgrades as valid entities for improved pathological recognition [77];

(e) *clinical*—there appear to be no published accounts in which a gastroenterologist necessarily had to rely, ultimately and crucially, on the pathologist's *sub-classification* of the relevant mucosal biopsy in order to facilitate diagnosis, treatment, or offer a prognosis for the patients concerned;

(f) *generalised usage*—finally, given the failure of this attempted reclassification, it seems to follow that more recently revised classifications of Marsh were based, however, on these sub-divisions, offering no further decisive clarity. In fact, they could be said to increase complexity and interpretational difficulties. For example, from a review of relevant papers published over the last decade, it is abundantly clear that these recent contenders for the job have not surfaced either as being more useful, more acceptable, or more easily employed. The original classification is as simple as could be.

7.3. The "Normal" Mucosa

Finally, we come to the interpretation of the 'normal' (Marsh Stage 0) mucosa. One problem concerns origins of specimens—from referred, symptomatic patients or apparently healthy individuals. There *are* differences—but which nowadays are rarely considered or explored (see last paragraph: Immunological Function of Mucosa, above). Second, 'normality' is no longer defined, although from early times, villi were seen as long, pencil-shaped structures 350–600 μm in height [9].

Overriding those relevant considerations, however, is the recognition that 'normal' mucosae, viewed histologically, may be consistent with gluten sensitivity, harbouring abnormalities requiring additional but difficult technologies for detection, including immunofluorescence of anti-TG antibodies on epithelial and microvascular basement membranes [78]; transmission EM detection of necrotic enterocytes [79,80], or assays of fatty acid binding protein as presumptive indicator of cell death [72].

7.4. Failures in Understanding the Marked Hypertrophic Remodelling Response

The problems arising from the sub-classification of the Marsh III lesion stem from the continuing belief that mucosal flattening strips every single villus down to the crypt-villus border, supposedly considered the end-stage of a progressive, atrophic process. There is no morphologic evidence for that presumption. The changes that involve most of the mucosa (excepting epithelium) represent the effects of considerable remodelling, embodying a vast hypertrophic response in terms of the upward growth and enlargement of the inter-villous ridges, and their amalgamation with partially reduced villi to create irregular mosaic plateaus over the mucosal surface, with height elevations of ~200 μm.

The hypertrophic response is further exemplified by the vast increase in the size of the crypts, their infiltration by a population of large IEL, and the increased dynamic of the ascending enterocyte column in its movement towards the surface. The lamina also swells to twice its volume due to extravasation of plasma fluid through the inflamed capillaries, and great increases in the bulk of infiltrating cells. This is a complex epithelial-mesenchymal response indeed, and a markedly dynamic hypertrophic response to gluten.

It seems that this end-phase of mucosal flattening is not generally well understood. As a result, random sections through the mosaic plateaus create a variety of appearances which histologically are invariably taken to represent stunted or branched villi. Surface microscopy, however, does not reveal the presence of any villi, so these structures seen two-dimensionally merely reflect the many possibilities on offer when a mosaic plateau is observed in any random section.

This state-of-affairs is scarcely helped by current, expert guidelines [81,82] whose authors collectively provide no incisive practical outcomes from the literature. The guidelines signally fail to engender the vital cooperative understandings required between pathologist and clinician regarding mucosal interpretation. In fact, these guidelines do not confidently explore the full spectrum of mucosal abnormalities of gluten-induced mucosal change, being more at ease with "atrophy" and the flat lesion. As a result (a) they tend to dismiss all other preliminary phase transitions as "non-specific"; (b) rely on traditional definitional criteria—that is, "atrophy"—resulting in a flat mucosa and (c) are hesitant to recommend a gluten-free diet without that latter criterion, despite a very large literature to the contrary [31,32,69–72,80,83].

There is a pressing need to reconstruct biopsies with computerised programmes, using either the systems of indices and matrices employed in computer-assisted design, or by employing 3-D printing. Such approaches would further expand our understandings of the mucosa, and its internal changes, especially where the remodelled microvasculature is concerned. If we knew more about the effects of gluten on the small vessels and how they influence the hypertrophic responses throughout the mucosa, we might be in a more enviable position to understand how these changes come about—both in their association with flattening as much as with regrowth. There is much to be re-remembered from the past, organised from the present, and planned for the future [15].

8. Afterword

Ptolemy may have been a little disgruntled when his geocentric theory was overtaken by the more ambitious heliocentric-based Copernican view of the universe. Yet it hardly seems time to declare that celiac disease has become so universalised that the intestinal tract has been side-stepped and no longer plays a central role in furthering insights into the disease: that seems to us to be a misleading—if not premature—conclusion.

From all this it should be clearly understood that:

1.   there are no (immuno)histologically unique diagnostic features for celiac disease that "absolutely" distinguish it from other mucosal enteropathies or more importantly, disease-control biopsies;

2. the spectre of the "normal" mucosa, but which is consistent with true gluten sensitivity, remains a difficult problem to deal with, including its redefinition;

3. there is considerable overlap between the populations of celiac intraepithelial lymphocyte (IEL) and controls (Figure 2)—regardless of the identifying technique used;

4. IEL populations do not comprise two separate populations (bimodal), but represent graded biological outcomes (to luminal antigens), analogous to height, weight, blood pressure or acid secretion (Figure 3);

5. additionally detailed studies of the dose-response characteristics of the $CD3^-$ innate pool of IEL, and their $CD127^+$ and $CD127^-$ components may bring new insights to diagnosis and mucosal interpretation;

6. ROC curve analysis (Figure 4 and Table 2) provides usable answers which overcome the immense numerical overlapping between IEL populations, including $CD3^+$ and $\gamma\delta^+$ cells, and removes to a great extent the inherent uncertainty, engendered with numerical counts, as to where to draw the cut-off;

7. log-transformation of the skewed celiac data does not produce means which materially differ from the numerical means (data not shown). Together, these results confirm that histopathologists do not need to log-transform their numerical counts, and that IEL counts in routine hematoxylin and eosin (H&E)sections can now be seen as a very easy and resourceful way of defining one's cut-off, provided receiver-operating characteristic (ROC) curve analysis is additionally carried out;

8. there is a vast cavern between high-level research still needed in continued interrogations of the mucosal response to gluten ingestion, and the somewhat more unsophisticated approaches deployable at histopathological level during routine diagnostic service work.

Notwithstanding those difficulties, the tracing of the historical development of our understandings of the structure and functioning of the small intestinal mucosa is a truly fascinating story. Our own view is that the mucosa still occupies a very central role in diagnosis and, together with related research, into its response to gluten peptides.

There is a long list of historic figures who have welded the story of the intestinal mucosa into one which still causes dissent, re-evaluation, and the pull of additional research initiatives. That is the true nature of investigative science, and there will surely be more advances to clarify, and to strengthen our grasp on this important field of gluten-induced hypersensitivity reactions within the intestinal mucosa.

Conflicts of Interest: The authors declare no conflict of interest.

References

1. Gee, S. On the Coeliac Affection. *St. Bartholomew's Hosp. Rep.* **1888**, *24*, 17–20.
2. Shiner, M. Jejunal biopsy tube. *Lancet* **1956**, *1*, 85. [CrossRef]
3. Crosby, W.; Kugler, H. Intraluminal biopsy of the small intestine. The intestinal biopsy capsule. *Am. J. Dig. Dis.* **1958**, *5*, 217–222.
4. Wood, I.; Doig, R.; Motteram, R.; Hughes, A. Gastric Biopsy: Report on fifty-five biopsies using a new flexible gastric biopsy tube. *Lancet* **1949**, *1*, 18–21. [CrossRef]
5. Paulley, J. Observations on the aetiology of idiopathic steatorrhoea: Jejunal and lymph node biopsies. *Br. Med. J.* **1954**, *2*, 1318–1321. [CrossRef] [PubMed]
6. Dicke, W.; Weijers, H.; van der Kamer, J. Coeliac disease. II—The presence in wheat ofa factor having a deleterious effect in cases of celiac disease. *Acta Paediatr.* **1953**, *42*, 34–42. [CrossRef]
7. Haas, S. The value of the banana in the treatment of celiac disease. *Am. J. Dis. Child.* **1924**, *28*, 421–437. [CrossRef]
8. Anderson, C. Histological changes in the duodenal mucosa in celiac disease: Reversibility during treatment with a gluten-free diet. *Arch. Dis. Child.* **1960**, *35*, 419–427. [CrossRef] [PubMed]

9. Booth, C.; Stewart, J.; Holmes, R.; Brackenbury, W. *Dissecting Microscope Appearances of Intestinal Mucosa*; Intestinal Biopsy (Ciba Foundation Study Group No. 14); Wolstenholme, G., Cameron, M., Eds.; Churchill: London, UK, 1962; pp. 2–23.

10. Cocco, A.; Dorhmann, M.; Hendrix, T. Reconstruction of normal jejunal biopsies: Three-dimensional histology. *Gastroenterology* **1966**, *51*, 24–31. [PubMed]

11. Loehry, C.; Creamer, B. Three-dimensional structure of the human small intestinal mucosa in health and disease. *Gut* **1969**, *10*, 6–12. [CrossRef] [PubMed]

12. Toner, P.; Carr, K.; Ferguson, A.; Mackay, C. Scanning and transmission electron microscopic studies of human intestinal mucosa. *Gut* **1970**, *11*, 471–481. [CrossRef] [PubMed]

13. Creamer, B.; Leppard, P. Post-mortem examination of a small intestine in the coeliac syndrome. *Gut* **1965**, *6*, 466–471. [CrossRef] [PubMed]

14. Padykula, H.; Strauss, E.; Ladman, A.; Gardner, F. A morphological and histochemical analysis of the human jejunal epithelium in nontropicalsprue. *Gastroenterology* **1961**, *40*, 735–765. [PubMed]

15. Marsh, M.N.; Rostami, K. What is a normal intestinal mucosa? *Gastroenterology* **2016**, *151*, 784–788. [CrossRef] [PubMed]

16. Gowans, J.L.; Knight, E.J. The route of re-circulation of lymphocytes in the rat. *Proc. R. Soc. B* **1964**, *159*, 257–282. [CrossRef]

17. Crabbé, P.; Carbonara, A.; Heremans, J. The normal human intestinal mucosa as a major source of plasma cells containing γA-immunoglobulin. *Lab. Investig.* **1965**, *14*, 235–248. [PubMed]

18. Tomasi, T.; Tan, E.; Solomon, A.; Prendergast, R. Characteristics of an immune system common to certain external secretions. *J. Exp. Med.* **1965**, *121*, 101–125. [CrossRef] [PubMed]

19. Crabbé, P.; Nash, D.; Bazin, H.; Eyssen, H.; Heremans, J. Antibodies of the IgA type in intestinal plasma cells of germfree mice after oral or parenteral immunization with ferritin. *J. Exp. Med.* **1969**, *130*, 723–738. [CrossRef] [PubMed]

20. Loft, D.; Marsh, M.N.; Sandle, G.; Crowe, P.; Garner, V.; Gordon, D.; Baker, R. Studies of intestinal lymphoid tissue. XII-Epithelial lymphocyte and mucosal responses to rectal gluten challenge in celiac sprue. *Gastroenterology* **1989**, *97*, 29–37. [CrossRef]

21. Ensari, A.; Marsh, M.N.; Morgan, S.; Lobley, R.; Unsworth, D.; Kounali, D.; Crowe, P.; Paisley, J.; Moriarty, K.; Lowry, J. Diagnosing coeliac disease by rectal gluten challenge: A prospective study based on immunopathology, computerized image analysis and logistic regression analysis. *Clin. Sci.* **2001**, *101*, 199–207. [CrossRef] [PubMed]

22. Quiding-Järbrink, M.; Lakew, M.; Nordström, I.; Banchereau, J.; Butcher, E.; Holmgren, J.; Czerkinsky, C. Human circulating specific antibody-forming cells after systemic and mucosal immunizations: Differential homing commitments and cell surface differentiation markers. *Eur. J. Immunol.* **1995**, *25*, 322–327. [CrossRef] [PubMed]

23. Barratt, M.; Powell, J.; Allen, W.; Porter, P. Immunopathology of intestinal disorders in farm animals. In *Immunopathology of the Small Intestine*; Marsh, M.N., Ed.; Wiley: Chichester, UK, 1987; pp. 253–281.

24. Kantele, J.; Arvilommi, H.; Kontiainen, S.; Salmi, M.; Jalkanen, S.; Savilahti, E.; Westerholm, M.; Kantele, A. Mucosally activated circulating human B cells in diarrhea express homing receptors directing them back to the gut. *Gastroenterology* **1996**, *110*, 1061–1067. [CrossRef] [PubMed]

25. Ráki, M.; Fallang, L.; Brottveit, M.; Bergseng, E.; Quarsten, H.; Lundin, K.; Sollid, L. Tetramer visualisation of gut-homing gluten-specific T cells in the peripheral blood of celiac disease patients. *Proc. Natl. Acad. Sci. USA* **2007**, *104*, 2831–2836. [CrossRef] [PubMed]

26. Brottveit, M.; Ráki, M.; Bergsen, E.; Fallang, L.; Simonsen, B.; Løvik, A.; Larsen, S.; Løberg, E.M.; Jahnsen, F.L.; Sollid, L.M.; et al. Assessing possible celiac disease by an HLA-DQ2-gliadin tetramer test. *Am. J. Gastroenterol.* **2011**, *106*, 1318–1324. [CrossRef] [PubMed]

27. Douglas, A.; Crabbé, P.; Hobbs, J. Immunochemical studies of the serum, intestinal secretions and intestinal mucosa in patients with adult celiac disease and other forms of the celiac syndrome. *Gastroenterology* **1970**, *59*, 414–425. [PubMed]

28. Ferguson, A.; Murray, D. Quantitation of intraepithelial lymphocytes in human jejunum. *Gut* **1971**, *12*, 988–994. [CrossRef] [PubMed]

29. Batman, P.; Miller, A.; Harris, J.; Pinching, A.; Griffin, G. Jejunal enteropathy associated with human immunodeficiency virus infection: Quantitative histology. *J. Clin. Pathol.* **1989**, *42*, 275–281. [CrossRef] [PubMed]

30. Hayat, M.; Cairns, A.; Dixon, M. Quantitation of intraepithelial lymphocytes in human duodenum: What is normal? *J. Clin. Pathol.* **2002**, *55*, 393–395. [CrossRef] [PubMed]

31. Mahadeva, S.; Wyatt, J.; Howdle, P. Is a raised intraepithelial lymphocyte count with normal duodenal villous architecture clinically relevant? *J. Clin. Pathol.* **2002**, *55*, 424–428. [CrossRef] [PubMed]

32. Kakar, S.; Nehra, V.; Murray, J.; Dayharsh, G.; Burgart, L. Significance of intraepithelial lymphocytosis in small bowel biopsy samples with normal mucosal architecture. *Am. J. Gastroenterol.* **2003**, *98*, 2027–2033. [CrossRef] [PubMed]

33. Veress, B.; Franzén, L.; Bodin, L.; Borch, K. Duodenal intraepithelial lymphocyte-count revisited. *Scand. J. Gastroenterol.* **2004**, *9*, 138–144. [CrossRef]

34. Biagi, F.; Luinette, O.; Campanella, J.; Klersy, C.; Zambelli, C.; Villanacci, V. Intraepithelial lymphocytes in the villous tip: Do they indicate potential celiac disease? *J. Clin. Pathol.* **2004**, *57*, 835–839. [CrossRef] [PubMed]

35. Nasseri-Moghaddam, S.; Mofid, A.; Nouraie, M.; Abedi, B.; Pourshams, A.; Malekzadeh, R.; Sotoudeh, M. The normal range of duodenal intraepithelial lymphocytes. *Arch. Iran. Med.* **2008**, *11*, 136–142. [PubMed]

36. Siriweera, E.; Qi, Z.; Yong, J. Validity of intraepithelial lymphocyte counts in the diagnosis of celiac disease: A histopathological study. *Int. J. Celiac Dis.* **2015**, *3*, 136–142.

37. Guix, M.; Skinner, J.; Whitehead, R. Measuring intraepithelial lymphocytes, surface area, and volume of lamina propria in the jejunal mucosa of celiac patients. *Gut* **1979**, *20*, 275–278. [CrossRef] [PubMed]

38. Weibel, E.R. *Stereological Methods*; Academic Press: New York, NY, USA, 1979; Volume I.

39. Marsh, M.N.; Crowe, P.; Moriarty, K.; Ensari, A. Morphometric Analysis of Intestinal Mucosa: The measurement of volume compartments and cell volumes in human intestinal mucosa. *Methods Mol. Med.* **2000**, *41*, 125–145. [PubMed]

40. Marsh, M.N. Gluten, major histocompatibility complex, and the small intestine: A molecular and mmunobiologic approach to the spectrum of gluten sensitivity ('celiac sprue'). *Gastroenterology* **1992**, *102*, 330–354. [CrossRef]

41. Marsh, M.N. Grains of truth: Evolutionary changes in small intestinal mucosa in response to environmental antigenic challenge. *Gut* **1990**, *31*, 111–114. [CrossRef] [PubMed]

42. Doherty, M.; Barry, R. Gluten-induced mucosal changes in subjects without overt small-bowel disease. *Lancet* **1981**, *317*, 517–520. [CrossRef]

43. Egan-Mitchell, B.; Fottrell, P.; McNichol, B. Early or pre-coeliac mucosa: Development of gluten enteropathy. *Gut* **1981**, *22*, 65–69. [CrossRef] [PubMed]

44. Marsh, M.N. Studies of intestinal lymphoid tissue. XIII—Immunopathololgy of the evolving celiac sprue lesion. *Pathol. Res. Pract.* **1989**, *185*, 774–777. [CrossRef]

45. Maki, M.; Holm, K.; Koskimies, S.; Hallstgrom, O.; Visakorpi, J. Normal small bowel biopsy followed by celiac disease. *Arch. Dis. Child.* **1990**, *65*, 1137–1141. [CrossRef] [PubMed]

46. O'Mahony, S.; Vestey, J.; Ferguson, A. Similarities in intestinal humoral immunity in Dermatitis herpetiformis without enteropathy and in coeliac disease. *Lancet* **1990**, *35*, 1487–1490. [CrossRef]

47. Collin, P.; Helin, H.; Mäki, M.; Hallström, O.; Karvonen, A.-L. Follow-up of patients positive in reticulin and gliadin antibody tests with normal small-bowel biopsy findings. *Scand. J. Gastroenterol.* **1993**, *28*, 595–598. [CrossRef] [PubMed]

48. Niveloni, S.; Pedreira, S.; Sugai, E.; Vazquez, H.; Smecuol, E.; Fiorini, A. The natural history of gluten sensitivity: Report of two patients from a long-term follow-up of non-atrophic, first-degree relatives. *Am. J. Gastroenterol.* **2000**, *95*, 463–468. [CrossRef] [PubMed]

49. Marsh, M.N. Mucosal pathology in gluten sensitivity. In *Coeliac Disease*; Marsh, M.N., Ed.; Blackwell Scientific Publications: Oxford, UK, 1992; pp. 136–191.

50. Marsh, M.N.; Loft, D.; Garner, V.; Gordon, D. Time/dose responses of celiac mucosae to graded oral challenges with Frazer's fraction III of gliadin. *Eur. J. Gastroenterol. Hepatol.* **1992**, *4*, 667–674.

51. Mowat, A.; Ferguson, A. Intraepithelial lymphocyte counts and crypt hyperplasia measure the mucosal component of the graft-versus-host reaction in mouse small intestine. *Gastroenterology* **1982**, *83*, 417–423. [PubMed]

52. Bjarnason, I.; Peters, T.; Veall, N. A persistent defect in intestinal permeability in celiac disease demonstrated by a 51Cr-labelled EDTA absorption test. *Lancet* **1983**, *12*, 323–325. [CrossRef]
53. Marsh, M.N.; Bjarnason, I.; Shaw, J.; Ellis, A.; Baker, R. Studies of intestinal lymphoid tissue: XIV—HLA status, mucosal morphology, permeability and epithelial lymphocyte populations in first degree relatives of patients with coeliac disease. *Gut* **1990**, *31*, 32–36. [CrossRef] [PubMed]
54. Crowe, P.; Marsh, M.N. Morphometric analysis of small intestinal mucosa IV. Determining cell volumes. *Virchows Arch. A* **1993**, *422*, 459–466. [CrossRef]
55. Crowe, P.; Marsh, M.N. Morphometric analysis of small intestinal mucosa. VI—Principles in enumerating intra-epithelial lymphocytes. *Virchows Arch.* **1994**, *424*, 301–306. [CrossRef] [PubMed]
56. Marsh, M.N. Studies of intestinal lymphoid tissue. III—Quantitative studies of epithelial lymphocytes in small intestinal mucosa of control human subjects and of patients with celiac sprue. *Gastroenterology* **1980**, *79*, 481–492. [PubMed]
57. Marsh, M.N. Studies of intestinal lymphoid tissue. IV – The predictive value of raised mitotic indices among jejunal epithelial lymphocytes in the diagnosis of gluten-sensitive enteropathy. *J. Clin. Pathol.* **1982**, *35*, 517–525. [CrossRef] [PubMed]
58. Marsh, M.N.; Haeney, M. Studies of intestinal lymphoid tissue. VI—Proliferative response of small intestinal lymphocytes distinguishes gluten- from non-gluten-induced enteropathy. *J. Clin. Pathol.* **1983**, *76*, 149–160. [CrossRef]
59. Trier, J.; Browning, T. Epithelial-cell renewal in cultured duodenal biopsies in celiac sprue. *N. Eng. J. Med.* **1970**, *283*, 1245–1250. [CrossRef] [PubMed]
60. Watson, A.; Wright, N. Morphology and cell kinetics of the jejunal mucosa in untreated patients. *Clin. Gastroenterol.* **1974**, *3*, 11–31. [PubMed]
61. Mowat, A.; Ferguson, A. Hypersensitivity reactions in the small intestine: 6—Pathogenesis of the graft-versus-host reaction in the small intestinal mucosa of the mouse. *Transplantation* **1981**, *32*, 238–243. [CrossRef] [PubMed]
62. Elson, C.; Reilly, R.; Rosenberg, I. Small intestinal injury in the GvHR: An innocent bystander phenomenon. *Gastroenterology* **1977**, *72*, 886–889. [PubMed]
63. Marsh, M.N.; Hinde, J. Morphometric analysis of small intestinal mucosa. III—The quantitation of crypt epithelial volumes and lymphoid cell infiltrates, with reference to celiac sprue mucosae. *Virchows Arch.* **1986**, *409*, 11–22. [CrossRef]
64. Marsh, M.N.; Hinde, J. Inflammatory component of celiac sprue mucosa. I—Mast cells, basophils, and eosinophils. *Gastroenterology* **1985**, *89*, 92–101. [CrossRef]
65. Dhesi, I.; Marsh, M.N.; Kelly, C.; Crowe, P. Morphometric analysis of small intestinal mucosa. II—Determination of lamina propria volumes, plasma cell and neutrophil populations within control and coeliac disease mucosae. *Virchows Arch.* **1984**, *403*, 173–180. [CrossRef]
66. Dvorak, H.; Dvorak, A. Basophils, mast cells and cellular immunity in animals and man. *Hum. Pathol.* **1972**, *3*, 454–456. [CrossRef]
67. Ruitenberg, E.; Elgersma, A. Absence of intestinal mast cell response in congenitally athymic mice during Trichinella spiralis infection. *Nature* **1976**, *264*, 258–260. [CrossRef] [PubMed]
68. Befus, D.; Pearce, F.; Gauldie, J.; Horsewood, P.; Bienenstock, J. Mucosal mast cells: I—Isolation and functional characteristics of rat intestinal mast cells. *J. Immunol.* **1982**, *128*, 2475–2480. [CrossRef]
69. Schmidt, E.; Smyrk, T.; Faubion, W.; Oxentenko, A. Duodenal intraepithelial lymphocytosis with normal villous architecture in pediatric patients: Mayo Clinic experiences, 2000–2009. *J. Pediatr. Gastroenterol. Nutr.* **2013**, *56*, 51–55. [CrossRef] [PubMed]
70. Zanini, B.; Lanzarotto, F.; Villanacci, V.; Carabellese, N.; Ricci, C.; Lanzini, A. Clinical expression of lymphocytic duodenosis in "mild enteropathy" celiac disease and in functional gastrointestinal syndromes. *Scand. J. Gastroenterol.* **2014**, *49*, 794–800. [CrossRef] [PubMed]
71. Rostami, K.; Aldulaimi, D.; Holmes, G.; Johnson, M.; Robert, M.; Srivastava, A.; Flejou, J.F.; Sanders, D.S.; Volta, U.; Derakhshan, M.H.; et al. Microscopic Enteritis: The Bucharest Consensus. *World J. Gastroenterol.* **2015**, *21*, 2593–2604. [CrossRef] [PubMed]
72. Not, T.; Zivberna, F.; Vatta, S.; Quaglia, S.; Martelossi, S.; Villanacci, V.; Marzari, R.; Florian, F.; Vecchiet, M.; Sulic, A.M.; et al. Cryptic genetic gluten intolerance revealed by intestinal anti-transaminase antibodies and response to gluten-free diet. *Gut* **2011**, *60*, 1487–1493. [CrossRef] [PubMed]

73. Oberhuber, G.; Granditsch, G.; Vogelsang, H. The histopathology of celiac disease: Time for a standardized report scheme for pathologists. *Eur. J. Gastroenterol. Hepatol.* **1999**, *11*, 1185–1194. [CrossRef] [PubMed]

74. Dickson, B.; Streutket, C.; Chetty, R. Coeliac disease: An update for pathologists. *J. Clin. Pathol.* **2006**, *59*, 1008–1016. [CrossRef] [PubMed]

75. Marsh, M.N.; Johnson, M.; Rostami, K. Mucosal histopathology in celiac disease: A rebuttal of Oberhüber's sub-division of Marsh III. *Gastroenterol. Hepatol. Bed Bench* **2015**, *8*, 99–109.

76. De Andrés, A.; Camarero, C. Distal duodenum versus bulb: Intraepithelial lymphocytes have something to say about celiac disease diagnosis. *Dig. Dis. Sci.* **2015**, *60*, 1004–1009. [CrossRef] [PubMed]

77. Charlesworth, R.; Andronicus, N.; Scott, D.; McFarlane, J.; Agnew, L. Can the sensitivity of the histopathological diagnosis of celiac disease be increased and can treatment progression be monitored using mathematical modelling of histological section?—A pilot study. *J. Adv. Med. Sci.* **2017**, in press.

78. Kaukinen, K.; Peraaho, M.; Collin, P. Small-bowel mucosal transaminase 2-specific IgA deposits in celiac disease without villous atrophy: A prospective and randomized clinical study. *Scand. J. Gastroenterol.* **2005**, *40*, 564–572. [CrossRef] [PubMed]

79. Sbarbati, A.; Valletta, E.; Bertini, M.; Cipolli, M.; Morroni, M.; Pinelli, L.; Tatò, L. Gluten sensitivity and "normal" histology: Is the intestinal mucosa really normal? *Dig. Liver Dis.* **2003**, *35*, 768–773. [CrossRef]

80. Tosca, A.; Maglio, M.; Paparo, F.; Rapacciuolo, L.; Sannino, A.; Miele, E. Immunoglobulin A anti-tissue transglutaminase antibody deposits in the small intestinal mucosa of children with no villous atrophy. *J. Pediatr. Gastroenterol. Nutr.* **2008**, *47*, 293–398. [CrossRef] [PubMed]

81. Rubio-Tapia, A.; Hill, I.; Kelly, C.; Claderwood, A.; Murray, J. ACG guidelines: Diagnosis and management of celiac disease. *Am. J. Gastroenterol.* **2013**, *108*, 656–676. [CrossRef] [PubMed]

82. Ludvigsson, J.; Bai, J.; Biagi, F.; Card, T.R.; Ciacci, C.; Ciclitira, P.J.; Green, P.H.; Hadjivassiliou, M.; Holdoway, A.; van Heel, D.A.; et al. Diagnosis and management of adult celiac disease: Guidelines from the British Society of Gastroenterology. *Gut* **2014**, *63*, 1210–1228. [CrossRef] [PubMed]

83. Tursi, A.; Brandimarte, G. The symptomatic and histologic response to a gluten-free diet in patients with borderline enteropathy. *J. Clin. Gastroenterol.* **2003**, *36*, 13–17. [CrossRef] [PubMed]

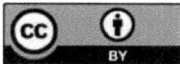

nutrients

MDPI

Review

The Low FODMAP Diet: Many Question Marks for a Catchy Acronym

Giulia Catassi, Elena Lionetti, Simona Gatti and Carlo Catassi *

Department of Pediatrics, Università Politecnica delle Marche, Via F. Corridoni 11, 60123 Ancona, Italy;
giulia.catassi@gmail.com (G.C.); mariaelenalionetti@gmail.com (E.L.); simona.gatti@hotmail.it (S.G.)
* Correspondence: c.catassi@univpm.it; Tel.: +39-071-596-23-64

Received: 29 December 2016; Accepted: 13 March 2017; Published: 16 March 2017

Abstract: FODMAP, "Fermentable Oligo-, Di- and Mono-saccharides And Polyols", is a heterogeneous group of highly fermentable but poorly absorbed short-chain carbohydrates and polyols. Dietary FODMAPs might exacerbate intestinal symptoms by increasing small intestinal water volume, colonic gas production, and intestinal motility. In recent years the low-FODMAP diet for treatment of irritable bowel syndrome (IBS) has gained increasing popularity. In the present review we aim to summarize the physiological, clinical, and nutritional issues, suggesting caution in the prolonged use of this dietary treatment on the basis of the existing literature. The criteria for inclusion in the FODMAPs list are not fully defined. Although the low-FODMAP diet can have a positive impact on the symptoms of IBS, particularly bloating and diarrhea, the quality of the evidence is lower than optimal, due to frequent methodological flaws, particularly lack of a proper control group and/or lack of blinding. In particular, it remains to be proven whether this regimen is superior to conventional IBS diets. The drastic reduction of FODMAP intake has physiological consequences, e.g., on the intestinal microbiome and colonocyte metabolism, which are still poorly understood. A low-FODMAP diet imposes an important restriction of dietary choices due to the elimination of some staple foods, such as wheat derivatives, lactose-containing dairy products, many vegetables and pulses, and several types of fruits. For this reason, patients may be at risk of reduced intake of fiber, calcium, iron, zinc, folate, B and D vitamins, and natural antioxidants. The nutritional risk of the low-FODMAP diet may be higher in persons with limited access to the expensive, alternative dietary items included in the low-FODMAP diet.

Keywords: low-FODMAP diet; irritable bowel syndrome; non-celiac gluten sensitivity; fermentable sugars; polyols; nutritional risk

1. Introduction

FODMAP, "Fermentable Oligo-, Di- and Mono-saccharides And Polyols", is a heterogeneous group of highly fermentable but poorly absorbed short-chain carbohydrates and polyols. The acronym FODMAP was first coined in 2005 by Gibson and Shepherd at Monash University in Melbourne, Australia, in a personal view article suggesting a link between the western lifestyle, the intake of FODMAP-rich foods, and susceptibility to Crohn's disease [1]. Soon after, the Australian group focused on the use of a low-FODMAP diet in the treatment of irritable bowel syndrome (IBS) [2], and in one of their most influential papers they showed that symptom improvement in patients with IBS and suspected non-celiac gluten sensitivity (NCGS) was not related to gluten avoidance, but to the concomitant reduction of FODMAP intake determined by the gluten-free diet (GFD). Interestingly, that study was double-blinded and placebo-controlled for the gluten challenge, but not for the reduction of dietary FODMAPs [3]. In recent years the putative role of FODMAPs in IBS has gained wide popularity in the general public and the subject has been addressed in books promoting the low-FODMAP diet and related recipes [4]. The recently revised British Dietetic Association (BDA) guidelines for the dietary management of IBS recommend the low-FODMAP diet as the second-line intervention in IBS patients [5]. A 2016 meta-analysis supports the efficacy of a low-FODMAP diet in the treatment of functional gastrointestinal symptoms [6]. Treatment with the low-FODMAP diet has also been advocated for diverticulitis [7], exercise-induced gastrointestinal symptoms [8], and inflammatory bowel diseases [9]. Although these studies indicate that a subgroup of patients with IBS may benefit from eating less highly fermentable sugars, i.e., the low-FODMAP diet [6], there are still several open questions regarding the physiology, the efficacy, and the safety of this dietary treatment.

In this paper the physiological, clinical, and nutritional issues suggesting caution in the prolonged use of the low-FODMAP diet will be summarized on the basis of the existing literature. The literature search was conducted in the PubMed MEDLINE and SCOPUS databases using the term "FODMAP" and "irritable bowel syndrome", and only articles in English were extracted. We identified 98 papers, and selected 17 prospective, intervention trials for analysis.

2. What Is FODMAP?

FODMAP is not a single entity, but a group of compounds, including oligosaccharides (fructans, fructo-oligosaccharides = FOS and galacto-oligosaccharides = GOS), disaccharides (lactose), monosaccharides (fructose), and polyols (sorbitol, mannitol, maltitol, xylitol, polydextrose, and isomalt). The list of dietary sugar alcohols (polyols) includes tens of compounds used widely and unpredictably by the food industry as thickeners and sweeteners. Lactose belongs to FODMAPs only in individuals showing non-persistence of high lactase levels, which is a highly variable percentage of subjects in different populations. On the other hand, lactulose is an orally administered, non-absorbable disaccharide that is used in the treatment of constipation, a problem affecting many patients with IBS, and should definitely be avoided in subjects undergoing the FODMAP exclusion.

The FODMAP definition is based on functional instead of biochemical characteristics: being poorly absorbable and highly fermentable in the intestine is the common denominator of FODMAPs. They might exacerbate IBS symptoms through various mechanisms, such as increasing small intestinal water volume, colonic gas production, and intestinal motility. Conversely, FODMAPs have important physiological effects: they increase stool bulk, enhance calcium absorption and modulate immune function, and decrease the levels of serum cholesterol, triacylglycerols, and phospholipids. They selectively stimulate the growth of some microbial groups such as *Bifidobacteria* (prebiotic effect) [10]. Due to their capacity to stimulate the growth of nonpathogenic intestinal microflora, FOS and GOS are increasingly included in food products and infant formulas [11]. Fermentation of small, fermentable carbohydrates in the colon results in the production of short-chain fatty acids (SCFAs = acetate, propionate, and butyrate) that have a trophic effect on the colonocyte metabolism by increasing energy production and cell proliferation, and protecting against colon cancer [12,13]. All of the above positive effects are obviously lost with the low-FODMAP diet.

The boundaries of a low-FODMAP diet are not perfectly known. The appreciable work of the Melbourne group produced some analytical tables on the food content of specific FODMAPs [14–16], however, (a) many commercial items are missing in this list; and (b) the content of FODMAPs in vegetables is highly variable, e.g., according to the degree of maturation [17]. Furthermore, the possible interactions between FODMAPs and other nutrients are still unclear.

Finally, how much is a "normal" and how much is a low FODMAP intake? This has not yet been defined in quantitative terms.

3. Efficacy of the Low-FODMAP Diet: What Is the Quality of the Evidence?

Table 1 reports the clinical trials that are available in the literature on the effect of a low-FODMAP diet in IBS patients [3,18–33]. In general, most studies and one meta-analysis [6] have shown that IBS symptoms, particularly bloating and abdominal pain, may benefit from this treatment. However, the quality of the evidence is lower than optimal in our opinion, due to frequent methodological flaws, particularly a lack of a proper control group and/or lack of blinding, as shown in the last column of Table 1. The finding that the low-FODMAP diet improves IBS symptoms in comparison with a normal diet does not prove that this treatment is superior to the conventional IBS dietary intervention, e.g., the restriction of high-fiber food, resistant starch, fresh fruit, coffee, tea, alcohol, fizzy drinks and sorbitol, as recommended by the British National Institute for Health and Care Excellence (NICE) guidelines [34].

Indeed, studies comparing the efficacy of the low-FODMAP diet vs. proper dietary advice for IBS did not show a clear-cut advantage of the low-FODMAP diet: (a) in a US trial, 40%–50% of patients reported adequate relief of their IBS with diarrhea symptoms with the low-FODMAP diet or a diet based on modified NICE guidelines, even though the low-FODMAP diet led to significantly greater improvement in individual IBS symptoms, particularly pain and bloating, compared with the NICE diet [31]; (b) in a Swedish study the severity of IBS symptoms was reduced in both the low-FODMAP and the conventional IBS diet groups, at the end of a four-week period of treatment [26].

Due to the lack of a biomarker of "FODMAP intolerance", the gold standard for proving the causal role of FODMAP, as well as other food intolerances/allergies, remains the double-blind placebo-controlled (DBPC) challenge. Three FODMAP challenge studies showed that high doses of fructose or fructans significantly worsen IBS symptoms [18,32,33]. Another randomized, DBPC study showed that gastrointestinal symptoms increased significantly after sorbitol and mannitol ingestion in patients with IBS compared to controls [14]. No DBPC challenge study is available for other FODMAPs or a mixed FODMAP-containing diet.

The duration of treatment with the low-FODMAP diet is rather short in the majority of published studies. This is a limitation for the evaluation of the low-FODMAP diet's long-term efficacy. IBS is a chronic/recurrent condition but this treatment is difficult to maintain over time, due to many food exclusions. In a recent follow-up study of patients with IBS or inflammatory bowel disorder (IBD) treated with the low-FODMAPs diet, only one-third were still adherent to the diet after a median follow-up of 18 months [35]. The inventors of the low-FODMAP diet suggest an "all-FODMAP" free diet for two months followed by a serial challenge with one FODMAP per week (so called FODMAP reintroduction plan) [4]. Not only is the rationale of this challenge unclear, given that the physiological effects of FODMAP are not expected to change in such a short period of time, but also unpractical, since the list of food to reintroduce on a weekly basis is extremely long.

Table 1. Clinical trials on the effect of low-FODMAP diet in IBS patients.

First Author, Year	Patients	n	Study Design	Diet Duration	Results	Comment on the Study Design
Shepherd et al. [18]	Patients with IBS	n = 25	Low-FODMAP diet followed by DBPC crossover challenge with fructose and fructane	2 weeks	70% of patients receiving fructose, 77% receiving fructans, and 79% receiving a mixture reported symptoms were not adequately controlled, compared with 14% receiving glucose	Only some FODMAPs were tested in this study
Staudacher et al. [19]	Consecutive patients with IBS	I = 43 C = 39	Low FODMAP vs. standard IBS diet	9 months	Improved satisfaction and IBS score in I group	Lack of randomization
Staudacher et al. [20]	Patients with IBS	I = 19 C = 22	RCT, Low FODMAPs vs. habitual diet	1 weeks	More patients in the intervention group reported adequate control of symptoms (68%) compared with controls (23%)	Lack of blinding
Biesiekierski et al. [3]	Patients with NCGS and IBS	n = 37	Low-FODMAP diet followed by DBPC crossover challenge with gluten	3 weeks	Improvement with low FODMAP diet, no change between gluten and placebo challenge	Lack of control and no blinding during the low FODMAP diet
De Roest et al. [21]	consecutive patients with IBS	n = 90	Open, low FODMAP diet	16 months	Improvement of pre-study symptom	Lack of control group
Halmos et al. [22]	Patients with IBS and controls	I = 30 C = 8	Randomized, crossover, low-FODMAP diet vs. typical Australian diet	3 weeks	Lower overall gastrointestinal symptom scores while on a diet low in FODMAPs	Lack of blinding
Pedersen et al. [23]	Patients with IBS	I₁ = 42 I₂ = 41 C = 40	Randomized, controlled trial comparing the low FODMAP diet, treatment with Lactobacillus GG or a control diet	6 weeks	Both the low FODMAP diet and treatment with Lactobacillus GG were similarly effective	Lack of blinding
Chumpitazi et al. [24]	Children with IBS	n = 33	Randomized, double-blind, crossover trial, children with Rome III IBS completed a one-week baseline period. They then were randomised to a low FODMAP diet or typical American childhood diet	2 days	Less abdominal pain occurred during the low FODMAP diet vs. typical diet	Complete blinding unlikely. Short duration of challenge (two days)
Whigham et al. [25]	Patients with IBS	n = 365	Evaluation of low FODMAP diet administered in a dietitian-led group education or traditional one-to-one education	6 weeks	Significant decrease in symptom severity from baseline to follow-up for both groups but no difference in symptom response between group and one-to-one education	Lack of a control group; no randomization
Böhn et al. [26]	Patients with IBS	I = 33 C = 34	Multi-center, parallel, single-blind study. Subjects were randomly assigned to for four weeks to a low-FODMAP or standard IBS diet	4 weeks	The severity of IBS symptoms was reduced in both groups during the intervention in both groups before vs. at the end of the four-week diet, without a significant difference between the groups	Single blinding

Table 1. *Cont.*

First Author, Year	Patients	n	Study Design	Diet Duration	Results	Comment on the Study Design
McIntosh K et al. [27]	Patients with IBS	I = 19, C = 18	Controlled, single blind study with randomization to a low or high-FODMAP diet for three weeks	3 weeks	The IBS severity symptom score (SSS) was reduced in the low-FODMAP diet group but not the high-FODMAP group	Single blinding
Peters et al. [28]	Patients with IBS	$I_1 = 25$, $I_2 = 24$, $I_3 = 25$	Consecutive patients were randomised to receive hypnotherapy, low-FODMAP diet or a combination	6 weeks	Improvements in overall symptoms were observed from baseline to week six for hypnotherapy, diet and combination with no difference across groups	No control group, no blinding
Laatikainen et al. [29]	Patients with IBS	$n = 87$	randomised double blind controlled cross-over study. Participants were supplied with both regular rye bread and low-FODMAP rye bread for four weeks	4 weeks	Many signs of IBS were milder on the low-FODMAP rye bread but no differences were detected in IBS-SSS or quality of life	Well-designed study; only rye FODMAPs were tested
Valeur et al. [30]	Patients with IBS	$n = 63$	Consecutive patients participating in a four-week FODMAP-restricted diet	4 weeks	Following the dietary intervention, IBS-SSS scores improved significantly	Lack of control group, and lack of blinding
Eswaran et al. [31]	Patients with IBS-D	$I_1 = 45$, $I_2 = 39$	Single-center, randomized-controlled trial comparing a low-FODMAP with the mNICE diet for four weeks.	4 weeks	40%–50% of patients reported adequate relief of their IBS-D symptoms with the low-FODMAP diet or a diet based on modified NICE guidelines. The low-FODMAP diet led to significantly greater improvement in individual IBS symptoms, particularly pain and bloating	Lack of blinding
Major et al. [32]	Patients with IBS	$n = 58$	Three-period, cross-over study with a single dose of high- or low-FODMAP drink	1 day	More patients reached the predefined symptom threshold after intake of inulin or fructose than glucose. Controls had lower symptom scores during the period after drink consumption, despite similar MRI parameters and breath hydrogen responses	Lack of blinding
Hustoft et al. [33]	Patients with IBS	$n = 20$	After three weeks of low-FODMAP patients were randomized and double-blindly assigned to receive a supplement of either FOS (FODMAP) or maltodextrin (placebo) for the next 10 days, followed by a three-week washout period before crossover	10 days	Irritable bowel syndrome symptoms consistently improved after three weeks of low FOMAP, and significantly more participants reported symptom relief in response to placebo than FOS	Only one type of FODMAP was investigated in this study

FODMAP: Fermentable Oligo-, Di- and Mono-saccharides And Polyols; IBS: Irritable bowel syndrome; IBS-D: Irritable bowel syndrome with diarrhea; RCT: randomized controlled trial; NCGS: non celiac gluten sensitivity; DBPC: double-blind placebo-controlled; I: intervention; C: control; SSS: severity symptom score; NICE: National Institute for Health and Care Excellence; FOS: fructo-oligosaccharides; GOS: galacto-oligosaccharides.

4. Is a Low-FODMAP Diet a Safe Approach?

The drastic reduction of FODMAP intake could have consequences that are still poorly understood on (a) the colonocyte metabolism (see Paragraph 2), (b) the intestinal microbiota, and (c) the nutritional status.

There is good evidence supporting the concept that the intestinal microbiota is perturbed in patients with IBS. Several recent studies have reported an increase in the relative abundance of Firmicutes, mainly *Clostridium* cluster XIVa, and Ruminococcaceae, together with a reduction in the relative abundance of *Bifidobacteria*. A lower diversity and a higher instability of the microbiota in IBS patients compared to controls have also been reported [36]. A low-FODMAP diet paradoxically does not correct these microbiota modifications, but induces similar changes, i.e., reducing the *Bifidobacteria* counts [20], and the total bacterial abundance [22], while increasing the abundance of Ruminococcaceae [36]. This dietary treatment induces decreased levels of fecal *Faecalibacterium prausnitzii* and total SCFAs/n-butyric acid [33]. Extensive analyses of microbiota composition, functionality, and fermentation products in relation to symptom generation are currently lacking. Finally, the long-term effects of the microbiota changes induced by the low-FODMAP diet, if any, remain to be determined.

A low-FODMAP diet imposes an important restriction of dietary choices due to the elimination of some staple foods, such as wheat derivatives, lactose-containing dairy products, many vegetables and pulses, and several types of fruits (Table 2).

Table 2. Common food that need to be excluded from the low-FODMAP diet.

Food Type	To be Excluded (High-FODMAP Content)
Cereals and their derivatives	Wheat, barley, rye
Legumes	All (lentils, beans, chickpeas, soy, peas)
Vegetables	Artichokes, asparagus, cauliflower, garlic, leeks, mushrooms, onions, scallions, shallots, snow peas
Fruit	Apples, apricots, Asian pears, blackberries, cherries, figs, jackfruit, mangoes, nectarines, peaches, pears, persimmon, plums, prunes, tamarillo, watermelon, white peaches, grape
Dairy products	Regular milk, ice cream, soft cheeses, yogurt

Despite the lack of studies on the long-term nutritional consequences of the low-FODMAP diet, possible risks of this treatment may be inferred from data available for other exclusion diets. As for cereal intake, the exclusion of wheat, rye, and barley is the same as the gluten-free diet (GFD) used for celiac disease treatment. Nutritional surveys have shown that subjects on a GFD may be at risk of reduced intake of fiber, calcium, iron, zinc, folate, and other B-group vitamins [37]. A deficient intake of dietary fiber may be expected to occur even more frequently on the low-FODMAP diet, due to a significant restriction of other fiber sources, such as fruit, vegetables, and legumes. The consequences of a fiber-poor diet may be particularly deleterious in subjects complaining of constipation as a manifestation of IBS. The restriction of lactose-containing dairy products may enhance the tendency to poor calcium availability since (a) these items are a primary source of calcium; and (b) the promoting effect of lactose on calcium absorption is lost [38,39]. A low-FODMAP diet may also be poor in natural antioxidants, such as flavonoids, carotenoids, and vitamin C contained in some FODMAP-rich vegetables (e.g., cauliflower, onion, garlic), or phenolic acid and anthocyanins present in fruits and blackberries. Wheat (which is excluded from the low-FODMAP diet) is a major source of phenolic acids, such as ferulic acid, caffeic acid, p-coumaric acid, p-hydroxybenzoic acid, vanillic acid, and protocatechuic acid [40]. Finally, the exclusion of dairy products in a low-FODMAP diet may favor a vitamin D deficiency [41].

We speculate that the nutritional risk of the low-FODMAP diet, in the long term, may follow an inverse socio-economic gradient, since persons with economical restraints may have limited access to many of the expensive, alternative dietary items included in the low-FODMAP diet (e.g., berries, exotic fruit, and pseudo-cereals).

5. Conclusions

The low-FODMAP diet can have a positive impact on the symptoms of IBS, particularly bloating and diarrhea. However, it remains to be proven whether this regimen is superior to conventional IBS diets. The drastic reduction of FODMAP intake could have physiological consequences on the colonocyte metabolism, the intestinal microbiota, and the nutritional status, which need further investigation. Based on our review, it might be helpful to consider the use of nutritional supplements to avoid possible deficiencies induced by a strict low-FODMAP diet over the long term.

Author Contributions: All authors conceived this work, G.C. performed the literature search and the data extraction, C.C. wrote the first draft of the manuscript, all authors critically revised the draft. All authors revised and approved the final version.

Conflicts of Interest: Carlo Catassi has received consultancy funds from Schär Company (Burgstall, BZ, Italy). Other authors declare no conflict of interest.

References

1. Gibson, P.; Shepherd, S.J. Personal view: Food for thought—Western lifestyle and susceptibility to Crohn's disease. The FODMAP hypothesis. *Aliment. Pharmacol. Ther.* **2005**, *21*, 1399–1409. [CrossRef] [PubMed]
2. Gibson, P.R.; Shepherd, S.J. Evidence-based dietary management of functional gastrointestinal symptoms: The FODMAP approach. *J. Gastroenterol. Hepatol.* **2010**, *25*, 252–258. [CrossRef] [PubMed]
3. Biesiekierski, J.R.; Peters, S.L.; Newnham, E.D.; Rosella, O.; Muir, J.G.; Gibson, P.R. No effects of gluten in patients with self-reported non-celiac gluten sensitivity after dietary reduction of fermentable, poorly absorbed, short-chain carbohydrates. *Gastroenterology* **2013**, *145*, 320–328. [CrossRef] [PubMed]
4. Shepherd, S.; Gibson, P. *The Complete Low FODMAP Diet: A Revolutionary Plan for Managing IBS and Other Digestive Disorders*, 1st ed.; The Experiment, LLC: New York, NY, USA, 2013.
5. McKenzie, Y.A.; Bowyer, R.K.; Leach, H.; Gulia, P.; Horobin, J.; O'Sullivan, N.A.; Pettitt, C.; Reeves, L.B.; Seamark, L.; Williams, M.; et al. British Dietetic Association systematic review and evidence-based practice guidelines for the dietary management of irritable bowel syndrome in adults (2016 update). *J. Hum. Nutr. Diet.* **2016**, *29*, 549–575. [CrossRef] [PubMed]
6. Marsh, A.; Eslick, E.M.; Eslick, G.D. Does a diet low in FODMAPs reduce symptoms associated with functional gastrointestinal disorders? A comprehensive systematic review and meta-analysis. *Eur. J. Nutr.* **2016**, *55*, 897–906. [CrossRef] [PubMed]
7. Uno, Y.; van Velkinburgh, J.C. Logical hypothesis: Low FODMAP diet to prevent diverticulitis. *World. J. Gastrointest. Pharmacol. Ther.* **2016**, *7*, 503–512. [CrossRef] [PubMed]
8. Lis, D.; Ahuja, K.D.; Stellingwerff, T.; Kitic, C.M.; Fell, J. Case Study: Utilizing a Low FODMAP Diet to Combat Exercise-Induced Gastrointestinal Symptoms. *Int. J. Sport. Nutr. Exerc. Metab.* **2016**, *26*, 481–487. [CrossRef] [PubMed]
9. Durchschein, F.; Petritsch, W.; Hammer, H.F. Diet therapy for inflammatory bowel diseases: The established and the new. *World. J. Gastroenterol.* **2016**, *22*, 2179–2194. [PubMed]
10. Staudacher, H.M.; Irving, P.M.; Lomer, M.C.; Whelan, K. Mechanisms and efficacy of dietary FODMAP restriction in IBS. *Nat. Rev. Gastroenterol. Hepatol.* **2014**, *11*, 256–266. [CrossRef] [PubMed]
11. Sabater-Molina, M.; Larqué, E.; Torrella, F.; Zamora, S. Dietary fructooligosaccharides and potential benefits on health. *J. Physiol. Biochem.* **2009**, *65*, 315–328. [CrossRef] [PubMed]
12. Andoh, A.; Tsujikawa, T.; Fujiyama, Y. Role of dietary fiber and short-chain fatty acids in the colon. *Curr. Pharm. Des.* **2003**, *9*, 347–358. [CrossRef] [PubMed]
13. Blachier, F.; Beaumont, M.; Andriamihaja, M.; Davila, A.M.; Lan, A.; Grauso, M.; Armand, L.; Benamouzig, R.; Tomé, D. Changes in the Luminal Environment of the Colonic Epithelial Cells and Physiopathological Consequences. *Am. J. Pathol.* **2017**, *187*, 476–486. [CrossRef] [PubMed]

14. Yao, C.K.; Tan, H.-L.; van Langenberg, D.R.; Barrett, J.S.; Rose, R.; Liels, K.; Gibson, P.-R.; Muir, J.G. Dietary sorbitol and mannitol: Food content and distinct absorption patterns between healthy individuals and patients with irritable bowel syndrome. *J. Hum. Nutr. Diet.* **2014**, *27*, S263–S275. [CrossRef] [PubMed]
15. Biesiekierski, J.R.; Rosella, O.; Rose, R.; Liels, K.; Barrett, J.S.; Shepherd, S.J.; Gibson, P.R.; Muir, J.G. Quantification of fructans, galacto-oligosaccharides and other short-chain carbohydrates in processed grains and cereals. *J. Hum. Nutr. Diet.* **2011**, *24*, 154–176. [CrossRef] [PubMed]
16. Muir, J.G.; Rose, R.; Rosella, O.; Liels, K.; Barrett, J.S.; Shepherd, S.J.; Gibson, P.R. Measurement of Short-Chain Carbohydrates in Common Australian Vegetables and Fruits by High-Performance Liquid Chromatography (HPLC). *J. Agric. Food Chem.* **2009**, *57*, 554–565. [CrossRef] [PubMed]
17. Liang, Z.; Sang, M.; Fan, P.; Wu, B.; Wang, L.; Duan, W.; Li, S. Changes of polyphenols, sugars, and organic acid in 5 Vitis genotypes during berry ripening. *J. Food Sci.* **2011**, *76*, C1231–C1238. [CrossRef] [PubMed]
18. Shepherd, S.J.; Parker, F.C.; Muir, J.G.; Gibson, P.R. Dietary triggers of abdominal symptoms in patients with irritable bowel syndrome: Randomized placebo-controlled evidence. *Clin. Gastroenterol. Hepatol.* **2008**, *6*, 765–771. [CrossRef] [PubMed]
19. Staudacher, H.M.; Whelan, K.; Irving, P.M.; Lomer, M.C. Comparison of symptom response following advice for a diet low in fermentable carbohydrates (FODMAPs) versus standard dietary advice in patients with irritable bowel syndrome. *J. Hum. Nutr. Diet.* **2011**, *24*, 487–495. [CrossRef] [PubMed]
20. Staudacher, H.M.; Lomer, M.C.; Anderson, J.L.; Barrett, J.S.; Muir, J.G.; Irving, P.M.; Whelan, K. Fermentable carbohydrate restriction reduces luminal bifidobacteria and gastrointestinal symptoms in patients with irritable bowel syndrome. *J. Nutr.* **2012**, *142*, 1510–1518. [CrossRef] [PubMed]
21. De Roest, R.H.; Dobbs, B.R.; Chapman, B.A.; Batman, B.; O'Brien, L.A.; Leeper, J.A.; Hebblethwaite, C.R.; Gearry, R.B. The low FODMAP diet improves gastrointestinal symptoms in patients with irritable bowel syndrome: A prospective study. *Int. J. Clin. Pract.* **2013**, *67*, 895–903. [CrossRef] [PubMed]
22. Halmos, E.P.; Christophersen, C.T.; Bird, A.R.; Shepherd, S.J.; Gibson, P.R.; Muir, J.G. Diets that differ in their FODMAP content alter the colonic luminal microenvironment. *Gut* **2015**, *64*, 93–100. [CrossRef] [PubMed]
23. Pedersen, N.; Andersen, N.N.; Végh, Z.; Jensen, L.; Ankersen, D.V.; Felding, M.; Simonsen, M.H.; Burisch, J.; Munkholm, P. Ehealth: Low FODMAP diet vs. Lactobacillus rhamnosus GG in irritable bowel syndrome. *World. J. Gastroenterol.* **2014**, *20*, 16215–16226. [CrossRef] [PubMed]
24. Chumpitazi, B.P.; Cope, J.L.; Hollister, E.B.; Tsai, C.M.; McMeans, A.R.; Luna, R.A.; Versalovic, J.; Shulman, R.J. Randomised clinical trial: Gut microbiome biomarkers are associated with clinical response to a low FODMAP diet in children with the irritable bowel syndrome. *Aliment. Pharmacol. Ther.* **2015**, *42*, 418–427. [CrossRef] [PubMed]
25. Böhn, L.; Störsrud, S.; Liljebo, T.; Collin, L.; Lindfors, P.; Törnblom, H.; Simrén, M. Diet low in FODMAPs reduces symptoms of irritable bowel syndrome as well as traditional dietary advice: A randomized controlled trial. *Gastroenterology* **2015**, *149*, 1399–1407. [CrossRef] [PubMed]
26. Whigham, L.; Joyce, T.; Harper, G.; Irving, P.M.; Staudacher, H.M.; Whelan, K.; Lomer, M.C. Clinical effectiveness and economic costs of group versus one-to-one education for short-chain fermentable carbohydrate restriction (low FODMAP diet) in the management of irritable bowel syndrome. *J. Hum. Nutr. Diet.* **2015**, *28*, 687–696. [CrossRef] [PubMed]
27. McIntosh, K.; Reed, D.E.; Schneider, T.; Dang, F.; Keshteli, A.H.; de Palma, G.; Madsen, K.; Bercik, P.; Vanner, S. FODMAPs alter symptoms and the metabolome of patients with IBS: A randomised controlled trial. *Gut* **2016**. [CrossRef] [PubMed]
28. Peters, S.L.; Yao, C.K.; Philpott, H.; Yelland, G.W.; Muir, J.G.; Gibson, P.R. Randomised clinical trial: The efficacy of gut-directed hypnotherapy is similar to that of the low FODMAP diet for the treatment of irritable bowel syndrome. *Aliment. Pharmacol. Ther.* **2016**, *44*, 447–459. [CrossRef] [PubMed]
29. Laatikainen, R.; Koskenpato, J.; Hongisto, S.M.; Loponen, J.; Poussa, T.; Hillilä, M.; Korpela, R. Randomised clinical trial: Low FODMAP rye bread vs. regular rye bread to relieve the symptoms of irritable bowel syndrome. *Aliment. Pharmacol. Ther.* **2016**, *44*, 460–470. [CrossRef] [PubMed]
30. Valeur, J.; Røseth, A.G.; Knudsen, T.; Malmstrøm, G.H.; Fiennes, J.T.; Midtvedt, T.; Berstad, A. Fecal Fermentation in Irritable Bowel Syndrome: Influence of Dietary Restriction of Fermentable Oligosaccharides, Disaccharides, Monosaccharides and Polyols. *Digestion* **2016**, *94*, 50–56. [CrossRef] [PubMed]

31. Eswaran, S.L.; Chey, W.D.; Han-Markey, T.; Ball, S.; Jackson, K. A Randomized Controlled Trial Comparing the Low FODMAP Diet vs. Modified NICE Guidelines in US Adults with IBS-D. *Am. J. Gastroenterol.* **2016**, *111*, 1824–1832. [CrossRef] [PubMed]

32. Major, G.; Pritchard, S.; Murray, K.; Alappadan, J.P.; Hoad, C.L.; Marciani, L.; Gowland, P.; Spiller, R. Colon Hypersensitivity to Distension, Rather Than Excessive Gas Production, Produces Carbohydrate-Related Symptoms in Individuals With Irritable Bowel Syndrome. *Gastroenterology* **2017**, *152*, 124–133. [CrossRef] [PubMed]

33. Hustoft, T.N.; Hausken, T.; Ystad, S.O.; Valeur, J.; Brokstad, K.; Hatlebakk, J.G.; Lied, G.A. Effects of varying dietary content of fermentable short-chain carbohydrates on symptoms, fecal microenvironment, and cytokine profiles in patients with irritable bowel syndrome. *Neurogastroenterol. Motil.* **2016**. [CrossRef] [PubMed]

34. The National Institute for Health and Care Excellence. *NICE Clinical Guidelines, No 61. Irritable Bowel Syndrome in Adults: Diagnosis and Management of Irritable Bowel Syndrome in Primary Care*; Last Updated: February 2015; National Collaborating Centre for Nursing and Supportive Care: London, UK; Royal College of Nursing: London, UK, February 2008.

35. Maagaard, L.; Ankersen, D.V.; Végh, Z.; Burisch, J.; Jensen, L.; Pedersen, N.; Munkholm, P. Follow-up of patients with functional bowel symptoms treated with a low FODMAP diet. *World J. Gastroenterol.* **2016**, *22*, 4009–4019. [CrossRef] [PubMed]

36. Rajilić-Stojanović, M.; Jonkers, D.M.; Salonen, A.; Hanevik, K.; Raes, J.; Jalanka, J.; de Vos, W.M.; Manichanh, C.; Golic, N.; Enck, P.; et al. Intestinal microbiota and diet in IBS: Causes, consequences, or epiphenomena? *Am. J. Gastroenterol.* **2015**, *110*, 278–287. [CrossRef] [PubMed]

37. Vici, G.; Belli, L.; Biondi, M.; Polzonetti, V. Gluten free diet and nutrient deficiencies: A review. *Clin. Nutr.* **2016**, *35*, 1236–1241. [CrossRef] [PubMed]

38. Infante, D.; Tormo, R. Risk of inadequate bone mineralization in diseases involving long-term suppression of dairy products. *J. Pediatr. Gastroenterol. Nutr.* **2000**, *30*, 310–313. [CrossRef] [PubMed]

39. Abrams, S.A.; Griffin, I.J.; Davila, P.M. Calcium and zinc absorption from lactose-containing and lactose-free infant formulas. *Am. J. Clin. Nutr.* **2002**, *76*, 442–446. [PubMed]

40. Brewer, M.S. Natural antioxidants: Sources, compounds, mechanisms of action, and potential applications. *Compr. Rev. Food Sci. Food Saf.* **2011**, *10*, 221–247. [CrossRef]

41. Gröber, U.; Reichrath, J.; Holick, M.F. Live Longer with Vitamin D? *Nutrients* **2015**, *7*, 1871–1880. [CrossRef] [PubMed]

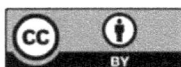

nutrients

MDPI

Editorial

Gluten-Free Diet Indications, Safety, Quality, Labels, and Challenges

Kamran Rostami [1], Justine Bold [2,*], Alison Parr [3] and Matt W. Johnson [4]

[1] Department of Gastroenterology, Milton Keynes University Hospital, Milton Keynes MK6 5LD, UK; kamran.rostami@nhs.net
[2] Allied Health and Social Sciences, Institute of Health and Society University of Worcester, Worcester WR2 6AJ, UK
[3] Freelance Nutrition Therapist, Manchester M33 5PD, UK; alison_parr@hotmail.com
[4] Department of Gastroenterology, Luton and Dunstable University Hospital, Luton LU4 0DZ, UK; matthew.johnson@ldh.nhs.uk
*   Correspondence: j.bold@worc.ac.uk; Tel.: +44-1905-855-391

Received: 23 July 2017; Accepted: 31 July 2017; Published: 8 August 2017

Abstract: A gluten-free diet (GFD) is the safest treatment modality in patient with coeliac disease (CD) and other gluten-related disorders. Contamination and diet compliance are important factors behind persistent symptoms in patients with gluten related-disorders, in particular CD. How much gluten can be tolerated, how safe are the current gluten-free (GF) products, what are the benefits and side effects of GFD? Recent studies published in *Nutrients* on gluten-free products' quality, availability, safety, as well as challenges related to a GFD are discussed.

Keywords: gluten-free diet; coeliac disease; non-coeliac gluten sensitivity

1. Editorial

Gluten-free diets hit centre stage in the early 1990s, and universally changed our food culture. Not only was there interest in coeliac disease (CD) [1], but there was also a resurgence of interest in the other gluten-related disorders [2,3]. Current evidence suggests that gluten and other wheat proteins play an important role in triggering symptoms in some people without CD [4]. There has been a rapid increase in dietary interest to use it as a treatment modality in the management of both irritable bowels syndrome (IBS) and functional bowel disorders. This strategy has evolved as a result of improvements in our understanding of how these grains induced pathogenicity [5,6]. The grains that contain gluten seem to have the potential of antigenicity, relating not only to the gluten itself [7] but also to their other proteins and additives. Junker et al. suggest that α-amylase/trypsin inhibitors (ATIs) in wheat represent strong activators of innate immune responses in monocytes, macrophages, and dendritic cells [8]. Therefore, a large proportion of the world's population is currently avoiding gluten-containing grains for a variety of different reasons; including sensitivities, intolerances, and allergic reactions (Figure 1).

Gluten intake, in particular prolamin, is a well-known triggering antigen that initiates adaptive T cells (Th1-mediated) immune response in individuals carrying HLA-DQ2 or HLA-DQ8 against small bowel cells. This in turn leads to an architectural distortion in CD. Epithelial cell damage is the first event to occur within the small bowel, leading to antigen increased intestinal permeability and malabsorption (even in the absence of severe inflammation). Some studies suggest gluten may affect diabetes development by influencing proportional changes in immune cell populations or by modifying the cytokine/chemokine pattern towards an inflammatory profile. Gluten-induced intestinal inflammation might in fact play a primary role in the pathogenesis of type 1 diabetes, by islet-infiltrating T cells expressing gut-associated homing receptors [9]. This is why untreated CD increases the risk for other autoimmune disorders and long-term complications.

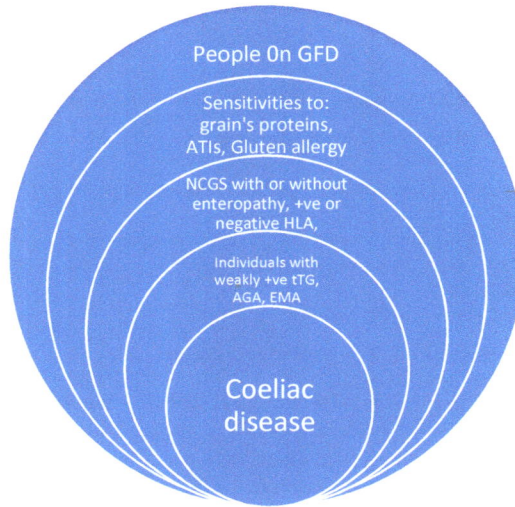

Figure 1. Gluten-related disorder, tTG: Tissue transglutaminase antibodies, AGA: Antigliadin antibodies, EMA: Endomysial antibodies, NCGS: Non-coeliac gluten sensitivity, ATIs: Amylase/trypsin inhibitors.

Gluten cannot be hidden in foods nowadays, as allergen labelling was introduced in the European Union (EU) in 2005. Now all wheat, rye, barley, and oat ingredients must be listed in the ingredients list. The amount of gluten capable of initiating an antigenic reaction has been estimated to be >20 mg/kg (or parts per million = ppm) of gluten, and contamination below 20 ppm is considered safe over a wide range of foods in daily consumption.

The EU gluten-free legislation published in 2009 and regulated in 2012 specifies two levels—gluten-free ($\leq$20 ppm/mg/kg) and low gluten (21–100 ppm/mg/kg), but in practice only the gluten-free standard is applied. If products do not have any gluten-containing ingredients, then an associated threshold would not be necessary.

2. How Do Gluten-Free Products Compare to a Normal Diet?

Coeliac disease was a difficult diagnosis to live with 20 years ago. This was largely due to the limited range of gluten-free products available to coeliac patients as well as the generally poor quality of these products.

Over recent years, the gluten-free food business has become a major industry and has gained enormous popularity with both coeliac and non-coeliac individuals, as there have been improvements in both the range of foods available and their overall palatability. Despite some concerns about potential side effects of GFD, the current evidence suggests that there is no need to be concerned as long as it proves beneficial in controlling symptoms and improving the quality of life. Some individuals consider GFD to be a very balanced and healthy diet, especially if gluten-free wholegrains are consumed, whilst others find it useful for weight control due to its restrictive nature.

GFD is not recommended for the general population, and there is no evidence that it is beneficial in non-symptomatic non-coeliac individuals. Instead, there are some concerns raised relating to its nutritional value. Recent studies suggest that GFDs might be a risk factor for metabolic syndrome [10]. They state that the nutritional composition of processed gluten–free food items may include high levels of lipids, sugars, and salt [11]. Saturni et al. report that a gluten-free diet may not guarantee adequate nutritional intake and that 20–38% of coeliac patients experience nutritional deficiencies that include proteins, dietary fibres, minerals, and vitamins [12]. It is unclear if persistent malabsorption syndrome accounts for some part of these deficiencies. For instance, secondary lactose intolerance might be one of the factors contributing toward vitamin D deficiency in CD [13].

Contrary to this, gluten-free substitute foods are not necessarily higher in sugar or lower in fibre according to Coeliac UK. There have been improvements in the quality of gluten-free products, such as the development of a broader range of fresh gluten-free items as well as products higher in fat, increasing palatability. There is, however, still room for improving the nutritional value and component qualities of gluten-free products.

It should be remembered that any treatment modality, including diet, might potentially have undesirable effects. Furthermore, this information, when available, should be highlighted to potential candidates [14]. If we compare the side effects of GF products with the drugs licenced to treat irritable bowel syndrome (IBS) and their enormous cost, a treatment with GFD is much less toxic and patients are able to tailor their personal dietary preferences with a little guidance [15]. Education is a key factor in achieving a much healthier dietary balance. A dietetic consultation or any consultation where food and diet are discussed should not entirely focus on the elimination of gluten, but also provide guidance for healthy choices based on the individual's needs.

Health professionals should also be mindful that a high sugar and fat content are not only found in some GF products, but are common in many other foods as well, indicating that the general population not on GFD is also exposed to a wide range of high calorie products and risks for metabolic syndrome. Ultimately, genetics and lifestyle factors, regardless of gluten intake, have the most significant influence in preventing or acquiring morbid obesity. Health professionals are most likely aware that the prevalence of obesity is unfortunately increasing in both coeliac and non-coeliac populations [16,17]. Once again, this highlights how education and the promotion of a healthier lifestyle is a public health priority for both the general population and gluten-sensitive individuals.

3. Cost and Availability

Gluten-free now constitutes a major food industry due to its popularity among not only CD patients but also individuals with other gluten-related conditions (Figure 1). The cost of living for patients following a GFD is much higher and it is quite challenging for people with a lower income to purchase the products without government support.

The products available to some in the UK on prescription may also not be easily available for purchase off-the-shelf, and it should be noted there is now a trend for GF prescription to be withdrawn, indicating that some patients are affected due to the lack of affordability. From a patient's perspective, the availability of GF products does not always square with accessibility, i.e., being at the shop shelf at the point of need. The government's support with prescription products has been a significant encouragement and support for patients, and withdrawing the prescription for the limited amount of permitted, prescribed food may result in reduced diet compliance, leading to increased complications and higher expenses for the healthcare system in the long term.

4. Safety and Contamination

Despite the availability of numerous GF products in the current market, maintaining a GFD is still challenging for many patients. Therefore, dietary transgressions of GFD is a major factor for refractory symptoms and persistently abnormal histology. Still, it should be noted that recently there have been substantial improvements in the commercial availability of a variety of GF products that offer a wide range of choices to gluten-sensitive people. Reassuringly, a recent study demonstrates that the safety profile of these products is improving thanks to quality assurance legislations. This recent study published in *Nutrients* analyses the contamination risk and changes in the gluten content of an impressive number of GF products (3141) from 1998 to 2016 [18,19]. The former is one of the largest published studies presenting data from food samples collected over an 18-year period.

The time period covers a lot of change in terms of the standard for gluten-free products in addition to the introduction of different methodologies for the analysis of gluten-free products, which may help to explain some of the idiosyncrasies in the data analysis and reporting over the period. The Codex standard for gluten-free changed in 2008, and was prefaced by agreement on the R5 Mendez method for the analysis of gluten in 2005–2016, endorsed by the Codex Committee on Methodology and Analysis. Eight useful food categories are identified, and the authors demonstrate that cereal-based foods for people with CD are becoming safer.

It is, however, concerning that in the period of 2013–2016 there were increases in the number of white flour samples with gluten contamination at 100 mg/kg—as this is such a staple food ingredient in gluten-free baking, contamination at this level can be problematic. Two different ELISA analyses were used in the study to determine the level of gluten contamination across the period of 1998–2016—one method was used from 1998–2001 and a different method was used from 2001–2016. The R5 ELISA Mendez method is mentioned as the type one methodology for the analysis of gluten in foodstuff in the Revised Codex Alimentarius standard (2008), but not in the EU legislation. Whilst both methods are recommended by the Codex Alimentarius and AOAC international, the reporting periods in the study do not mirror these time periods. As three periods have been used: 1998–2002, 2003–2008, and 2009–2016, perhaps it might have been beneficial to report particularly on the 1998–2001 period itself given that this period used a different ELISA technique.

The Italian study [19] includes 200 certified GF foods and many foods that are naturally gluten-free—such as buckwheat, quinoa, etc. These are rarely included in other studies, and there is a paucity of data on these products in the current literature. Therefore, assessing the safety of these products is another valuable part of this review that may improve the nutritional quality and the experience of a GF diet for gluten-sensitive individuals. The benefits of these products, as highlighted by the authors, is very informative for any professional giving dietary advice. particularly as they are wholegrain cereals, such food products are welcome additions to a GFD given the concerns about the high sugar content of some GF foods. The study provides statistical analysis, consideration of factors such as cost, and a categorisation of foods into types (and meal types). The Italian study reports some important findings, namely that four out of five oat samples tested were contaminated with gluten, as were several sample of buckwheat and lentils (the latter was unexpected and the authors state that the origin of the contamination is unknown). Sadly, the authors do not specify the individual brands, or whether the samples were certified as GF. Lunch and dinner foods were more contaminated compared to snack products. Hence, professionals working with coeliac patients should consider highlighting the importance of buying certified gluten-free oats and oats-based products.

Studies such as those mentioned above show the importance of ongoing regulation and control of certified GF foods as well as the importance of on-going policing of those foods. Interestingly, they show that cheaper foods have higher contaminations, suggesting that better control costs more. This indicates that patients with lower incomes might be exposed to a higher risk for contamination, particularly as many gluten-free prescriptions in the UK are now under threat.

5. Conclusions

Gluten, additives, and a range of other grain proteins have all been associated with a range of gastrointestinal and autoimmune disorders, particularly CD. Despite the concerns related to the content of some GF products, this modality of treatment is still the safest strategy available to coeliac patients and other gluten related disorders (GRD) patients. The concerns related to metabolic syndrome should not be limited to GFD and should include the modern lifestyle. Transgression related to high contents of gluten in GF products has been a culprit for refractory symptoms in CD patients. Reassuringly, a recent study has suggested that gluten contamination is uncommon or mild; however, it is occurring and needs both on-going and tighter regulation in order to protect those people who are sensitive to gluten.

Conflicts of Interest: The authors declare no conflicts of interest.

References

1. Catassi, C.; Ratsch, I.M.; Fabiani, E.; Rossini, M.; Coppa, G.V.; Giorgi, P.L.; Bordicchia, F.; Candela, F. Coeliac disease in the year 2000: Exploring the iceberg. *Lancet* **1994**, *343*, 200–203. [CrossRef]

2. Cooper, B.T.; Holmes, G.K.; Ferguson, R.; Thompson, R.A.; Allan, R.N.; Cooke, W.T. Gluten-sensitive diarrhea without evidence of celiac disease. *Gastroenterology* **1980**, *79*, 801–806. [PubMed]

3. Sapone, A.; Bai, J.C.; Ciacci, C.; Dolinsek, J.; Green, P.; Hadjivassiliou, M.; Kaukinen, K.; Rostami, K.; Sanders, D.; Schumann, M.; et al. Spectrum of gluten-related disorders: Consensus on new nomenclature and classification. *BMC Med.* **2012**, *10*, 13. [CrossRef] [PubMed]

4. Shahbazkhani, B.; Sadeghi, A.; Malekzadeh, R.; Khatavi, F.; Etemadi, M.; Kalantri, E.; Rostami-Nejad, M.; Rostami, K. Non-Celiac Gluten Sensitivity Has Narrowed the Spectrum of Irritable Bowel Syndrome: A Double-Blind Randomized Placebo-Controlled Trial. *Nutrients* **2015**, *7*, 4542–4554. [CrossRef] [PubMed]

5. Uhde, M.; Ajamian, M.; Caio, G.; Giorgio, R.; Indart, A.; Green, P.; Verna, E.; Umberto, V.; Alaedini, A. Intestinal cell damage and systemic immune activation in individuals reporting sensitivity to wheat in the absence of coeliac disease. *Gut* **2016**, *65*, 1930–1937. [CrossRef] [PubMed]

6. Di Liberto, D.; Mansueto, P.; D'Alcamo, A.; Lo Pizzo, M.; Lo Presti, E.; Geraci, G.; Fayer, F.; Guggino, G.; Iacono, G.; Dieli, F.; et al. Predominance of type 1 innate lymphoid cells in the rectal mucosa of patients with non-celiac wheat sensitivity: Reversal after a wheat-free diet. *Clin. Transl. Gastroenterol.* **2016**, *7*, e178. [CrossRef] [PubMed]

7. Dieterich, W.; Ehnis, T.; Bauer, M.; Donner, P.; Volta, U.; Otto Riecken, E.; Schuppan, D. Identification of tissue transglutaminase as the autoantigen of celiac disease. *Nat. Med.* **1997**, *3*, 797–801. [CrossRef] [PubMed]

8. Junker, Y.; Zeissig, S.; Kim, S.J.; Barisani, D.; Wieser, H.; Leffler, D.; Zevallos, V.; Libermann, T.; Dillon, S.; Freitag, T.; et al. Wheat amylase trypsin inhibitors drive intestinal inflammation via activation of toll-like receptor 4. *J. Exp. Med.* **2012**, *209*, 2395–2408. [CrossRef] [PubMed]

9. Antvorskov, J.C.; Josefsen, K.; Engkilde, K.; Funda, D.P.; Buschard, K. Dietary gluten and the development of type 1 diabetes. *Diabetologia* **2014**, *57*, 1770–1780. [CrossRef] [PubMed]

10. Tortora, R.; Capone, P.; De Stefano, G.; Imperatore, N.; Gerbino, N.; Donetto, S.; Monaco, V.; Capooraso, N.; Rispo, A. Metabolic syndrome in patients with coeliac disease on a gluten-free diet. *Aliment. Pharmacol. Ther.* **2015**, *41*, 352–359. [CrossRef] [PubMed]

11. Mariani, P.; Viti, M.G.; Montuori, M.; La, V.A.; Cipolletta, E.; Calvani, L.; Bonamico, M. The gluten-free diet: A nutritional risk factor for adolescents with celiac disease? *J. Pediatr. Gastroenterol. Nutr.* **1998**, *27*, 519–523. [CrossRef] [PubMed]

12. Saturni, L.; Ferretti, G.; Bacchetti, T. The gluten-free diet: Safety and nutritional quality. *Nutrients* **2010**, *2*, 16–34. [CrossRef] [PubMed]

13. Ojetti, V.; Nucera, G.; Migneco, A.; Gabrielli, M.; Lauritano, C.; Danese, S.; Assunta Zocco, M.A.; Nista, E.C.; Cammarota, G.; de Lorenzo, A.; et al. High prevalence of celiac disease in patients with lactose intolerance. *Digestion* **2005**, *71*, 106–110. [CrossRef] [PubMed]

14. Rostami, K.; Aldulaimi, D.; Rostami-Nejad, M. Gluten free diet is a cure not a poison! *Gastroenterol. Hepatol. Bed Bench* **2015**, *8*, 93–94. [PubMed]

15. Soubieres, A.; Wilson, P.; Poullis, A.; Wilkins, J.; France, M. Burden of irritable bowel syndrome in an increasingly cost-aware National Health Service. *Frontline Gastroenterol.* **2015**, *6*, 246–251. [CrossRef]

16. Tucker, E.; Rostami, K.; Prabhakaran, S.; Al-Dulaimi, D. Patients with coeliac disease are increasingly overweight or obese on presentation. *J. Gastrointestin. Liver Dis.* **2012**, *21*, 11–15. [PubMed]

17. Lobstein, T.; Jackson-Leach, R.; Moodie, M.L.; Hall, K.D.; Gortmaker, S.L.; Swinburn, B.A.; James, W.P.T.; Wang, Y. Child and adolescent obesity: Part of a bigger picture. *Lancet* **2015**, *385*, 2510–2520. [CrossRef]

18. Bustamante, M.A.; Fernandez-Gil, M.P.; Churruca, I.; Miranda, J.; Lasa, A.; Navarro, V.; Simon, E. Evolution of gluten content in cereal-based gluten-free products: An overview from 1998 to 2016. *Nutrients* **2017**, *9*, 21. [CrossRef] [PubMed]

19. Verma, A.K.; Gatti, S.; Galeazzi, T.; Monachesi, C.; Padella, L.; Baldo, G.D.; Annibalo, R.; Lionetti, E.; Catassi, C. Gluten contamination in naturally or labeled gluten-free products marketed in Italy. *Nutrients* **2017**, *9*, 115. [CrossRef] [PubMed]

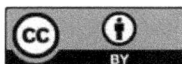

MDPI AG

St. Alban-Anlage 66

4052 Basel, Switzerland

Tel. +41 61 683 77 34

Fax +41 61 302 89 18

http://www.mdpi.com

Nutrients Editorial Office

E-mail: nutrients@mdpi.com

http://www.mdpi.com/journal/nutrients

www.ingramcontent.com/pod-product-compliance
Lightning Source LLC
Chambersburg PA
CBHW051836210326

41597CB00033B/5678